AT-RISK INFANTS

AT-RISK INFANTS

Interventions, Families, and Research

edited by

NICHOLAS J. ANASTASIOW, PH.D.
Thomas Hunter Professor
Special Education, Hunter College
Graduate Center, City University of New York
New York

and

SHAUL HAREL, M.D.
Director, The Institute for Child Development
and the Pediatric Neurology Unit
Division of Pediatrics
Tel Aviv Medical Center
University of Tel Aviv
Associate Professor of Pediatrics
Sackler Faculty of Medicine
University of Tel Aviv
Israel

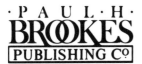

·P·A·U·L·H·
BROOKES
PUBLISHING C°

Baltimore • London • Toronto • Sydney

Paul H. Brookes Publishing Co.
P.O. Box 10624
Baltimore, Maryland 21285-0624

Typeset by Brushwood Graphics, Inc., Baltimore, Maryland.
Manufactured in the United States of America by
The Maple Press Company, York, Pennsylvania.

Library of Congress Cataloging-in-Publication Data
Anastasiow, Nicholas J.
　At-risk infants : interventions, families, and research / Nicholas J. Anastasiow,
Shaul Harel.
　　　p.　　cm.
　Includes bibliographical references and index.
　ISBN 1-55766-104-9
　1. Child development deviations—Prevention—Congresses.　2. Infants—Family
relationships—Congresses.　3. Infants—Health risk assessment—Congresses.
4. Parenting.　I. Harel, Shaul.　II. Title.
　[DNLM: 1. Child Development Disorders—etiology.　2. Child Development
Disorders—prevention & control.　3. Infants, Low Birth Weight.　4. Infant. Premature. WS 350.6 A534a]
RJ134.A52　1993
618.92—dc20
DNLM/DLC
for Library of Congress
92-16167
CIP

Contents

Contributors

Adriana A. Alcantara, M.A.
University of Illinois at Urbana-Champaign
Department of Psychology
Neuroscience Program and Beckman Institute
405 North Mathews
Urbana, Illinois 61801

C. Robert Almli, Ph.D.
Departments of Psychology and Psychiatry
Programs in Occupational Therapy
Developmental Neuropsychobiology Laboratory
Washington University School of Medicine
4567 Scott Avenue, Box 8066
St. Louis, Missouri 63110

Nicholas J. Anastasiow, Ph.D.
Thomas Hunter Professor
Hunter College
695 Park Avenue
New York, New York 10021
and
Program in Educational Psychology
Graduate Center
City University of New York
New York, New York 10036-8099

Brenda J. Anderson, M.S.
University of Illinois at Urbana-Champaign
Department of Psychology
Beckman Institute
405 North Mathews
Urbana, Illinois 61801

Janette Atkinson, M.D.
University of Cambridge
Visual Development Unit
22 Trampington Street
Cambridge CB2 1QA
ENGLAND

Carol J. Claflin, Ph.D.
Johnson County Community College
Psychology Department
12345 College
Overland Park, Kansas 66210-1299

Esther Dromi, Ph.D.
School of Education
University of Tel Aviv
Ramat Aviv, Tel Aviv 69978
ISRAEL

Aviva Fatal, M.D.
Department of Neurobiology
The Weizmann Institute of Science
Rehovot
ISRAEL

Tiffany Field, Ph.D.
Professor
Pediatrics, Psychology, and Psychiatry
Touch Research Institute
University of Miami Medical School
P.O. Box 016820
Miami, Florida 33101

William T. Greenough, Ph.D.
University of Illinois at Urbana-Champaign
Department of Psychology
Neuroscience Program and Beckman Institute
405 North Mathews
Urbana, Illinois 61801

Robin L. Hansen, M.D.
Associate Professor of Clinical Pediatrics
Department of Pediatrics
School of Medicine
University of California, Davis
2516 Stockton Boulevard
Sacramento, California 95817

Gloria L. Harbin, Ph.D.
Frank Porter Graham Child Development Center
The University of North Carolina at Chapel Hill
NCNB Bank Plaza
Suite 300
Chapel Hill, North Carolina 27514

Shaul Harel, M.D.
Director
The Institute for Child Development
  and the Pediatric Neurology Unit
Division of Pediatrics
Tel Aviv Medical Center
University of Tel Aviv
and
Associate Professor of Pediatrics
Sackler Faculty of Medicine
University of Tel Aviv
Tel Aviv 65211
ISRAEL

Nicholas Hawrylak, M.C.
University of Illinois at Urbana-Champaign
Neuroscience Program and Beckman Institute
405 North Mathews
Urbana, Illinois 61801

Christoph M. Heinicke, Ph.D.
Professor
Department of Psychiatry
University of California at Los Angeles
760 Westwood Plaza
Los Angeles, California 90024

Ariel Jaffa, M.D.
Department of Obstetrics and Gynecology "A"
Serlin Maternity Hospital
Tel Aviv Medical Center
University of Tel Aviv
Tel Aviv 65211
ISRAEL

Miriam Kutai, M.D.
The Institute for Child Development
  and the Pediatric Neurology Unit
Division of Pediatrics
Tel Aviv Medical Center
University of Tel Aviv
Tel Aviv 65211
ISRAEL

Yael Leitner, M.D.
The Institute for Child Development
  and the Pediatric Neurology Unit
Division of Pediatrics
Tel Aviv Medical Center
University of Tel Aviv
Tel Aviv 65211
ISRAEL

Laurence B. Leonard, Ph.D.
Audiology and Speech Sciences
1353 Heavilon Hall
Purdue University
West Lafayette, Indiana 47907-1353

Samuel J. Meisels, Ph.D.
Professor and Research Scientist
Center for Human Growth and Development
University of Michigan
300 North Ingalls
Ann Arbor, Michigan 48104

Harvey B. Sarnat, M.D., F.R.C.P. (C)
Professor of Pediatrics (Neurology) and Pathology
  (Neuropathology)
University of Washington
School of Medicine
Children's Hospital and Medical Center
Neurology/Neuropathology, CH-49
4800 Sand Point Way N.E.
Seattle, Washington 98105

Anat Scher, Ph.D.
School of Education
Haifa University
Haifa 31905
ISRAEL

Jack P. Shonkoff, M.D.
Professor of Pediatrics
Chief, Division of Developmental and Behavioral
  Pediatrics
University of Massachusetts Medical School
Department of Pediatrics
55 Lake Avenue North
Worcester, Massachusetts 01655

Anita M. Sirevaag, Ph.D.
Department of Histology and Neurobiology
Karolinska Institute
P.O. Box 60400
S-104 01 Stockholm
SWEDEN

Avraham Steinberg, M.D.
Center for Medical Ethics
Hebrew University—Hadassah Medical School
  and Department of Pediatrics
Shaare Zedek Medical Center
P.O. Box 3235
Jerusalem 91031
ISRAEL

Emanuel Tirosh, M.D.
Hannah Koushy Child Development Center
Bnai Zion Medical Center and
  the Faculty of Medicine
P.O. Box 4940
Haifa 31048
ISRAEL

Edith Tal-Posener, M.D.
The Institute for Child Development
    and the Pediatric Neurology Unit
Division of Pediatrics
Tel Aviv Medical Center
University of Tel Aviv
Tel Aviv 65211
ISRAEL

Abraham Tomer, M.D.
The Institute for Child Development
    and the Pediatric Neurology Unit
Division of Pediatrics
Tel Aviv Medical Center
University of Tel Aviv
Tel Aviv 65211
ISRAEL

Gordon L. Ulrey, Ph.D.
Associate Clinical Professor
Department of Psychiatry
School of Medicine
University of California, Davis
2516 Stockton Boulevard
Sacramento, California 95817

Christopher S. Wallace
University of Illinois at Urbana-Champaign
Neuroscience Program and Beckman Institute
405 North Mathews
Urbana, Illinois 61801

Ivan Jeanne Weiler, Ph.D.
University of Illinois at Urbana-Champaign
Department of Psychology
Neuroscience Program and Beckman Institute
405 North Mathews
Urbana, Illinois 61801

Ginger S. Withers
University of Illinois at Urbana-Champaign
Neuroscience Program and Beckman Institute
405 North Mathews
Urbana, Illinois 61801

Ephraim Yavin, Ph.D.
Department of Neurobiology
The Weizmann Institute of Science
P.O. Box 26
Rehovot 76100
ISRAEL

Preface

IN 1974, PHYSICIAN AND PEDIATRIC NEUROLOGIST SHAUL HAREL HAD A DREAM OF A WORKSHOP that would bring together professionals from a variety of fields to share their expertise on how best to remedy the state of at-risk infants. Infants who are in at-risk states fall into three categories: 1) those born with known genetic disorders, such as Down syndrome, who must be worked with early in life to achieve their potential; 2) those born prematurely or with low birth weight who are subject to acquiring disabling conditions through their immaturity at birth and/or by the procedures used to save their lives; and 3) those endangered by environmental factors, such as those born to adolescent mothers, particularly those living in poverty, who may not have had prenatal care, adequate nutrition, or family support; those born to substance-abusing parents, particularly mothers; and those born to families who live in economic poverty or to disorganized or abusive families.

Dr. Harel was well aware that individuals from a wide set of professions would be needed to combine their expertise to improve the at-risk state of these infants. In Israel, he enlisted the help of Dr. N. Bogair, under whose patronage the workshop could be held. Dr. Harel also enlisted the help of two colleagues—a physician, Yehuda Shapira, and a psychologist, Galiya Rabinovitz—to help plan a multidisciplinary workshop on the at-risk infant, to be held in Israel.

While in the United States, Dr. Harel enlisted a child development psychologist, Nicholas Anastasiow, and a pediatrician, the late Leo Stern, to serve as locaters and organizers of the workshop strands. The first workshop was held in 1979, with very positive results. The organizers were able to bring together a multidisciplinary team of speakers and audience members, and the papers presented were published by Excerpta Medica as *The At Risk Infant* (1980).

The healthy exchange of ideas across disciplines opened new areas of research and intervention. Furthermore, it increased the participants' mutual respect and stimulated cooperation among professionals across disciplines.

Following the success of the first workshop, many of those in attendance pressed for a second one, which was held in Jerusalem in 1984. The papers from that conference were published by Paul H. Brookes Publishing Co. as *The At-Risk Infant: Psycho/Socio/Medical Aspects* (1985).

Those who had learned the advantages of working across disciplines called for a third workshop. Due to political conditions in the Middle East, the workshop was postponed until the summer of 1991. Whereas the first two workshops investigated potential causes of and remedies for infants in at-risk states, the third workshop combined the research of those who work with animals and those who work with human beings. It was clear that basic animal research conducted between 1976 and 1991 has much to offer as the scientific foundation for early intervention for infants at risk for developmental problems.

Of the papers presented at the 1991 conference, those selected for this book were the ones that can serve as guideposts for what is known and should be implemented, as well as for what is unknown and needs to be addressed in future research. In many ways, it will determine future activities in the field. Clearly, Dr. Harel's basic assumption was correct. This work requires the cooperation and energies of individuals from a variety of professions who not only must work together, but also learn from one another's work.

THE BOOK

This book is divided into three major sections: Interventions, Families, and Research.

The first section opens with Anastasiow's paper, which is a summary and overview of the impact of early intervention programs and longitudinal studies of individuals without disabilities. This paper is followed by Sternberg's thoughtful examination of the moral and ethical issues involved in conducting research with infants. The author concludes, "When in doubt, err in favor of life" (p. 17).

In the next chapter, Dromi presents an overview of the prelinguistic communication sequence that leads to speech. This work is important not only for those who would facilitate language development, but also for those who work with individuals with severe disabilities who may learn to use these precursors of speech as aids to communication. Leonard focuses his chapter on the uses of intervention approaches with children with language disorders or disabilities. Atkinson's chapter presents her and her colleagues' work in developing assessment tools to determine visual impairments in infants. She discusses various aspects of visual abilities that should be assessed. The section concludes with Shonkoff's overview of his own longitudinal study with at-risk infants, and he speculates as to future needs for research and service delivery programs.

The second section deals with the families of at-risk infants. Claflin and Meisels present an overview of the impact of low birth weight infants on their families and provide useful information about instruments developed to measure the stress and impact on the family. Field reports on her work with infant massage with at-risk infants and efforts to sensitize families to the needs of these children.

Heinicke summarizes his research and that of others regarding how to reduce the potential pathology in the at-risk infant and his or her family. He describes his work with families aimed at improving their overall functioning. Harbin concludes this section with her view of how research and theory have modified practice in the early intervention field and what these changes will mean for public policy.

The final section deals with basic research with human and animal subjects. The relevance of including research with animals is that the researcher can examine the impact of the environment on brain functioning in experimentation. This research could not morally be conducted with human beings. However, their research has given us major insights into the course of development of the brain, the nature of early plasticity, and the brain's openness to environmental experiences.

The section begins with human data reported by Hansen, who explores the myths and realities of substance abuse as it affects the infants of users. This chapter is followed by Almli's review of research on the impact of invasive procedures used with low birth weight infants, focusing on the Cyclic Spontaneous Movement Patterns as a measure of the integrity of the premature nervous system.

In his chapter, Tirosh discusses respiration habituation and behavioral excitability (temperament); his research indicates the value of determining different neonatal characteristics. Harel and his colleagues examine the impact of intrauterine growth on outcomes at birth.

Sarnat's work with animals has influenced many researchers who work with human beings, as Almli acknowledges in his chapter. He reports his findings from studies on factors that influence the development of the central nervous system. The section closes with Greenough and his colleagues summarizing their early research findings on environmental influences on the developing brain, as well as his current research confirming the profound impact the environment has on brain development. His work has major implications for those who work with at-risk infants and would remedy their state.

In this book, professionals who work to prevent at-risk states from occurring, those who attempt to ameliorate at-risk states after birth, and those who work with infants and children with disabilities and their families will find useful information and thoughtful ideas to assist them in their efforts.

REFERENCES

Harel, S. (1980). *The at-risk infant*. Amsterdam: Excerpta Medica.

Harel, S., & Anastasiow, N. (Eds.). (1985). *The at-risk infant: Psycho/socio/medical aspects*. Baltimore: Paul H. Brookes Publishing Co.

Acknowledgments

THE THIRD AT-RISK INFANT WORKSHOP WAS CONDUCTED UNDER THE AUSPICES OF THE FOLlowing organizations:

- Israel Academy of Sciences and Humanities
- Israeli Association of Child Development Centers
- Israeli Society of Pediatric Neurology
- Municipality of Tel Aviv/Yafo—Hospitals and Public Health Department
- National Commission to Prevent Infant Mortality, USA
- National Institute of Child Health and Human Development (NICHD), Center for Research for Mothers and Children, USA
- National Institute of Neurological Disorders and Stroke, Developmental Neurology Branch, National Institute of Health, USA
- Sackler Faculty of Medicine, Tel Aviv University

With deep gratitude, we acknowledge the financial support of the following:

- ALIN—Israel Society for Crippled Children
- Hachamov Bros. Investment and Real Estate
- The Harris Foundation, Chicago, Illinois
- International Ltd. Tours and Congresses
- Israel Academy of Sciences and Humanities
- Ministry of Health, Israel
- Ministry of Science and Technology, Israel
- Municipality of Tel Aviv/Yafo
- National Institute of Health, USA
- Tikva Layeled—The Foundation of Cerebral Palsy Children in Israel

Our work is dedicated not only to the children and families who have helped us learn about at-risk conditions and their remedy, but also to the late Dr. N. Bogair, whose strong support and patronage led to the development and presentation of the first and second workshops and whose spirit was strongly felt at the third; and to Arthur Slater-Hammel, distinguished researcher in the field of motor skills. The senior editor gratefully acknowledges Slater-Hammel's intellectual and emotional support and friendship, as well as the desk on which part of this book was written and all of it was assembled.

We also wish to express our gratitude to the very competent staff of the Paul H. Brookes Publishing Co., particularly Melissa A. Behm and Roslyn Sassani Udris.

Section I

INTERVENTIONS

Chapter 1

The Effects of Early Intervention

NICHOLAS J. ANASTASIOW, PH.D.
Hunter College, New York, New York

TWO KINDS OF QUESTIONS ARE ASKED ABOUT intervention: Does it improve the disability now? Will it make any difference in the long run (when the child is an adult)? Both of these questions are addressed in the sections that follow. The first set of data addresses the latter question through the long-term results of longitudinal studies conducted within a variety of populations. The second set of data is from studies of children with disabilities or those who are at risk for disabilities.

Longitudinal studies either follow individuals from pre-term and infancy to 30 years of age, or follow children and adolescents to middle adulthood. An overview of the major results of these studies will be presented, as they provide clues of factors that lead to adult success. These factors are usually defined as the ability to work and the ability to establish intimate relationships (Vaillant & Milofsky, 1980). The studies offer insight into important variables that lead to success with individuals who do not have disabilities. It is assumed that the same factors would apply to the population of persons with disabilities, as societies have fairly uniform expectations as to the manner in which healthy adults function (Vaillant & Vaillant, 1981).

The longitudinal studies are surprisingly similar in their identification of the elements that lead to success for ordinary people in Western societies and the aspects of success

for those reared in adverse environmental conditions.

These studies have been conducted in both Europe and the United States with populations that vary from the Kauai study (Werner & Smith, 1992), in which the sample consisted primarily of Americans of Asian background, to delinquents in Boston (Glueck & Glueck, 1968; Vaillant & Milofsky, 1980; Vaillant & Vaillant, 1981), children reared in orphanages in England (Rutter, 1987), the college privileged (Vaillant & Milofsky, 1980; Vaillant & Vaillant, 1981), children whose parents are divorced (Cherlin et al., 1991), ordinary people (Block, 1971), adolescent mothers (Furstenberg, Brooks-Gunn, & Morgan, 1987), and many others eloquently summarized by Werner and Smith (1992).

The major finding of these studies is stated by Kolvin, Miller, Scott, Gazonts, and Fleeting (1990) in their long-term follow up of the Newcastle-on-Thames 1000 family study. "What seems to matter in the long run is the quality of physical and emotional care. Lack of money, poor housing, large families, cognitive limitations and adverse life events can be overcome by good care" (p. 179).

Garmezy (1991) summarizes three factors related to positive outcome that he found in his studies of the economically poor and children of parents who suffer from some form of psychopathology: 1) warmth, cohesion, and the presence of a caring adult; 2) positive child temperament, positive response to others, and cognitive skills; and 3) the presence of a source of external support (p. 321). The same set of variables was found by Werner and Smith (1992). In essence, as stated in the Newcastle study, healthy outcomes are a product of the individual and the environment.

Longitudinal studies tell us that being at risk, or vulnerable to risk, is a relative state, a complex interaction of constitutional factors and life circumstances. Resilience is the result of interactions or transitions of both, and is governed by protective factors within the child, the family environment, and the larger social context (Werner & Smith, 1992). The balance between intrinsic and extrinsic factors change with life stage cycles, which are more appropriately called developmental tasks (Vaillant & Milofsky, 1980), the sex of the child, and the family and culture into which he or she is born.

These findings will help to dispel some misconceptions and provide alternative intervention schemata that may help other children develop resiliency by using potential buffers (Werner & Smith, 1992) in their environment. It will also highlight the current emphasis on the family and its major role in intervention.

It is important to note that the long-term impact of lower social class appears to hold up in cross-sectional studies but not in longitudinal studies, as indicated by the Newcastle study cited above and by Vaillant and Milofsky (1980). As Vaillant and Milofsky state, "Life is not painted in primary colors nor is it mastered in a task completion" (p. 1357).

These studies are telling us that development is a process in which the individual participates in his or her own development from the very beginning: balancing, mediating, choosing among internal strengths and weaknesses and aspects of the environment's strengths and weaknesses.

The long-term followup of special education students conducted by Affleck, Edgar, Levine, and Kortering (1990) found positive results in a variety of reports on special education in the United States. For example, in a study conducted with a cross-categorical population in Colorado, 67% of the students who graduated

from high school were employed. In a study in Vermont, 66% of the students were employed, and in Virginia, 41% were employed. In their own study, broken down by categories, they found that 67% of persons with neurological impairments, 67% of those with learning disabilities, 62% of those with behavioral disorders, 37% of those with mild disabilities, 49% of those with severe disabilities, and 56% of those with sensory impairments were employed. These are impressive results, even though they could be higher. What was missing from the learning or education of the students was an emphasis on life plans (goal setting, independent learning, self-evaluation, adjustment, job coaching), that is, not merely educational plans but also individual plans to become productive and independent adults.

The next major set of data of a longitudinal nature is on children reared in economic poverty, summarized by Anastasiow (1986). The earlier expectation was that at least 50% of the children exposed to poverty would inevitably be at high risk for failure in school, work, and relationships. The current conclusion is that what was missing from those interventions were the factors identified by Garmezy (1991) and succinctly summarized by Rutter (1989). "We need to focus on those protective factors, that is, [to] promote self esteem and self efficacy, which are probably the key ingredients of any intervention project" (p. 50).

A major move has been made in the United States to follow the advice of Rutter and others to focus on personal as well as educational skills and, in addition, to provide transition services that emphasize life and job skills, such as how to behave in an interview and how to get along with one's employer and co-workers. Major curricula have been developed to meet these needs (Bellamy, Rhodes, Mank, & Albin, 1988; Falvey, 1989; Ford et al., 1989; O'Neil, Gothelf, Cohen, Lehman, & Woolf, 1991).

PRENATAL CARE AND EARLY CHILDHOOD INTERVENTION STUDIES

A point well described by Mencher and Gerber (1983) is that the question is not whether to intervene with children with disabilities, but rather how to identify the primary handicap, see if it is influenced by other handicaps, and determine its location. For instance, is the problem a central auditory processing deficit, a disruption in peripheral visual functioning, or a condition that has failed to promote optional reciprocal communication? These examples are for hearing impairments, although the principle applies to other handicapping conditions as well.

As Mencher and Gerber state, "Management will begin with an assessment of the strengths of the child and then assist these strengths to develop through training and experience . . . with the family the primary vehicle for management" (pp. 2–3).

We need not repeat that the effects of early intervention and prevention are positive, and most interventionists find support in the animal literature concerning the malleability of development during the time of central nervous system plasticity early in life (see Sarnat, chap. 15, this volume; and Greenough et al., chap. 16, this volume).

As reported elsewhere (Anastasiow, 1990), only 30% of the brain is mature at birth. It then proceeds through a series of gene-programmed maturational stages throughout life (Lecours, 1975). It is commonly held that this immaturity of the central nervous system allows for openness to experience. Learnings can be recorded in an area of the brain before that area is fully mature. This openness is very positive in learning about the world, as not all social information is passed through genes. The openness also has a negative aspect in that the brain can be influenced by noxious substances and negative environmental events. It is clear that the brain will mature and develop structures whether or not the environment provides experiences for the development of species-expected structures (e.g., learning to communicate through speech or sign language, or not learning to communicate due to child neglect or abuse and lack of caregiver–child interactions that normally would lead to learning the language of the culture).

A most encouraging result from animal studies is that if a particular area of the brain is damaged, another section may assume its function early in life (see Sarnat, chap. 15, this volume). Thus early interventionists realize that to improve a disability, or perhaps remediate it, action must be taken early in life, before the brain becomes fully mature (Anastasiow, 1986; Westlake & Kraiser, 1991).

TYPES OF INTERVENTION

Many individuals think of types of intervention in terms of where they occur, that is, in the home, the classroom, or the larger community. The home is being given increased importance as an effective place for infant and child intervention (Shonkoff & Hauser-Cram, 1987), whereas the community is now seen as the most appropriate place for intervention with those having severe and profound disabilities (Falvey, 1989; Peck, 1991).

The first type of intervention is *prevention*, which can take place through genetic counseling, prenatal care, and informing the expectant mother about toxic substances and positive health care practices. Genetic counseling will provide the expectant parents with a probability statement as to the risk of having a child with a disability. Prenatal care may detect a problem that can be treated in order to prevent a disability from occurring.

The second type is *diagnostic procedures*, which, after the child is born, seek to determine whether a disability exists, and, if so, what the appropriate treatment should be. Diagnosis usually follows some kind of screening.

Third is *corrective procedures*, which are intended to improve the functioning of the individual with a disability by means of a prosthetic device such as a hearing aid.

The fourth type of intervention is *compensation*, which is an effort to offset a weakness by providing an enriched environment and possibly stimulate the child's other senses in order to assist him or her in functioning.

Fifth is *circumvention*, which involves finding means of providing alternative sensory input for a child with a disability. For example, circumvention might involve providing early rich haptic experiences for the visually impaired child.

The last type of intervention is *remediation*,

which is an attempt to prevent the occurrence of secondary deficits and to fill gaps in development (Boothroyd, 1983).

An intervention program may include all or some of the strategies listed above.

THE AT-RISK INFANT: GENERAL INTERVENTION

In spite of criticism, early intervention is effective in improving the lives of children with many types of disabilities (Meisels & Shonkoff, 1990; Shonkoff & Hauser-Cram, 1987; Upshur, 1990; Westlake & Kaiser, 1991). Now, according to Bricker (1990), the most prevalent questions among interventionists are as follows: Which strategies are most effective with a particular population? Where should the process take place? Who should be involved? It has been documented that "at-risk states" can sometimes be cured (Harel & Anastasiow, 1984; Parmelee, 1985; Werner & Smith, 1982), and functioning can be improved in most cases. Even for a person with severe physical and central nervous system damage, intervention can improve his or her life. The field has now come to use the term *handicap* to refer to conditions that prevent an individual with disabilities from gaining access to a building or place of employment. Now, the phrase commonly used to describe the individual is a *person with a disability or disabilities*. The following is a brief examination of different categories of risk or disability and some findings on intervention.

Biological and In Utero Risk

Incidents of genetic risk in the United States now account for less than 1% of the children classified as disabled (Anastasiow, 1986). Through genetic counseling, many risks can be identified before pregnancy. Prospective parents can obtain a probability statement on the chances of their producing a child with a disability. Alpha fetal protein tests, sonography, and amniocentesis can assist in identifying fetuses with disabilities (Batshaw & Perret, 1992). Genetic counseling gives the parents options to not bear children, adopt, or to take the risk of having a child with disabilities. If a disability is discovered through the aforemen-

tioned tests during pregnancy, the parents must then decide whether to have the child or to abort the fetus. Essentially, any of these issues involve both ethical and political issues (Peck, 1991).

Today, in the 1990s, there are few cures for genetically linked disabilities. In some limited experiments, however, a missing gene has been injected into the bloodstream to compensate for the deficiency and prevent the disability from developing (Angier, 1991). While these are new and controversial procedures, there will probably be more of them as gene therapy advances.

Thyroid conditions and phenylketonuria can lead to disabilities if they are not detected, but screening at birth and early treatment are effective means of prevention. Unfortunately, not all genetic conditions can be treated so readily.

However, education and prenatal care can do much to reduce the number of premature and low birth weight babies (conservative estimates run as high as 60%–80%). For example, teenage mothers under 16 can have healthy full-term babies if they are provided with good prenatal care and a support system in the environment (Field, 1989). Health education can encourage women to have the recommended inoculations, particularly for measles, in order to prevent the damage that rubella can do to the fetus. It can also help them to avoid toxic substances such as alcohol, and thereby eliminate the risk of fetal alcohol syndrome, and to eliminate the use of drugs such as heroin, which can be so devastating to the unborn child.

In the United States, the major concern has been to *save* low birth-weight infants after they are born rather than to first *prevent* low birth weight. Currently, little federal money is provided for prenatal care of women living in economic poverty. Many European countries (e.g., Finland and Sweden) have made major investments in the prevention of low birth weight, which reduces the amount that would otherwise be spend on low birth-weight infants. The death rate among infants of the economically poor is extremely high, and this contributes to a much higher infant mortality rate in the United States than in other industrialized nations. If a 2- or 3-pound baby survives, the outlook for his or her cognitive and social abilities is not very positive (Als, Duffy, McAnulty, & Badian, in press). The medical interventions necessary to save their lives often interfere with later functioning. In addition, many of these premature infants have disorders such as lung dysplasia. The medical procedures used to save the lives of very small babies appear to be overstimulating and may have a negative impact on the neural pathways under development, by readying the child for environmental learning while receiving stimulation before the brain is organized to receive it (Als et al., 1991). Many researchers are turning their attention to this group (see Hansen & Ulrey, chap. 11, this volume).

IMPROVEMENT VERSUS CURE

Visual, Hearing, and Physical Disabilities

If a child is born with a sensory disability, it is unlikely that the disability will be cured. Sensory damage is generally irreversible for most disabled children. However, early intervention can improve the child's functioning markedly, by focusing on whatever residual functioning remains and emphasizing sensory stimulation in areas that are not impaired—that is, finding the strengths. In addition, early intervention that provides alternative stimulation tends to prevent the development of noxious secondary behaviors that can develop in the absence of sensory input. These secondary behaviors (often called self-stimulation, behavior disorders, or, now in the United States, challenging behaviors) fail to develop when early input is provided to the infant (Murphy, 1983).

The classic case is the work of Selma Fraiberg (1965). Her research with the visually impaired demonstrated that the autistic like behaviors formerly associated with institutionalized blind infants could be prevented through touch and haptic stimulation. She also found that this physical stimulation was needed during the critical stage of 2–3 months and also from 7 to 9 months, when the infant-caregiver attachment system develops.

Fraiberg's work raised the question of risk factors that the trainer may introduce into therapeutic interventions by interfering with the normal progression of the attachment system, which seems to be essential in the development of the self-system (Bretherton & Walters, 1985).

Research has indicated that there is a need for all interventionists to be concerned with the normal developmental programs of the human being, and to orient intervention toward assisting the child with disabilities to develop in a normal progression (Rutter, 1989). This progression appears in the following manner:

1. Attachment system (0–3 years)
2. Autonomy (2–3 years)
3. Self efficacy (2–3 years)
4. Self confidence (3–5 years)
5. Learning how to learn (0–3 years)
6. Cognitive and language skills (0–6 years)

In addition, linguists have now alerted interventionists to the nonverbal gestures, cries, specific hand movements, eye contact, and emotional expressions that are all precursors of language development (Bates, 1979). The sequence of development of the nonverbal communication systems should not be overridden by other intervention strategies, but rather encouraged to develop (Murphy, 1983). It should be kept in mind that the attainment of developmental tasks by ordinary people is still the basis on which one is judged to be delayed or on target for development.

Studies indicate that most physical disabilities occurring at birth, usually with damage to the central nervous system as well, cannot be cured. However, a marked improvement can often be effected through exercise, massage, prosthesis, and appropriate positioning techniques so that the child with a disability can learn as part of his or her own efforts (Krajicek, 1991). Many children with disabilities are not mentally retarded, and delays in their development may be the results of environmental inaccessibility. Many individuals with severe physical disabilities can learn to live independently and function normally in the work force if appropriate interventions are available to assist their development and barriers are removed from schools and work places (O'Byren & Joyce, 1983).

It has been demonstrated that early intervention with the hearing impaired can improve residual hearing. If there is no residual hearing, and signing is introduced at an early age, the child will learn sign language in a normal manner, develop normal intelligence, and not develop the tone of voice and facial expressions that many find unpleasant (Klima & Bellegi, 1979).

Infants with hearing impairments appear to use hand movement as signs in much the same way that normal hearing infants use babbling (Petitte & Marentelle, 1991). The trainer needs to reinforce these signs just as a caregiver reinforces the babbling sounds that appear to be part of the language of the culture, such as mama and dada. As Linden, Kankkunen, and Tjellstrom (1983) indicate, nothing was found inherent in a hearing deficit that should create additional social and psychological deficits.

Severe and Profound
Extremely Low Functioning

A major change in curriculum and treatment strategies is occurring in the field of the severely and profoundly disabled which has long been dominated by orthodox Skinnerian approaches (Gaylord-Ross & Browder, 1991). It is now recognized that many of these individuals will never attain symbolic functioning (speech or American sign language), but they can discover, and need to discover, the following: 1) that they are persons, 2) that there are other persons, 3) that they (persons with disabilities) have needs, 4) that these needs can be met by other persons, and 5) that they can meet some of their needs themselves (Murphy & Byrne, 1983, p. 355). An integral part of the revision of the work with the severe and profound is the acceptance of Murphy and Byrne's sequence and the recognition of the sequence of nonverbal behaviors that lead to speech. The nonverbal communication system appears to be genetically programmed (Bates, 1979) and can be stimulated by the environment, as trainers recognize their occurrence and stimulate continuation (Murphy & Byrne, 1983). It is important to recognize these behaviors in an in-

dividual who is barely responsive, because recognition and training assist the severely and profoundly disabled in making meaningful requests through nonverbal communication and learning how to learn, in spite of their cognitive limitations. That is to say, they can learn how to request help for needs they cannot meet, by eye contact, gesture, hand pressure, pointing, and non-speech sounds.

In the training of these individuals in the United States, there has been a shift from schools to the setting in which the person will function. This approach is often referred to as *functionalism*. The main point is that while gestures may occur, if the individual is not trained to use them to elicit, to reject, and to communicate in general, they will disintegrate into what appears to be random bizarre movement. Training must occur early in life, or the individual will not be able to control his gestures easily. As Kevin Murphy (1983) writes, "Delayed intervention leads to an almost insuperable task of trying to shift the children's focus of attention from themselves to the world around them" (p. 6). The noxious stereotypic behaviors of self-rocking, self-abuse, and head banging appear to be products of self-exploration and self-stimulation that develop in the absence of extrapersonal (other person) stimulation as a consequence of sensory deprivation (Murphy, 1983). Murphy also believes that self-stimulation stimulates the pleasure area of the brain, the limbic systems (preoptic, hypothalamus), which accounts for their continuation in spite of the physical damage that results from head banging and so forth. Murphy has attempted to flood the individual with vibrations during these self-stimulation episodes. These vibrations appear to stop the self-stimulation behavior, and the trainer immediately offers an appropriate alternative stimulation. It will be interesting to see if this technique will prove successful.

Technological advances have also been made in home and portable oxygen devices, feeding tubes, respiratory ventilators, gastrostomy tubes, sonic location devices for the blind, and many other devices that allow the child to be kept at home as well as improving his or her life chances (Krajicek, 1991).

Major progress has been made with the mildly retarded through regular preschool experience (Anastasiow, 1986). Many of these children develop enough in cognitive functioning to be placed in regular education classes. In the United States, there are new curricula that follow the normal developmental sequence in small steps for this population—for example, *The Carolina Curriculum for Infants and Toddlers with Special Needs* (Johnson-Martin, Jens, Attermeier, & Hacker, 1991) and *The Carolina Curriculum for Preschoolers with Special Needs* (Johnson-Martin, Attermeier, & Hacker, 1990).

Play, as Lerner (1986) indicates, is the human species' specific way of learning. As the educational aspect of play is rediscovered, it is being added to most intervention programs as a strategy for learning as well as assessment (Linder, 1990; Rabinovitz & Harel, 1985). Encouragement of children to request, explore, manipulate objects, and raise questions is replacing strict behavioral lessons that have little or no generalization effects.

Interventionists have again discovered that the behavior systems of human beings are primarily affective, and the relation to secure attachment is primary (Villant & Milofsky, 1980). Children need to explore, to exercise their innate curiosity, to fulfill their motivations, to manipulate the environment, and to play with things they choose. Through these activities, they learn and learn how to learn. Once these processes are in operation, the child is ready to learn how to read, to work, to become intimate, and to achieve the balance of intimacy and work that we call mental health (Vaillant & Vaillant, 1981).

Perhaps the best example in the field of retardation is the work with the population with Down syndrome (Guralnick & Bricker, 1987; Upshur, 1990). It should be recognized that there are many different types of children with Down syndrome, some having special health needs. However, the intervention efforts with these children and their families have been outstandingly successful. In the past, children with Down syndrome were frequently institutionalized, and they rarely developed more than a small vocabulary in that setting. Now most are reared at home and receive the necessary medical and educational treatment from birth, including early intervention programs. Under these conditions, they usually achieve IQs in the 60s. In one case in Hawaii, a child with Down syndrome was placed in an infant program, proceeded onto regular education, and graduated from high school (S. Furuno, personal communication, July, 1990). Those who work with this population have reversed what was the typical pattern of the child with Down syndrome, which was a drop in IQ scores as he grew older. Guralnick and Bricker (1987) have reported that recent studies indicate that this drop has been stopped, a truly remarkable achievement.

Although researchers may use a variety of terms to describe what they consider crucial, the construct underlying all these research efforts is the need for the infant-caregiver joint-attention interaction/transaction, or what others call the infant–caregiver attachment system (Sroufe, 1985). For all people, including the disabled and those at risk, the foundation of adult mental health—the ability to work and to play—arises out of the strengths of the early childhood environment. As Werner and Smith (1992) point out, 60%–80% of all successful adults and 70% of the failures can be identified from data gathered in the first 2 years of life. These findings are supported by Vaillant and Milofsky (1980) and Vaillant and Vaillant (1981).

As stated earlier, the Newcastle 1000 family study says it best. "What seems to matter in the long run is the quality of physical and emotional care in childhood. Lack of money, poor housing, large families, cognitive limitations, adverse life events can be overcome by good care" (Kolvin et al., 1990, p. 176).

REFERENCES

Afflek, J.Q., Edgar, E., Levine, P., & Kortering, L. (1990, December). Postschool status of students classified as mildly mentally retarded, learning disabled, or non-

handicapped: Does it get better with time? *Education and Training in Mental Retardation*, 315–324.

Als, H., Duffy, F.H., McAnulty, G.B., & Badian, N.

(in press). Continuity of neurobehavioral functioning in preterm and full term newborns. In M. Bornstein & N. Krasnegor (Eds.), *Continuity in development*. Hillsdale, NJ: Lawrence Erlbaum Associates.

Anastasiow, N.J. (1986). *Development and disability: A psychobiological analysis for special educators*. Baltimore: Paul H. Brookes Publishing Co.

Anastasiow, N.J. (1990). Implications of the neurobiological model for early intervention. In S. Meisels & J. Shonkoff (Eds.), *Handbook of early intervention* (pp. 196–216). New York: Cambridge University Press.

Angier, N. (1991, July 29). Doctors' success treating a blood disease by altering genes. *New York Times*, p. 16.

Bates, E. (1979). On the evolution of symbols. In E. Bates (Ed.), *The emergence of symbols* (pp. 3–32). New York: Academic Press.

Batshaw, M.L., & Perret, Y.M. (1992). *Children with disabilities: A medical primer* (3rd ed.). Baltimore: Paul H. Brookes Publishing Co.

Bellamy, G.T., Rhodes, L.E., Mank, D.M., & Albin, J.M. (1988). *Supported employment: A community implemented guide*. Baltimore: Paul H. Brookes Publishing Co.

Block, J. (1971). *Lives through time*. Berkeley: Bancroft Books.

Boothroyd, A. (1983). Assessment and intervention from a developmental perspective. In G.T. Mencher & S.E. Gerber (Eds.), *The multihandicapped hearing impaired child* (pp. 117–338). New York: Grune and Stratton.

Bretherton, M., & Walters, L. (Eds.). (1985). Growing points of attachment theory and research. *Monographs of the Society of Research in Child Development, 50* (1-2, Serial No. 309).

Bricker, D. (1990). *Early education of at-risk and handicapped infants and preschool children*. Glenview, IL: Scott, Foresman.

Cherlin, A.J., Furstenberg, F. Jr., Chase-Lansdale, P.L., Kiernan, K., Robins, P.K. Morrison, D., & Teitler, J.O. (1991, June). Longitudinal studies of effects of divorce on children in Great Britain and the United States. *Science, 752*, 1386–2388.

Falvey, J. (1989). *Community-based curriculum: Instructional strategies for students with severe handicaps* (2nd ed.). Baltimore: Paul H. Brookes Publishing Co.

Field, T. (1989). Interaction coaching for high risk infants and their parents. *Prevention in Human Series, 1*, 8–54.

Ford, A., Schnorr, R., Meyer, L., Davern, L., Black, J., & Dempsey, P. (Eds.). (1989). The *Syracuse community-referenced curriculum guide for students with moderate and severe disabilities*. Baltimore: Paul H. Brookes Publishing Co.

Fraiberg, S. (1965). *The magic years*. New York: Scribner.

Furstenberg, F., Brooks-Gunn, J., & Morgan, S.D. (1987). *Adolescent mothers in later life*. Cambridge, MA: Cambridge University Press.

Garmezy, G.N. (1991, March-April). Resiliency and vulnerability to adverse developmental outcomes associated with poverty. *American Behavioral Scientist, 24*, 416–430.

Gaylord-Ross, R., & Browder, D. (1991). Functional assessment: Dynamic and domain properties. In L.H. Meyer, C.A. Peck, & L. Brown (Eds.), *Critical issues in the lives of people with severe disabilities* (pp. 45–66). Baltimore: Paul H. Brookes Publishing Co.

Glueck, S., & Glueck, E. (1968). *Delinquents and non-delinquents in perspective*. Cambridge, MA: Harvard University Press.

Guralnick, M.J., & Bricker, D.D. (1987). The effectiveness of early intervention for children with cognitive and general development delays. In M.J. Guralnick & F.C. Bennett (Eds.), *The effectiveness of early intervention for at-risk and handicapped children* (pp. 115–174). New York: Academic Press.

Harel, S., & Anastasiow, N.J. (Eds.). (1985). *The at-risk infant: Psycho/socio/medical aspects*. Baltimore: Paul H. Brookes Publishing Co.

Johnson-Martin, N.M., Jens, K.G., Attermeier, S.M., & Hacker, B.J. (1991). *The Carolina curriculum for infants and toddlers with special needs* (2nd ed). Baltimore: Paul H. Brookes Publishing Co.

Johnson-Martin, N.M., Attermeier, S.M., & Hacker, B. (1990). *The Carolina curriculum for preschoolers with special needs*. Baltimore: Paul H. Brookes Publishing Co.

Klima, E.S., & Bellegi, U. (1979). *The signs of language*. Cambridge, MA: Harvard University Press.

Kolvin, I., Miller, F.J., Scott, D. McI., Gazonts, S.K.M., & Fleeting, M. (1990). *Continuities of deprivation? The Newcastle 1,000 family study*. Adyershot, England: Avebuun/Gover.

Krajicek, M.J. (1991). *Handbook for the care of infants and toddlers with disabilities and chronic conditions*. Lawrence, KS: Learner Managed Designs.

Lecours, A.R. (1975). Myelogenetic correlates of the development of speech and language. In E.H. Lenneberg & E. Lenneberg (Eds.), *Foundations of language development* (Vol. 1, pp. 121–135). New York: John Wiley & Sons.

Lerner, R.M. (1986). *The nature of human plasticity*. New York: Cambridge University Press.

Linden, G., Kankkunen, A., & Tjellstrom, A. (1983). Multi handicaps and ear malformations in hearing impaired children. In G.T. Mencher & S. Gerber (Eds.), *The multiple handicapped hearing impaired child* (pp. 67–82). New York: Grune & Stratton.

Linder, T. (1990). *Transdisciplinary play-based assessment: A functional approach to working with young children*. Baltimore: Paul H. Brookes Publishing Co.

Meisels, S., & Shonkoff, J. (1990). *Handbook of early intervention*. New York: Cambridge University Press.

Mencher, G.T., & Gerber, S. (Eds.). (1983). *The multiple handicapped hearing impaired child*. New York: Grune & Stratton.

Mitgang, D.E., Horiuchi, C.N., & Fanning, P.N. (1985). A report to the Colorado statewide follow up of special education students. *Exceptional Children, 53*, 551–561.

Murphy, K. (1983). The educator-therapist and deaf, multiply disabled children: Some essential criteria. In G.T. Menscher & S. Gerber (Eds.), *The multihandicapped child* (pp. 13–76). New York: Grune & Stratton.

Murphy, K., & Byrne, D. (1983). Selection of optimal modalities as avenues of learning in deaf, blind, multiply disabled children. In G.T. Mencher & S. Gerber (Eds.), *The multihandicapped child* (pp. 355–396). New York: Grune & Stratton.

O'Byren, D., & Joyce, D. (1983). Language intervention with the severely handicapped. *Journal of Special Education, 19*(1), 7–9.

O'Neil, J., Gothelf, C., Cohen, S., Lehman, L., & Woolf, S.B. (1991). *A curriculum approach to support the tran-*

sition to adulthood of adolescents with dual sensory impairments. Albany: New York State Education Department, Department of Special Education. (ERIC Document Reproduction Service, No. ED 333 693-697)

Parmelee, A. (1985). Sensory stimulation in the nursery. *Developmental & Behavioral Pediatrics, 6,* 242–243.

Peck, C.A. (1991). Linking values and science in social policy decisions affecting citizens with severe disabilities. In L.H. Meyer, C.A. Peck, & L. Brown (Eds.), *Critical issues in the lives of people with severe disabilities* (pp. 1–15). Baltimore: Paul H. Brookes Publishing Co.

Petitte, L.A., & Marentelle, P. (1991, March). Babbling in the manual mode: Evidence of ontogeny of language. *Science, 251,* 2493–2495.

Rabinovitz, G., & Harel, S. (1985). Educational and health planning for infants and toddlers: Guidelines for an ecological model for early infancy (397–401). In S. Harel & N.J. Anastasiow (Eds.), *The at-risk infant: Psycho/socio/medical aspects.* Baltimore: Paul H. Brookes Publishing Co.

Rutter, M. (1987). Psychosocial resilience and protective mechanisms. *American Journal of Orthopsychiatry, 57,* 316–331.

Rutter, M. (1989). Pathways from childhood to adult life. *Journal of Child Psychology and Psychiatry, 30,* 23–51.

Shonkoff, J.P., & Hauser-Cram, P. (1987). Early intervention for disabled infants and their families. *Pediatrics, 80,* 650–658.

Sroufe, L.A. (1985). Attachment classifications from the perspective of infant-caregiver relationships. *Child Development, 56,* 1–14.

Sroufe, L.A., & Rutter, M. (1985). The domain of developmental psychopathology. *Child Development, 55,* 1184–1199.

Upshur, C. (1990). Early intervention as prevention. In S. Meisels & J. Shonkoff (Eds.), *Handbook of early intervention* (pp. 633–650). New York: Cambridge University Press.

Vaillant, G., & Milofsky, M. (1980, November). Natural history of male psychological health: Empirical evidence of Erikson's model of the life cycle. *American Journal of Psychiatry, 137*(11), 1348–1359.

Vaillant, G., & Vaillant, C. (1981, November). Natural history of male psychological health: Work as a positive predictor of mental health. *American Journal of Psychiatry, 138*(11), 1433–1440.

Werner, E., & Smith, R. (1982). *Vulnerable and invincible.* New York: McGraw-Hill.

Werner, E., & Smith, R. (1992). *Overcoming the odds: High risk children from birth to adulthood.* Ithaca: Cornell University Press.

Westlake, C.R., & Kaiser, A.P. (1991). Early childhood services for children with severe disabilities: Research, values, policy, and practice. In L.H. Meyer, C.A. Peck, & L. Brown (Eds.), *Critical issues in the lives of people with severe disabilities* (pp. 429–458). Baltimore: Paul H. Brookes Publishing Co.

Chapter 2

Ethical Issues
in Early Intervention

Avraham Steinberg, M.D.
*Hebrew University—Hadassah Medical School
and Shaare Zedek Medical Center, Jerusalem, Israel*

One of the most difficult and debated ethical dilemmas in modern medicine concerns the care of critically ill newborns and babies born with severe disabilities. Rapid advances in neonatology have brought about a significant reduction in neonatal mortality. The availability of sophisticated resuscitative measures, hyperalimentation, and complicated surgical procedures have produced a significant improvement in the survival rate of neonates. However, the increased rate of survivors, many with markedly decreased quality of both physical and mental life, and the enormous economic and emotional burdens on the survivors, their families, and the entire society, have engendered many new ethical dilemmas. These ethical issues concern a significant number of neonates— about 1% of premature infants, and about 1.5% of neonates born with major anomalies.

In earlier times, the question was: "Can we save the life of a newborn with a severe defect?" Today the questions are: "Should we?" or "How far should we intervene?" Many issues are involved that require resolution including medical, legal, ethical, religious, psychosocial, and sociocultural issues. A multitude of books, monographs, reviews, and articles have been published discussing the various aspects of this problem.

The major ethical questions concerning newborns with disabilities include moral rights, the value of life versus quality of life, and the scarcity of resources.

MORAL RIGHTS

Are the moral rights of a newborn different from those of an older child or an adult? Is it morally justified to differentiate between a poor quality of life in a newborn and the same quality of life in an older child? Is the decision to forego life-sustaining treatment in a neonate easier only because the newborn cannot object, or because a psychological bond with the baby has not yet been established? Is there a justifiable inherent moral distinction between newborns and adult?

Western societies demand that a healthy newborn be respected as a human being with potential personhood, and his or her rights be strictly protected. Infanticide is no less a crime than the murder of an adult person, and abusing or neglecting a neonate is as reprehensible as committing these offenses against older children or adults. Therefore, a newborn with a disability should have the same rights as an older person with a disability. Thus, one who treats a child or an adult with an illness or de-

13

fect must do the same for the neonate. However, there is no obligation to prolong the dying process of a newborn with a structural or metabolic defect that is incompatible with life. In this regard, a nonviable newborn is similar to a dying adult for whom "heroic" measures need not be applied. Supportive care, however, including nutrition and hydration, are required to the very end. Active euthanasia or abandonment of the newborn should be prohibited by all means.

VALUE OF LIFE
VERSUS QUALITY OF LIFE

The value of life versus the quality of life is an ongoing debate, the pros and cons of which are beyond the scope of this chapter. However, it should be pointed out that in the case of a newborn with a disability, an additional ethical dilemma concerns the inability of newborns to exercise autonomous decision-making capacity, and there is no way to ascertain *their* definition of quality of life. Since quality of life can almost never be universally defined, a "slippery slope" consequence (i.e., applying the concept of "quality of life" arbitrarily, hence letting die or killing less and less severely affected newborns with no clear way to draw a line) of arbitrarily applied definitions of this concept ought to be seriously considered. How is a decision to withhold treatment from a newborn with a disability different from a decision of Spartans to let babies die on the hillside if they were females, disabled, or sick? Tiny, premature babies have a high frequency of mental and physical disabilities. Should we let *all* babies die because so many eventually have a poor quality of life? Should a baby with Down syndrome and duodenal atresia not be operated on and be allowed to die because many persons with Down syndrome also have mental retardation? Is it the expected percentage and degree of abnormality and disability that counts? If so, what is the "magic" number, and by whom should it be determined when the patient (i.e., newborn baby) is incapable of making his or her own decision?

SCARCITY OF RESOURCES

The treatment and rehabilitation of newborns with severe defects are costly. A large team of experts is necessary to provide such care. Many of these patients also require repeated hospitalizations, surgical procedures, technical devices, medications, and special education facilities.

Nonetheless, as weighty as these considerations might be, it is immoral to jeopardize the constitutional rights of individuals with disabilities from equal access to adequate health care. The problem of scarce resources cannot morally justify the sacrifice of the life and well-being of individuals with disabilities. If modern society does not wish to resemble Sparta as far as its public health policy is concerned, it must allocate adequate economic and emotional support to the indigent.

Defects in newborns can be divided into two major groups: 1) defects that are currently fatal and incurable; and 2) defects that are nonfatal but cause significant suffering, both mental and physical, to the child, the family, and society.

It seems as though the determining factor in the decision of whether to treat or not to treat a newborn with a severe defect depends on its chances for viability in accordance with the scientific knowledge and technical capabilities available at that time. Therefore, an anencephalic newborn should not be treated beyond the administration of food and fluids, since any treatment for such a baby is futile. On the other hand, a newborn baby who has a chance for survival, even if the expected quality of life is poor, should be treated the same way as one treats an older child or an adult with a similar degree of disability. Whatever conclusions are reached for an adult person in regard to "do not resuscitate" should also apply to the neonate.

To illustrate some of these ethical issues, the situation of a newborn with meningomyelocele (MMC) and a premature baby is presented.

MENINGOMYELOCELE (MMC)

The medical literature amply documents divergence of opinion as to whether or not such patients should be treated medically and/or surgically. All concerned are ambivalent and uncomfortable about these decisions.

Since the 1970s, the attitudes of physicians toward a neonate with a neural tube defect have undergone significant philosophical and therapeutic changes. Before adequate surgical and rehabilitative therapy was available for this defect, nearly all babies with MMC died. In the early 1960s, a vigorous, aggressive, and nonselective therapeutic approach was adopted, recommending immediate and comprehensive treatment of all such babies. In the early 1970s, various selection criteria for nontreatment were developed because of significant residual disabilities. These criteria were widely accepted, but not universally. In the latter part of the 1980s these criteria were challenged on medical as well as on moral and legal grounds (Noetzel, 1989).

Clearly, many ethical positions are influenced by personal emotions, convictions, and biases. However, as in all branches of medicine, good ethics start with good facts. Ethical arguments are irrelevant if they are based on false or inaccurate data. A prerequisite for reaching sound decisions is a complete and accurate knowledge of the diagnosis, short- and long-term prognosis, and the therapeutic alternatives.

In the case of MMC, the diagnosis is straightforward and poses no difficulties. The surgical procedure of closing the defect is simple, safe, and lifesaving in that it prevents the often fatal complication of meningitis. However, the moral dilemma in these cases is the uncertainty of the long-term medical and psychological sequelae.

Undoubtedly, the quality of life of a patient born with MMC is far from optimal. The patient may suffer from a variety of complications such as hydrocephalus, paraplegia, orthopedic problems, bladder and bowel dysfunction, and neurodevelopmental problems, including mental retardation, learning disabilities, and convulsions.

Selection criteria for treatment were developed in an attempt to distinguish between babies who might do well following surgery and those who would remain severely disabled.

These criteria are based on anticipated major adverse medical factors heralding physical disabilities or anticipated mental retardation in the very early stages of life. Lorber (1972) initiated this approach, which was then modified by other investigators. Lorber's criteria for nontreatment included hydrocephalus at birth; complete paraplegia, with a lesion at the level of the first lumbar vertebra or above; and associated major congenital anomalies. Newborns with two or more of these adverse factors were then selected for nontreatment (Lorber, 1972).

Many studies support the prognostic value of these criteria for *most* infants (Gross, Cox, Tatznek, Polley, & Barnes, 1983; Lorber & Salfield, 1981; Stark & Drummong, 1973). However, recent studies have shown that the "selected in" babies, even according to strict criteria, may still have significant residual disabilities, and the "selected out" babies may do surprisingly well physically, and particularly mentally. For example, more than 20% of Lorber's own patients who were "selected out" eventually had completely normal intelligence.

Most children born with MMC and hydrocephalus were assumed to have mental retardation eventually because of a congenital defect in the architecture of the brain (polymicrogyria), which often accompanies this anomaly. This assumption was proven to be wrong. Several investigators (Mapstone et al., 1984) found a low degree of correlation between hydrocephalus, the level of the lesion, and the outcome. Only complications of treatment, particularly post-shunt ventriculitis, correlated more closely with mental retardation.

Approximately 30% of all cases of MMC are accompanied by some degree of retardation. However, there are no definite predictors of retardation, including severe hydrocephalus (Noetzel, 1989). Most patients with MMC, when treated, are capable of meaningful human relationships, and many are of normal intelligence. Such patients are able to walk with assistive devices, attend regular schools, and achieve bowel and bladder control (Freeman, 1984). Recent technological advances have significantly improved almost every aspect of the care of infants and children with MMC. Therefore, many pessimistic statements that ascribe a very poor prognosis to most patients with MMC have not been substantiated.

Another erroneous assumption was that almost all babies with MMC would die within a short period of time if this condition was not surgically corrected. Several studies have shown that babies with a severe untreated lesion do not always succumb immediately, and some studies even reported a 10%–30% survival rate of children selected for nontreatment (Noetzel, 1989). This outcome is probably due to the natural development of granulation tissue, which seals the defect.

There is little doubt that untreated surviving babies will suffer more than those surgically treated. Thus, all selection criteria are of only statistical importance. In individual cases, false-positive *and* false-negative fallacies are unavoidable.

The Spina Bifida Association of America issued an *Amicus Curiae* brief which stated:

> Since we have found it virtually impossible to predict at birth which infants with meningomyelocele will become competitive, ambulatory and intellectually able, we have not relied on arbitrary guidelines to determine which children should or should not be treated. On the contrary, we believe that all such children should be treated, and we feel that our data show this philosophy to be correct. (Stenbock, 1984)

Thus, great caution needs to be exercised in applying statistical data in difficult life and death decisions for individual patients. Based on the known data concerning MMC babies, today almost *all* such babies should be operated on.

EXTREMELY LOW BIRTH WEIGHT

The prognosis for premature infants has substantially improved with the development of perinatal and neonatal intensive care. During the 1980s, physicians and ethicists debated the ethical and medical advisability of saving and treating *low* birth weight neonates, namely those born with birth weights below 2500 grams. They then argued about *very low* birth weight babies, namely those born below 1,500 grams. Today, in the 1990s, no one disputes the well-established policy to treat these babies vigorously. Rather, the current debate concerns

extremely low birth weight babies, or micronates, namely those below 1,000 grams and particularly below 750 grams, or babies born with a gestational age below 26 weeks. Management of these babies remains controversial among ethicists who debate whether or not intensive care of these smallest premature infants is justified. Two major issues are addressed: 1) mortality, and 2) morbidity, including intraventricular bleeding with resultant severe brain damage, retinopathy of prematurity with resultant blindness, and bronchopulmonary dysplasia with severe chronic lung disease. If the mortality rate is very high, the prolonged, very expensive, and futile intensive care will consume and drain a large amount of scarce medical resources, thus denying care for other patients with better chances of survival. If the rate of significant morbidity is high, is it morally justified to save these babies?

The answer to these questions is uncertain, since we find conflicting and changing statistical data. Studies still dispute the prognosis of these infants. In 1981, one study found no survivors from birth weights below 700 grams (Britton, Fitzhardinge, & Ashby, 1981), and a survey of 23 centers in 1983 demonstrated a mortality rate approaching 90% at gestational age below 26 weeks (Sell, 1986). In 1987, the survival rate was reported to have increased over 50%. Seventy-one percent of all deaths in this study occurred within 48 hours of birth, and late death beyond 28 days was uncommon (Ferrara et al., 1989). This fact considerably weakens the argument regarding the consumption of scarce resources. At follow up, only 23% of survivors were impaired, leading to the conclusion that survival with good outcome is attainable at gestational ages and birth weights previously considered incompatible with life (Ferrara et al., 1989).

Recent reviews of published survival rates of very small premature babies from various countries revealed survival rates of 0%–16.7% for infants born at 23 weeks of gestation, 4%–31% for those born at 24 weeks, 13.5%–66% for those born at 25 weeks, and 10%–63% for those born at 26 weeks. Birth weight survival rates at weights of 500–599 grams ranged from 5% to 20%; at 600–699 grams, from 32% to

41%; and at 700–799 grams, from 33% to 61% (Hack & Fanaroff, 1989). This wide range of survival rates from different sources requires explanation and casts significant doubt on the scientific validity concerning prognosis of small newborns. The numbers vary because of differences in the medical and surgical capabilities of the reporting centers, the inclusion of criteria of the subjects in the study groups, the number of babies included, the length of follow up, the grading and definition of morbidity, the departmental policy on the aggressiveness of treatment, and the influence of socioeconomic factors on the long-range development of the infants. This tremendous variation was substantiated in a recent meta-analysis of outcome of surviving very low birth weight infants (Escobar, Littenberg, & Petitti, 1991).

There are also uncertainties as to the extent of morbidity and its severity, since reported incidence of severe neurological sequelae, or any degree of residual neurodevelopmental damage, varies significantly. Hence, there are no reliable scientific data concerning morbidity or mortality of tiny newborns. Moreover, there are still very few early prognostic markers for survival and for significant morbidity in *individual* babies. One can certainly debate the

definition of low quality of life, what is an "acceptable" quality of life, and who decides for the non-autonomous newborn whether he should live or die. Even the definition of futility is variable (Sprung & Steinberg, 1990; Youngner, 1988). Moreover, it is also well documented that early intervention and preventive measures are beneficial in improving the quality of life for many defective and premature infants. Therefore, it seems a reasonable conclusion that an individual baby who has a chance for survival should be treated as vigorously as necessary.

CONCLUSION

Difficult moral issues and treatment decisions regarding newborns with disabilities require careful consideration. Only in extreme cases where the available therapeutic options are unequivocally futile should one consider nontreatment. Whenever uncertainties exist, life must be favored. The rule of thumb should be: "When in doubt, err in favor of life." Therefore, scrupulous respect for all human life is required. Otherwise, a slippery slope process might lead to irreversible, undesired, and immoral actions and consequences.

REFERENCES

Britton, S.B., Fitzhardinge, P.M., & Ashby, S. (1981). Is intensive care justified for infants weighing less than 801 grams at birth? *Journal of Pediatrics, 99*, 937–943.

Escobar, G.J., Littenberg, B., & Petitti, D.B. (1991). Outcome among surviving very low birthweight infants: A meta-analysis. *Archives of Diseases in Childhood, 66*, 204–211.

Ferrara, T.B., Hoekstra, R.E., Gaziano, E., Knox, G.E., Couser, R.J., & Fangman, J.J. (1989). Changing outcome of extremely premature infants: Survival and follow-up at a tertiary center. *American Journal of Obstetrics and Gynecology, 161*, 1114–1118.

Freeman, J.M. (1984). Early management and decision making for the treatment of myelomeningocele: A critique. *Pediatrics, 73*, 564–566.

Gross, R.H., Cox, A., Tatznek, R., Polley, M., & Barnes, W.A. (1983). Early management and decision making for the treatment of myelomeningocele. *Pediatrics, 72*, 450–458.

Hack, M., & Fanaroff, A.A. (1989). Outcome of extremely-low-birth-weight infants between 1982 and 1988. *New England Journal of Medicine, 321*, 1642–1647.

Lorber, J. (1972). Spina bifida cystica: Results of treatment of 270 consecutive cases with criteria for selection for

the future. *Archives of Diseases in Childhood, 47*, 854–873.

Lorber, J., & Salfield, S.A.W. (1981). Results of selective treatment of spina bifida cystica. *Archives of Diseases in Childhood, 56*, 822–830.

Mapstone, T.B., Rekate, H.L., Nulsen, F.E., et al. (1984). Relationship of CSF shunting and IQ in children with myelomeningocele: A retrospective analysis. *Child's Brain, 11*, 112–118.

Noetzel, M.J. (1989). Myelomeningocele: Current concepts of management. *Clinics in Perinatology, 16*, 311–329.

Sell, E. (1986). Outcomes of very very low birth weight infants. *Clinics in Perinatology, 13*, 451–460.

Sprung, C.L., & Steinberg, A. (1990). Acquired immunodeficiency syndrome and critical care. *Critical Care Medicine, 18*, 1300–1302.

Stark, G.D., & Drummond, M. (1973). Results of selective early operation in myelomeningocele. *Archives of Diseases in Childhood, 48*, 676–683.

Stenbock, B. (1984, February). Baby Jane Doe in the courts. *Hastings Center Report*, 13–19.

Youngner, S.J. (1988). Who defines futility? *Journal of the American Medical Association, 260*, 2094–2095.

Chapter 3

The Development of Prelinguistic Communication
Implications for Language Evaluation

ESTHER DROMI, PH.D
University of Tel Aviv, Tel Aviv, Israel

IT IS COMMONLY BELIEVED THAT LANGUAGE development begins when an infant starts to utter the first comprehensible words. Parents throughout the world eagerly await this developmental achievement that for normal children is documented at 12–18 months of age (Dromi, 1987). Our present-day scientific understanding of the normal course of language development indicates that the emergence of the first words are strongly dependent on the child's more general communicative and cognitive skills that are developed very early in life and are established throughout the prelinguistic stage (Bates, 1979; Bruner, 1975). New findings on the course of early communicative development in normal infants shape our goals for clinical assessment and determine the procedures for evaluating communicative competence among very young children who are "at risk" for language acquisition. In this chapter, current findings on the normal development of communication during infancy are summarized, and a model is outlined for the assessment of communicative abilities during the prelinguistic stage in young hearing impaired sub-

jects, or in other populations of preverbal children with disabilities (e.g., mentally retarded, autistic, specific language impaired).

THE STUDY OF PRELINGUISTIC COMMUNICATION

The study of prelinguistic communication covers quite a wide range of research topics. This review focuses on the following areas: 1) the establishment of eye contact and the demonstration of mutual gaze between mothers and infants, 2) the structure of turn taking in prespeech vocalizations, 3) the emergence of intentional communication, and 4) the development of symbolic gestural expression.

Eye Contact and Mutual Gaze

Infants' capacity to control the flow of visual stimuli, to maintain visual fixation, and to divert from too-familiar or too-intense visual inputs has been documented from birth (Fantz, 1966). During the first few months of life, infants apply their visual capacity in two separate domains: the domain of social interchanges

This chapter describes a model that was conceptualized in my research project entitled "Language Intervention for Preschool Hearing Impaired Children." The project is funded by the Israeli Ministry of Education and the National Council of Micha. I wish to thank the members of the research team: D. Ben Yzhak, H. Ben Shachar, S. Beni-Noked, E. Guralnik, V. Himel, A. Sandbank, A. Plaut, N. Zohar, and D. Ringwald-Frimerman, for their invaluable contribution to this work.

and the domain of physical objects. Stern (1974) documented a dyadic structure of gaze behaviors between mothers and infants during the first few weeks of life. He suggested that both mother and infant actively participate in social-interactive exchanges through the establishment of eye contact and mutual gaze. Initially, the infant looking at the mother's eyes represents a response to her solicitation attempts, yet gradually the infant becomes more and more competent in initiating visual exchanges independently.

During the first 6 months of life, infants are observed scanning and visually exploring the world of objects around them (Sugarman, 1987). At this initial phase, however, they cannot interrupt a sequence of visual scanning of objects in order to socially interact with the mother. If such an interruption occurs, for instance when the mother lifts the child or places her face between him or her and the explored object, the infant reveals a loss of interest in the object as he or she starts to interact with the adult (D'Odrico & Levorato, 1990).

During the second half of the first year of life, the infant can be observed focusing on discrete components of the visual stimuli in the physical environment. For example, the infant can be seen looking at a specific clock or a familiar picture which is hanging on the wall, or focusing for a very short period of time on a specific piece of furniture in the room. This phenomenon has been described by Newson (1978) as a "referential look," where the infant's visual behavior becomes a means for conveying personal interest in discrete elements of reality, in contrast to the earlier global, or diffuse scanning, of the environment.

A substantial visual attainment is documented at about 9 months of age, when the infant starts to incorporate social interactions into sequences of object scanning and manipulation (D'Odrico & Levorato, 1990). At this level, infants begin to demonstrate their ability to alternate their gaze between an object of interest and a communicative partner and vice versa (Masur, 1990). This developmental attainment is highly significant for a later important achievement of establishing "joint atten-

tion" between the infant and the adult, either when the infant initiates it or when the adult does so. In many instances, when joint attention is obtained, the adult provides a label for the object or event which is of mutual visual interest (Bruner, 1975). This behavior strongly enhances efficient lexical learning.

Prespeech Vocalizations

New evidence on preverbal productions has recently challenged the traditional view that vocal behaviors during infancy are discontinuous with respect to true speech. In several research programs, continuities rather than discontinuities have been reported between prespeech vocalizations and meaningful speech (Oller, 1986; Smith, Brown-Sweely, & Stoel-Gammon, 1989).

From a very early age, infants are recorded to produce vocalizations of various acoustic qualities. Infants several weeks old are involved in bidirectional vocal turntaking with their caregivers. At birth, or shortly after birth, newborns are able to match visual models of articulatory movements (Meltzoff & Moore, 1983). At 1–3 months of age, infants develop the ability to sporadically produce reciprocal imitations of cooing sounds corresponding to their repertoire of spontaneous productions (Uzgiris, 1984). Imitations of verbal sounds become systematic at 4–8 months, with a growing tendency of the mother to imitate the infant's sounds and to establish reciprocal vocal play.

In a series of investigations of mother-infant vocal exchanges, Papoušek and Papoušek (1989) revealed that in spontaneous mother-infant interactions during the second, third, and fifth months of life, over half of the child's voiced noncry vocalizations were either imitated by the mother or were imitations of segments from the mother's previous productions. The proportion of mother–infant matches equalled the proportion of infant–mother matches, thus emphasizing the reciprocal nature of interaction in which each partner takes turns modelling and matching.

Veneziano (1988) also reported a high level of sonoric similarity between the mother's and the child's adjunct productions during the pre-linguistic stage. She argued that the mothers' imitations of the child's vocalizations help the child to assimilate the particular phonological characteristics of his or her mother tongue. According to this theory, the child's initial relatively large repertoire of speech sounds will be gradually reduced as he or she identifies those vocalizations which are imitated by the mother as true sounds of the target language. Eventually, only the imitated vocalizations will remain in the child's linguistic system, and will turn to function as true words in the child's productive lexicon. (A similar claim has been made by Locke [1986].)

Several researchers have noted that toward the end of the prelinguistic stage, children's vocalizations are often associated with specific communicative functions. The most ambitious attempt to describe the evolution of sound-function parallels was that of Carter (1979). In her son's verbal productions, Carter recorded vocalizations which were clearly associated with identified communicative intents. She termed these consistent sound-function correlates "s/m morphemes," claiming that these morphemes would eventually develop into true words. Thus, at some time before learning that words constitute labels for specific objects, Carter argues, children may point at various objects and consistently vocalize the same sound (e.g., "o/§o/§o/" or "dze/§dze/§dze/"), indicating that they realize speech sounds stand for objects and serve a declarative function. During the same time, when the infant wants to manipulate the mother or other adults, he or she might use another sound (e.g., "M/ M/ M/" or "DA/ DA/ DA/") in a request intonation to indicate that he or she demands an action. These vocalizations are often interpreted by the listeners as requests for action or as imperatives.

Intentional Communication

The emergence of intentional communication prior to the recording of the first comprehensible words was heavily investigated during the 1970s and 1980s (Bates, Camaioni, & Volterra, 1979; Bruner, 1975; Harding, 1983; Harding &

Golinkoff, 1979; Ninio & Bruner, 1978; Sugarman, 1978, 1983). Studies which examined communicative intents from within the framework of "speech act" theory (Austin, 1962; Searle, 1969) indicated that the prelinguistic stage is divided into two distinct developmental phases with regard to communicative intentions: the perlocution phase and the illocution phase.

During the first few months of life, termed by Bates et al. (1979) as the *perlocution* phase, infants are not yet able to produce identifiable communicative intentions and their acts are interpreted by the adults who observe them. Most of the infants' behaviors, such as cries, sneezes, kicks, vocalizations, and smiles, generate interpretative reactions in the mothers. As infants develop cognitively and physically, their behaviors become more and more controlled and goal-oriented; they start to look at, move toward, and reach for objects. Even at this more advanced level, however, mothers can only infer from what they see what the child is doing, and what he or she might want (Harding, 1983).

Intentional communication, however, requires much more than inferences made by the observer or the listener. Intentional communication refers to the reciprocal ability of the organism to generate signals that another person can comprehend, and to understand signals that were purposefully produced by another person (Harding, 1983). Only in the second phase of the prelinguistic stage, termed by Bates et al. (1979) as the phase of *illocution*, at about the age of 9–12 months old, do infants start to overtly signal to others their communicative intents through gestures, vocalizations, and contrastive intonation patterns.

Two distinct communicative functions have been described by Bates and colleagues (1979) to emerge at this phase: proto-declarative and proto-imperative. *Proto-declarative* is a function of a descriptive nature, usually manifested by pointing and vocalizing (e.g., pointing to different objects and vocalizing "da/ da/ da/" as if naming the pointed objects). The proto-imperative is a function of manipulating and controlling others' behaviors (e.g., reaching for an empty bottle while whining "U/ U/ U/" in a request intonation for an adult to fill the bottle and hand it to the child to drink).

Sugarman (1978) provided an interesting explanation for the transition from the perlocution to the illocution phase of the prelinguistic stage. She argued that during the first few months of life, an infant's object-oriented behaviors and person-oriented behaviors are completely separated from one another. During this phase the infant's improvement of his or her schemes for object manipulation, as well as his or her social schemes, are conducted along parallel tracks. A qualitative shift in the infant's behaviors is observed around 10–12 months of age, when the infant starts to *coordinate* the object and the social schemes. (Note: a similar claim has been made with reference to the development of visual skills during the first year of life.)

Prior to this coordination (in the perlocution phase), if the infant fails to obtain a desired object which is near the mother but out of reach, he or she will stop efforts at some point and move ahead to another goal without signalling to the mother that her help is needed. However, when the infant becomes able to coordinate object and social schemes (in the illocution phase), if he or she seeks to obtain an object that cannot be reached, the infant will signal to the mother by crying, shifting his or her gaze between the mother and the desired object, and showing, reaching, or pointing that some help is required.

An important prerequisite for the establishment of reference and the acquisition of conventional speech is the ability to initiate and participate in a communicative collaboration (Ninio & Bruner, 1978). During the second half of the prelinguistic stage, infants show their ability to initiate such collaboration, and to respond to adults' initiations of communicative exchanges. A major attainment that is a prerequisite for lexical learning is that of establishing shared topics or targets of attention. In his work on the transition from communication to language, Bruner (1975) discussed the relation between the developmental achievements of "joint action" and "joint attention" and the emergence of referential speech. *Joint atten-*

tion refers to the ability of one person to follow another person's line of visual regard, which leads to a concurrent focusing of the two persons on an external object of reference. *Joint action* refers to the collaborative efforts of two participants in performing a task together (e.g., building a tower of blocks, turning pages in a picture book, playing with a ball).

Prior to the emergence of meaningful speech, infants start to point at objects, a behavior which signals to the mother the topic of interest. They also begin to respond to the mother's pointing and to follow her line of regard. Joint attention then becomes a reciprocal activity. When the infant points at a toy (or lifts it), the mother looks at it and might also label it; when the mother points at a picture or an object and also labels it, the infant focuses his or her visual gaze on it, establishing reference.

Symbolic Gestural Expression

Recent research on the emergence of symbolic gesture in normally developing prelinguistic children has produced a number of important findings which further indicate that the first comprehensible words are strongly tied to pre-existing general cognitive and communicative functions. Prior to the emergence of their first words, a large proportion of children produce meaningful gestures (Acredolo & Goodwyn, 1990; Caselli, 1990). Toward the end of the prelinguistic stage, sequences of gestures appear, and the gestural system is gradually replaced by conventional words.

Gestures may be classified into two major subgroups: deictic and referential. Deictic gestures are conventional signals that refer to external objects and events. These gestures express communicative intention that can be understood only through the extralinguistic context in which they are produced. The three most frequently recorded deictic gestures are *showing, giving*, and *pointing*, which emerge in that sequence.

Referential gestures denote a precise referent and have a semantic content which does not change according to context. Examples of referential gestures are: *bye bye, bravo, dancing, no, sleep, hat, phone, hungry*. Caselli (1990) found that early referential gestures are initially embedded within everyday social routines. Gestures are decontextualized gradually and are then produced by the child spontaneously in different contexts. Similar processes of decontextualization have been described for both early gestures and early words (Bates, 1979; Caselli, 1990).

The comprehensive body of data on prelinguistic developments in the visual, vocal, communicative, and gestural domains supports the position that continuity rather than discontinuity exists between precursors of speech and conventional language. Studies in the different areas show that in the normally developing child, prelinguistic achievements are synchronized in the four domains reviewed. A qualitative shift is observed around the ages of 9–12 months in the communicative abilities of infants. This shift is characterized by the emergence of intentional communication, which seems to be a prerequisite for the emergence of speech.

THE ASSESSMENT OF COMMUNICATIVE SKILLS IN THE PRELINGUISTIC STAGE

Against the rich theoretical background that was summarized above for normally developing children, a clinical model has been constructed for the evaluation of communication in prelinguistic hearing-impaired subjects.

Four aspects of prelinguistic communication are examined: 1) the structure of discourse, 2) the range of communicative functions, 3) the modalities of expression, and 4) the language addressed to the child. The empirical testing of this model on a population of prelinguistic hearing-impaired children at the ages of 6 months to 4 years old is in its planning stages.

The Structure of Discourse

In the assessment of the structure of discourse, evaluation takes place on whether the child is participating in visual, vocal, and/or gestural communicative interchanges. The child is also observed to see if he or she initiates interactions with adults (e.g., mother and clinician) or

responds to adults' initiations. By counting the number of turns in observed interactions, the extent to which child–adult interchanges are elaborated and balanced are examined. In addition, the means are specified by which the child signals to the adult that he or she is no longer interested in the communicative collaboration.

Data on the structure of adult–child discourse interactions are obtained from a 30-minute spontaneous play session of the mother with the child. The means used by each participant in the visual, vocal, and gestural domains are examined. Direct inspection of the child's interaction patterns with the adult–clinician during the evaluation session also provides information on the structure of discourse in adult–child interchanges.

Communicative Functions

The second assessment index consists of the range of communicative intents observed in the spontaneous behavior of the child. The taxonomy of communicative functions that is used in this analysis is presented in Table 1.

Information on the range of communicative functions and the frequency of their use is obtained through the analysis of the video-recorded play sessions, and through the clinician's direct testing of the child's communicative behaviors during spontaneous play. Parent interviews are also used for gathering information on the extent of application of the different functions at home, in the natural environment of the child.

Modes of Expression

In this analysis, the nature of the child's vocalizations and manual expressions are assessed. The repertoire of speech sounds produced by the child is recorded, and the level of manual expression is analyzed, distinguishing between deictic and referential gestures and sign productions. The analysis of sign productions is restricted to those hearing-impaired infants who are born to deaf parents and hence acquire sign language as a mother tongue, or to children who are educated in rehabilitation programs, which utilize the simultaneous communication mode of instruction (i.e., speech

Table 1. Communicative functions in the prelinguistic stage

Function	Definition
1. Prerequisite behaviors	The child evidences: 1) coordination of object and social schemes, 2) joint action, and 3) joint attention.
2. Proto-declaratives	The child points and vocalizes for labelling objects.
3. Proto-imperatives	The child uses gestures and vocalizations for manipulating and controlling the adult's activities.
4. Interactions	The child shows interest in environmental stimuli and takes part in interactional games.
5. Heuristic and informative behaviors	The child uses gestures or vocalizations as a heuristic for gathering information (e.g., shows an object to the adult and await the adult's response of naming it).
6. Responses	The child responds to gestural or verbal requests or simple instructions and sometimes imitates adult vocalizations and gestures.
7. Symbolic representation	The child produces referential gestures, and shows symbolic activities with objects (e.g., rings and speaks over the phone, throws a ball, brushes own hair).

and sign) (Dromi & Ringwald-Frimerman, 1990; Ringwald-Frimerman, 1990). No reference is made here to the analysis of conventional sign productions, as it does not directly follow from the review of the literature cited above. (The interested reader is referred to Newport [1982, 1984] and to Petitto [1988, 1990] for detailed reports on sign language acquisition. These reports strongly indicate great similarities in underlying processes of language learning in the two modalities of speech and sign [Dromi, 1989].)

The analysis of gesture production is rooted in Caselli's distinction between deictic and referential gesturing. The production and response to pointing, which is the most developed deictic gesture, is examined and the diverse forms of referential gestural expression are tested. Finally, the idea that referential sequences are produced and consistent speech sounds are embedded within these sequences is also looked at.

Data on modes of expression are obtained from the video recording of mother–child interactions, from the clinician's direct inspection during the assessment sessions, and from a structured questionnaire in which parents are requested to indicate what kind of communicative and noncommunicative behavior(s) are produced by the child within specific, highly

familiar, daily life contexts. The parents' questionnaire was constructed in Italy by Camaioni, Caselli, Longobardi, and Volterra (1990) to evaluate prelinguistic behaviors in normally developing infants. It was translated into Hebrew and adapted for use with hearing–impaired subjects. The questionnaire presents a given set of options for child responses in each of five contexts: 1) asking for food, 2) picture book telling, 3) looking for a familiar adult or a family pet, 4) the "peekaboo" game, and 5) looking for a desired toy. Parents' reports helped us determine the level of gesture production by each child.

Language Exposure and Language Comprehension

A complete evaluation of prelinguistic communication must include reference to the language addressed to the child. Levels of language exposure and language comprehension are distinguished as being two distinct psycholinguistic phenomena. *Exposure* refers to the language produced by the adult with no requirement for any response by the child, whereas *comprehension* refers to those parts of the linguistic input that require the child's motor or verbal responses. At the exposure level, it is determined if the linguistic model for the child is rich and productive. In other words, the language addressed to the child should reveal a diversity of simple syntactic constructions: declarative sentences, interrogatives, and negatives. At the comprehension level, testing is performed to see if the child responds to a few linguistic terms (nouns and verbs) that are frequently used in everyday situations (e.g., ball, airplane, car, doll, spoon, sleep, eat, jump, sit). Children at the prelinguistic stage are expected to respond to simple routine instructions which are produced in natural contexts (e.g., "give me," "throw the ball," "put it in the box"). Tests are performed to see if the parents provide such instructions and whether the child responds to them.

Data on the language addressed to the child are obtained from the video recording of the spontaneous play session, and by direct testing of the child's responses to simple instructions during the clinical evaluation sessions.

SUMMARY

This chapter reviews an infant's normally developing communication at the prelinguistic stage and illustrates a model for the clinical evaluation of prelinguistic communicative skills among young hearing-impaired, and other language impaired, populations. The model pinpoints four different aspects of communication that can be assessed even before first words emerge. The significance of mother–child dyadic interactions in the prelinguistic stage is emphasized, calling for clinical procedures which focus on the adult–child dyadic interactions rather than only on the child. We propose the usage of three procedures for data collection: 1) video recordings of spontaneous mother–child play, 2) direct testing by the clinician during evaluation sessions, and 3) parents' interviews or reports that can be obtained through structured questionnaires.

REFERENCES

Acredolo, L.P., & Goodwyn, S.W. (1990). Sign language among hearing infants: The spontaneous development of symbolic gestures. In V. Volterra & C.J. Erting (Eds.), *From gesture to language in hearing and deaf children* (pp. 68–78). Berlin: Springer-Verlag.

Austin, J.L. (1962). *How to do things with words.* Cambridge, MA: Harvard University Press.

Bates, E. (1979). *The emergence of symbols: Cognition and communication in infancy* (pp. 111–132). New York: Academic Press.

Bates, E., Camaioni, L., & Volterra, V. (1979). The acquisition of performatives prior to speech. In E. Ochs & B.B. Schieffelin (Eds.), *Developmental pragmatics.* New York: Academic Press.

Bruner, J. (1975). The ontogenesis of speech acts. *Journal of Child Language, 2,* 1–19.

Camaioni, L., Caselli, M.C., Longobardi, E., & Volterra, V. (1990). *Construction and validation of a parent report instrument for assessing communicative and linguistic development in the second year of life.* Paper presented at the Fifth International Congress for the Study of Child Language, Budapest, Hungary.

Carter, A.L. (1979). Prespeech meaning relations: an outline of one infant's sensorimotor morpheme development. In P. Fletcher & M. Garman (Eds.), *Language acquisition: Studies in first language development* (pp. 71–92). Cambridge: Cambridge University Press.

Caselli, M.C. (1990). Communicative gestures and first words. In V. Volterra & C.J. Erting (Eds.), *From gesture to language in hearing and deaf children* (pp. 56–68). Berlin: Springer-Verlag.

D'Odrico, L., & Levorato, M.C. (1990). Social and cognitive determinants of mutual gaze between the mother and infant. In V. Volterra & C.J. Erting (Eds.), *From gesture to language in hearing and deaf children* (pp. 9–17). Berlin: Springer-Verlag.

Dromi, E. (1987). *Early lexical development.* Cambridge: Cambridge University Press.

Dromi, E. (1989). *The significance of input and interaction for children who learn language under exceptional circumstances.* Paper presented at the Tenth Biannual Meeting of ISSBD, Jyvaskula, Finland.

Dromi, E., & Ringwald-Frimerman, D. (1990). *The effects of input characteristics on lexical learning by hearing impaired children.* Paper presented at the Fifth International Congress for the Study of Child Language, Budapest, Hungary.

Fantz, R.L. (1966). Pattern discrimination and selective attention as determinants of perceptual development from birth. In L. Kidd and G. Rivoire (Eds.), *Perceptual development in children* (pp. 143–173). New York: International University Press.

Harding, C.G. (1983). Setting the stage for language acquisition: Communication in the first year. In R.L. Golinkoff (Ed.), *The transition from prelinguistic to linguistic communication* (pp. 93–111). Hillsdale, NJ: Lawrence Erlbaum Associates.

Harding, C.G., & Golinkoff, R.L. (1979). The origins of intentional vocalizations in prelinguistic infants. *Child Development, 50,* 33–40.

Locke, J.L. (1986). The linguistic significance of babbling. In B. Lindblom & R. Zetterstrom (Eds.), *Precursors of early speech* (pp. 143–160). Stockholm: Stockton Press.

Masur, E.F. (1990). Gestural development, dual-directional signaling and the transition to words. In V. Volterra & C.J. Erting (Eds.), *From gesture to language in hearing and deaf children* (pp. 18–31). Berlin: Springer-Verlag.

Meltzoff, A.N., & Moore, M.K. (1983). Newborn infants imitate adult facial gestures. *Child Development, 54*, 702–709.

Newport, E.L. (1982). Task specificity in language learning? Evidence from speech perception and American Sign Language. In E. Wanner & L. Gleitman (Eds.), *Language acquisition: The state of the art* (pp. 450–486). Cambridge: Cambridge University Press.

Newport, E.L. (1984). Constraints on learning: Studies in the acquisition of American Sign Language. *Papers and Reports on Child Language Development, 23*, 1–22.

Newson, J. (1978). Dialogue and development. In A. Lock (Ed.), *Action, gesture and symbol* (pp. 31–42). London: Academic Press.

Ninio, A., & Bruner, J. (1978). The achievement and antecedents of labelling. *Journal of Child Language, 5*, 1–15.

Oller, D.K. (1986). Metaphonology and infant vocalizations. In B. Lindblom & R. Zetterstrom (Eds.), *Precursors of early speech* (pp. 21–35). Stockholm: Stockton Press.

Papoušek, M., & Papoušek, H. (1989). Form and function of vocal matching in interactions between mothers and their precanonical infants. *First Language, 9*, 137–158.

Petitto, L.A. (1988). "Language" in the prelinguistic child. In F.S. Kessel (Ed.), *The development of language and language researchers: Essays in honor of Roger Brown* (pp. 187–218). Hillsdale, NJ: Lawrence Erlbaum Associates.

Petitto, L.A. (1990). The transition from gesture to symbol in American Sign language. In V. Volterra & C.J. Erting (Eds.), *From gesture to language in hearing and deaf children* (pp. 153–161). Berlin: Springer-Verlag.

Ringwald-Frimerman, D. (1990). *The relationship between Simultaneous Communication input characteristics and lexical learning processes of hearing impaired preschool children who are educated in a simultaneous communication framework.* Master's thesis. School of Education, Tel Aviv University.

Searle, J.R. (1969). *Speech acts.* Cambridge, England: Cambridge University Press.

Smith, B.L., Brown-Sweely, S., & Stoel-Gammon, C. (1989). Prelinguistic phonetic contingency: Data from Down syndrome. *First Language, 9*, 175–191.

Stern, D.N. (1974). Mother and infant at play: the dyadic interaction involving facial, vocal, and gaze behaviors. In M. Lewis & L. Rosenblum (Eds.), *The effects of infants on its caregiver* (pp. 187–213). New York: John Wiley & Sons.

Sugarman, S. (1978). Some organizational aspects of preverbal communication. In I. Markova (Ed.), *The social context of language* (pp. 5–27). New York: John Wiley & Sons.

Sugarman, S. (1983). Empirical versus logical issues in the transition from prelinguistic to linguistic communication. In R.L. Golinkoff (Ed.), *The transition from prelinguistic to linguistic communication* (pp. 133–143). Hillsdale, NJ: Lawrence Erlbaum Associates.

Sugarman, S. (1987). *Piaget's construction of the children's reality.* Cambridge: Cambridge University Press.

Uzgiris, I.C. (1984). Imitation in infancy: Its interpersonal aspects. In M. Perlmuter (Ed.), *Parent child interaction and parent child relations in child development.* Hillsdale NJ: Lawrence Erlbaum Associates.

Veneziano, E. (1988). Vocal-verbal interaction and the construction of early lexical knowledge. In M. Smith & J. Locke (Eds.), *The emergent lexicon* (pp. 110–145). New York: Academic Press.

Chapter 4

Intervention Approaches for Young Children with Communicative Disorders

LAURENCE B. LEONARD, PH.D.
Purdue University, West Lafayette, Indiana

T HE FOCUS OF THIS CHAPTER IS EARLY LAN- guage intervention, with special emphasis placed on children clinically labeled "specifically language-impaired." This is a rather heterogeneous group of children who exhibit a significant deficit in language learning ability, yet have normal hearing, score at age level on nonverbal tests of intelligence, show no signs of frank neurological impairment, and come from homes where language stimulation is more than adequate (Johnston, 1988; Leonard, 1979, 1989).

Given the current state of knowledge, the accurate identification of language disorders in such children cannot take place until well after the first year of life. Consequently, intervention typically does not begin until an age at which some very important language milestones have already been achieved by normally developing children. For example, by 8 weeks of age, normally developing infants can distinguish the prosody or intonation of the surrounding language from the prosody of another language (Mehler et al., 1988). By 18 weeks of age, infants can identify which of two silent videorecordings of a person producing vowels is the one that matches an audiorecorded vowel (Kuhl & Meltzoff, 1988). At the age of 6 months, children show evidence of forming categories needed for later object naming, such as the category "bird" (Colombo, O'Brien, Mitchell, Roberts, & Horowitz, 1987). By 7 months of age, they show a sensitivity to the acoustic cues that correlate with major syntactic boundaries (Hirsh-Pasek et al., 1987). For example, children at this age show a listening preference for material that contains pauses at clause and phrase boundaries rather than in the middle of the clause or phrase. Indeed, by 10 months, children are so attuned to the language to which they are exposed that they begin to lose their ability to perceive phonetic distinctions that are not phonemic in their language, while of course not losing any of their ability to perceive distinctions that are relevant (Werker, 1989).

Evidence of this sort is sobering for those responsible for the identification of language problems in children. Each month that passes could well represent a possible opportunity to remove or apply some external factor, or to foster some compensatory skill.

The possibility of missed opportunities is especially great in children with specific language impairment. Because these children do not show clear evidence of other types of handicap, and because many normally developing children can be a bit slow in their language development, it is very easy to miss these children.

IDENTIFYING CHILDREN WITH SPECIFIC LANGUAGE IMPAIRMENT

Fortunately, thanks to a number of recent studies, criteria have been established for judging a child to be at risk for a language disorder, even when all else appears relatively intact. For example, after a systematic program of research, Rescorla (1989) and her colleagues concluded that a child is at risk for a language disorder if, at the age of 24 months, he or she has a production vocabulary of fewer than 50 words or produces no word combinations.

In Rescorla's procedure, the clinician presents the parent with a carefully selected printed list of approximately 300 words and asks the parent to indicate which words the child produces. The parents may also add any words not on the list that the child says. The parents are also asked if their child produces any word combinations, such as "more cookie" and so on, and are requested to provide a few examples. Rescorla found that 90% of children who showed clinically significant scores on standardized tests had in fact failed to acquire 50 words and produced no word combinations at 24 months of age. In contrast, approximately 90% of children who showed age-appropriate scores on the standardized tests produced more than 50 words and/or used word combinations at 24 months. Work is currently underway to confirm initial impressions that Rescorla's criteria are successful in predicting which children continue to show language difficulties at 3 years of age. A more comprehensive inventory has been developed that also shows good reliability and validity (Dale, 1991; Dale, Bates, Reznick, & Morisset, 1989).

Apart from expressive vocabulary size and ability to produce word combinations, two other factors may be helpful in the early identification of language impairment. Thal, Tobias, and Morrison (1991) identified a group of children who at approximately 2 years of age were in the lowest 10% of their age group in number of words produced. A detailed assessment of

their language and communication at this age and 1 year later revealed the best outcomes for those children who initially had higher language comprehension scores and an ability to express "symbolic" gestures, such as making a drinking gesture with a toy cup.

Although the research reviewed above is encouraging, it nevertheless suggests that we must wait until a child reaches at least 24 months of age before considering him or her to be at risk for a language disorder. There is one additional factor, however, that may allow us to lower this age: evidence of familial aggregation in specific language impairment. Examples of two recent findings are provided in Tables 1 and 2.

In the first example, from Tallal, Ross, and Curtiss (1989), it can be seen that the percentage of specifically language-impaired children whose parents had a history of language problems was higher than the percentage seen for a group of control children. Comparable percentage differences were also seen when siblings were examined. Although these findings are generally typical of other recent findings, the percentages for the control group seem somewhat high. This could be due to the fact that the definition of "affected" family member was quite broad, including a history of academic problems which may or may not have been directly linked to a language problem.

In the example summarized in Table 2, from Tomblin (1989), the definition of "affected" family member was restricted to a diagnosed problem of spoken language comprehension and/or production. As can be seen, the percentages are lower for the parents of the controls than seen in the last study, and the differences between the parents of the specifically language-impaired children and the parents of the control children are even larger. Again, the results

Table 1. Percentage of parents with history of language problems

Group	Mothers	Fathers
SLI[a]	33	18
Control	13	8

Adapted from Tallal, Ross, and Curtiss (1989).
[a]Specifically language-impaired children.

Table 2. Percentage of parents with history of language problems

Group	Mothers	Fathers
SLI[a]	20	19
Control	4	3

Adapted from Tomblin (1989).

[a]Specifically language-impaired children.

for the siblings resembled those seen for the parents. A reasonable conclusion that can be drawn from findings such as these is that although the actual evidence for a language disorder won't be impressive until 24 months, a positive family history of language problems can probably be considered a risk factor.

INTERVENTION

Assuming that a child with a clear problem in language development has been identified, intervention proceeds in a manner not unlike that seen with children who are at risk for a range of developmental problems. For example, the two basic models of intervention are those commonly used elsewhere, involving a home-based or center-based approach. (Often, a combination of these models is used.) The home-based approach involves a discussion with the parents regarding how the previous week or month went. The clinician then works with the child, seeking appropriate next steps to facilitate the child's language learning, and assessing the child's responses and progress. The final step involves working with the parents on the new activity they are to use with their child, ensuring that the parents understand and feel comfortable with it. In the center-based model, there are often larger group activities in which the goals are more general and small group or individual activities in which the goal is highly specific to the child's language needs.

Regarding the content of language intervention, there are several different aspects of language that warrant attention. These include: 1) the lexicon, that is, words and their meanings; 2) pragmatics, or the social use of language; 3) phonology, or the sound system of the language, including articulation; 4) syntax,

which pertains to word combining and word order in constructing sentences; and 5) morphology, which involves the use of grammatical suffixes, prefixes, and function words. Even the last of these, morphology, emerges in the speech of normally developing children before the age of 30 months. For this reason, all of these aspects of language are likely to receive attention during early intervention.

The procedures that are effective in teaching language to young children with specific language impairments should be considered now. It should be added, however, that although these procedures are being discussed in the context of children with specific language impairment, most of them have also been used with other types of children who are at risk for language disorders. Some of these procedures are more commonly seen during individual activities, others can be easily incorporated into group activities. All can be administered by clinicians, but several can be performed by parents. Emphasis will be placed on procedures that focus on language production skills.

The review is restricted in one other important way. The only procedures included are those for which there is evidence that the observed gains can be attributed to intervention with some degree of confidence. Investigations providing evidence of this type include: 1) the use of a no-treatment control group or a comparison group that received treatment unrelated to the linguistic features of interest; 2) the use of a single-subject design in which experimental control can be demonstrated, such as a multiple baseline design or alternating treatments design; 3) the use of statistical estimation to evaluate observed gains relative to those expected from maturation; and 4) the use of a nonsense form whose acquisition could not be due to extra-experimental sources.

Imitation-Based Procedures

Until the mid 1970s, the dominant treatment approach for children with language impairments was one that made significant use of elicited imitation. That is, the clinician produces the exact sentence or phrase required of the child, and the child is asked to repeat it. Although imitation-based approaches have consistently resulted in clear language gains by the children, such approaches have not been adopted as frequently in recent years. Nevertheless, examples can be found in the literature. For example, elicited imitation has been used to teach new words to children (Olswang, Bain, Dunn, & Cooper, 1983), and imitation has been incorporated into more comprehensive intervention programs to teach two- and three-word utterances (e.g., "boy eat cake") (Warren & Kaiser, 1986).

Modeling Procedures

A second type of procedure involves the use of modeling. The child observes someone (the model) produce examples of utterances containing the linguistic form serving as the focus of intervention. The child is not asked to imitate the modeled utterances. However, he is instructed that the model will be talking in a special way. At this point, specific modeling approaches differ. In some approaches, the child only observes, while in others, the child is asked to take turns producing examples of the target pattern once the observation period is over. Recent evidence (Weismer & Murray-Branch, 1989) corroborates earlier studies indicating that modeling results in clear language gains.

Incidental Language Teaching

A third type of intervention procedure is called "incidental language teaching." This procedure resembles the approaches just described in that the language targets used in intervention are preselected by the clinician. However, incidental language teaching is quite different in other respects. In particular, it must be conducted in a more naturalistic setting, such as free play. The clinician arranges the setting to increase the likelihood that the child will initiate some form of communication. When the child indicates interest in the activity or object in question, the clinician shows attention and, as necessary, provides the child with increasingly specific cues for production of the target form. Natural contingencies are applied to the child's production of the target. For example,

following the child's successful production of the utterance "want block," the clinician gives the child the requested object. Although the bulk of work with this procedure has focused on children with more general developmental disabilities, successful application of this procedure can also be seen in the literature on specific language impairment (Warren, McQuarter, & Rogers-Warren, 1984).

Adaptations of Expansion

Another procedure that requires the child to be the initiator is expansion. This approach has its origins in the literature on normal language development, in which it was reported that mothers often responded to their young children's telegraphic utterances (e.g., "Gina daddy") with a more complete and grammatical rendition (e.g., "Yes, Gina is going with daddy"). Reported gains using this basic form of expansion with children with specific language impairments have been minimal. However, an adaptation of expansion has been found to be successful with these children (Schwartz, Chapman, Terrell, Prelock, & Rowan, 1985). In this adaptation, the adult, rather than the child, initiates the communication. For example, in teaching a child to use word combinations that specify the location of an object, the following interchange might occur:

Adult: What's this?
Child: Block.
Adult: What's the block in?
Child: Truck.
Adult: The block is in the truck.

Focused Stimulation Procedures

There are many intervention procedures that differ from one another in certain details but are similar in that they provide the child with concentrated exposure to particular linguistic forms. These are often called "focused stimulation" procedures (Leonard, 1981). Perhaps the most straightforward example can be seen in lexical treatment studies (e.g., Leonard et al., 1982) in which the clinician introduces a new object during play and says its name several times per session. In other types of focused stimulation procedures, the clinician tells the child a story that contains numerous examples of the target form, and the clinician and child then act out the story, each taking the role of one of the characters (Brooks & Benjamin, 1989). A range of focused stimulation approaches have been found to be effective.

GENERALIZATION AND MAINTENANCE

Effective language intervention implies more than the use of a linguistic feature in a narrowly defined context. Most investigators do not regard intervention as successful unless, at a minimum, the child is able to use the feature in untrained sentences in a task that resembles the ones used during intervention. However, a number of researchers have made the requirement stiffer: The child must use the feature in new sentences during conversational speech (Warren & Kaiser, 1986). Furthermore, because gains made in intervention do not mean very much if they don't last, a number of investigators have made efforts to determine whether the higher levels of performance are maintained at least 1 month later (e.g., Warren et al., 1984). The results using criteria such as these have been encouraging.

CATCHING UP OR NOT LOSING GROUND?

One final question is yet to be addressed. The fact that children with specific language impairments make gains during intervention that exceed those made without treatment does not necessarily mean that within a few months or years they will be on par with their normally developing peers. Longitudinal and follow-up studies have demonstrated not only that linguistic features emerge at a later age in the speech of children with specific language impairments, but that the period from emergence to mastery of these features is also protracted. Consequently, without intervention, these children fall even further behind their peers across time. Thus, intervention may actually permit children with specific language impairments to catch up, or it may have the more modest effect of allowing the children to begin to progress at a normal rate, so as not to fall further behind over time.

Of these two possibilities, the truth seems to fall somewhere in between. On the one hand, studies that make use of standardized tests to assess progress frequently report gains in standard scores and language quotients that are closer to the norm than before treatment began (Cole & Dale, 1986). Such large post-test gains do not appear attributable to a regression toward the mean because they are seen for tests on which the pre-test scores of children with specific language impairments were at or near the norm, as well as for tests on which the children performed very poorly.

On the other hand, the jury is still out on whether children receiving early intervention will ever reach a level of language ability that can be regarded as socially or educationally adequate. Early language intervention is still a relatively new enterprise. Consequently, the children who have received such services have not yet reached an age that permits evaluation of the long-term effects of early intervention. It is known, however, that many children with specific language impairments who received intervention only as they approached school age managed to close some of the gap, although even years later these children show language scores and achieve academic levels that are well below average. One can only hope that for the new generation of children who do receive early services, the outcome is more favorable.

REFERENCES

Brooks, A., & Benjamin, B. (1989). The use of structured role play therapy in the remediation of grammatical deficits in language delayed children: Three case studies. *Journal of Childhood Communication Disorders, 12*, 171–186.

Cole, K., & Dale, P. (1986). Direct language instruction and interactive language instruction with language delayed preschool children: A comparison study. *Journal of Speech and Hearing Research, 29*, 366–374.

Colombo, J., O'Brien, M., Mitchell, D., Roberts, K., &

Horowitz, F. (1987). A lower boundary for category formation in preverbal infants. *Journal of Child Language, 14*, 383–385.

Dale, P. (1991). The validity of a parent report measure of vocabulary and syntax at 24 months. *Journal of Speech and Hearing Research, 34*, 565–571.

Dale, P., Bates, E., Reznick, S., & Morisset, C. (1989). The validity of a parent report instrument of child language at twenty months. *Journal of Child Language, 16*, 239–250.

Hirsh-Pasek, K., Nelson, D., Jusczyk, P., Cassidy, K., Druss, B., & Kennedy, L. (1987). Clauses are perceptual units for young infants. *Cognition, 26*, 269–286.

Johnston, J. (1988). Specific language disorders in the child. In N. Lass, L. McReynolds, J. Northern, & D. Yoder (Eds.), *Handbook of speech-language pathology and audiology* (pp. 685–715). Toronto: B.C. Decker.

Kuhl, P., & Meltzoff, A. (1988). Speech as an intermodal object of perception. In A. Yonas (Ed.), *Perceptual development in infancy* (pp. 235–266). Hillsdale, NJ: Lawrence Erlbaum.

Leonard, L. (1979). Language impairment in children. *Merrill-Palmer Quarterly, 25*, 205–232.

Leonard, L. (1981). Facilitating linguistic skills in children with specific language impairment. *Applied Psycholinguistics, 2*, 89–118.

Leonard, L. (1989). Language learnability and specific language impairment in children. *Applied Psycholinguistics, 10*, 179–202.

Leonard, L., Schwartz, R., Chapman, K., Rowan, L., Prelock, P., Terrell, B., Weiss, A., & Messick, C. (1982). Early lexical acquisition in children with specific language impairment. *Journal of Speech and Hearing Research, 25*, 554–564.

Mehler, J., Jusczyk, P., Lambertz, G., Halsted, N., Bertoncini, J., & Amiel-Tison, C. (1988). A precursor of language acquisition in young infants. *Cognition, 29*, 143–178.

Olswang, L., Bain, B., Dunn, C., & Cooper, J. (1983). The effects of stimulus variation on lexical learning. *Journal of Speech and Hearing Disorders, 48*, 192–201.

Rescorla, L. (1989). The Language Development Survey: A screening tool for delayed language in toddlers. *Journal of Speech and Hearing Disorders, 54*, 587–599.

Schwartz, R., Chapman, K., Terrell, B., Prelock, P., & Rowan, L. (1985). Facilitating word combination in language-impaired children through discourse structure. *Journal of Speech and Hearing Disorders, 50*, 31–39.

Tallal, P., Ross, R., & Curtiss, S. (1989). Familial aggregation in specific language impairment. *Journal of Speech and Hearing Disorders, 54*, 167–173.

Thal, D., Tobias, S., & Morrison, D. (1991). Language and gesture in late talkers: A 1-year follow-up. *Journal of Speech and Hearing Research, 34*, 604–612.

Tomblin, J.B. (1989). Familial concentration of developmental language impairment. *Journal of Speech and Hearing Disorders, 54*, 287–295.

Warren, S., & Kaiser, A. (1986). Generalization of treatment effects by young language-delayed children: A longitudinal analysis. *Journal of Speech and Hearing Disorders, 51*, 239–251.

Warren, S., McQuarter, R., & Rogers-Warren, A. (1984). The effects of mands and models on the speech of unresponsive language-delayed preschool children. *Journal of Speech and Hearing Disorders, 49*, 43–52.

Weismer, S., & Murray-Branch, J. (1989). Modeling versus modeling plus evoked production training: A comparison of two language intervention methods. *Journal of Speech and Hearing Disorders, 54*, 269–281.

Werker, J. (1989). Becoming a native listener. *American Scientist, 77*, 54–59.

Chapter 5

The Cambridge Assessment
and Screening of Vision
in High-Risk Infants and Young Children

JANETTE ATKINSON,
University of Cambridge, United Kingdom

A NUMBER OF NEW CLINICAL METHODS were devised during the late 1970s and through to the 1990s that enabled a quantitative assessment of vision in infants and young children (Atkinson, 1985, 1989a). Many of these methods, which have been developed out of research paradigms, require no extensive verbal capacity or fine motor skills on the part of the child. However, to succeed on these tests there is the minimum requirement that the child be in an appropriate state to regard the visual display. This chapter describes various new ideas and tests incorporated into the latest test battery in the Visual Development Unit in Cambridge. These new tests have initially been used to gauge the time course of normal development of brain mechanisms underlying spatial vision. They have also proved very useful in diagnosing and assessing abnormal visual development.

THE STUDY POPULATIONS

The pediatric vision problems examined here vary widely in their severity. They can be divided along a dichotomy separating:

1. Those involving mild defects resulting in only mild or no visual disability for most everyday visual tasks (e.g., strabismus, monocular amblyopia, refractive errors)
2. Major defects causing a severe disabling impairment ranging from partial sight to complete blindness and lack of functional vision (e.g., cataracts and cortical blindness)

Fortunately, children in developed countries with severe visual impairment are rare (although estimates of prevalence vary widely between 2 per 10,000 and 3 per 1,000 depending on definition), whereas mild visual disabilities

This work is supported by the Medical Research Council of Great Britain, the Wellcome Trust, and by a grant from the East Anglia Regional Health Authority. Many past and present members of the Visual Development Unit have been involved in the research described here, in particular Oliver Braddick, John Wattam-Bell, Shirley Anker, Bruce Hood, Joss Smith, and Frank Weeks. Dr. David Allen, Shirley Anker, Bill Bobier, Jackie Day, Kim Durden, Carol Evans, Dr. Fiona Griffith, Ann MacIntyre, Dr. Michael Mair, Elizabeth Pimm-Smith, Claire Towler, and John Wattam-Bell have assisted in carrying out the screening and follow-up. I thank Mr. P.G. Watson, consultant ophthalmologist, and members of the Department of Community Health, Cambridge Health Authority, for their support, and many general practitioners and health visitors for their co-operation. Dr. Sue Atkinson, and Dr. Oliver Braddick, together with myself, jointly designed the study and Dr. Sue Atkinson administered a parallel screening programme in Bristol. Tony Moore, consultant ophthalmologist, collaborated with members of the VDU in the early onset of strabismus study. Drs. Janet Rennie, Cliff Roberton, and Heather Coughtrey collaborated with the VDU in the VLBW study.

are very common. The prevalence of strabismus, amblyopia, and significant refractive error in preschool children is estimated to be between 2% and 10% depending on population and definition. It has been estimated that 20,000 children born each year within the United Kingdom will become strabismic in the preschool years, with most becoming so in the first 2 years of life (Medical Research Council Annual Report, 1988/89).

The extent of disability resulting from the common visual defects of strabismus (commonly called "squint") and amblyopia is controversial. For example, many people have noted that strabismus carries with it a whole range of possible consequences (many unmeasured and unquantifiable), and is associated with difficulties of social interactions and communication and visuomotor and cognitive deficits. Others have considered strabismus in isolation a defect but not a disability (Social Paediatric and Obstetric Research Unit, 1991). This controversy runs throughout the pediatric vision literature and stems from lack of detailed research on pediatric visual disability. The concept of visual disability has not been clearly defined in an age-specific way for infants and children, leading to a lack of clear guidelines for definitions of partial sight and blindness. There is also a lack of knowledge about the interdependencies of visual development with motor, cognitive, and social development, and whether developmental problems in different domains are correlated or causally linked in individual children.

In addition, recent studies of dyslexia have suggested that visual defects (e.g., poor control of convergence, abnormal eye movements, defects of the transient visual system) can play a significant role in the syndrome. While many would be unhappy in calling "dyslexia" a visual defect, it is obviously a prevalent pediatric disability which can be associated with certain visual disorders for which there may be visual precursors in infancy. Visual dyslexia can be considered a severe disability in educational terms, but a mild one in terms of everyday functional vision.

The clinical populations discussed here can also be divided into two groups:

1. Those with a visual defect in isolation (i.e., with largely normal motor, cognitive, and social development)
2. Those with more than one major defect including vision (i.e., multiple disabilities), of which the largest group consists of those with cerebral palsy

In a recent report in the United Kingdom (Royal National Institute for the Blind, 1990), the second group is referred to as multihandicapped visually impaired (MHVI). It has been estimated that there are 21,000 children with visual impairments in the United Kingdom and a conservative estimate would suggest that close to 6,000 children age birth to 19 years would be classified as MHVI. The latter figure is likely to be an underestimation because of the difficulties with both assessment and diagnosis of children under 2 years.

Given these estimates of pediatric visual defects, attempts must be made to assess abnormality by comparison with normative data concerning various aspects of vision.

VISUAL ASSESSMENT IN CAMBRIDGE, U.K.

Between the late 1970s and early 1990s the Visual Development Unit in the University of Cambridge has built up a repertoire of assessment methods in research and adapted them for vision assessment in clinical pediatric patients and in "high risk" groups where there is a high probability of visual defect.

Children assessed in the Unit vary a great deal along both dichotomies outlined earlier (mild/severe disability and visual only/MHVI). This means that the tests have to be practically robust for a range of development from the normal to the severely neurologically impaired and for children with and without accompanying behavioral, motor, cognitive, and emotional problems. Several tests have proved extremely robust and valuable for clinical testing and will be briefly reviewed.

Assessment of Acuity

The Forced Choice Preferential Looking Method (FPL) (Dobson & Teller, 1978; Lewis & Maurer, 1986; Teller, Morse,

Borton, & Regal, 1974; Van Hof-van Duin & Mohn, 1986) has been used to assess resolution acuity in all infants and children who can turn their head and/or eyes to the left and right and are not able to understand or participate in a visual matching task (e.g., the Cambridge Crowding Cards—see below). The Cambridge FPL acuity set-up is automated and fixed in position with the stripe patterns electronically displayed (Atkinson & Braddick, 1982a; Atkinson, Braddick, & Moar, 1977; Atkinson, Braddick, & Pimm-Smith, 1982; Atkinson, Wattam-Bell, Pimm-Smith, Evans, & Braddick, 1986). The observer is "forced" to choose at the end of each presentation which side the child "preferred" and to then make a "blind" choice (the micro-computer generates a random sequence of pattern presentation on the left or right monitor for each trial). The advantage of this automated version compared to cards acuity (McDonald et al., 1975) is speed of testing, robustness of the apparatus, and inability on the part of the observer to cheat! The disadvantages of the automated set-up compared with the cards are its fixed position, making it suitable only for a clinical unit; and its relative cost (around $6,000 or £3000). Recently, a project was carried out comparing the use of automated FPL set-ups with both the Teller Cards and the Keeler Cards (see ABCDEFV below).

The Cambridge Crowding Cards (CCC)
This test has been devised to enable an estimate to be made in preschool children of letter recognition acuity, comparable to Snellen acuity. The test is a modification of the Sheridan Gardiner single letter test. The CCC test is a multiple letter test—the center letter must be matched to one of five letters shown on a display card. The letter to be matched is surrounded at a set distance by four other letters (from a different subset), which produces a crowding effect—reduced acuity compared to single letter acuity. In addition to giving a Snellen equivalent, the test has a number of other advantages over other preschool tests. It is normalized for a 3 meter viewing distance, which is more practical than 6 meter viewing for preschool children. The display letters (used in matching) are large and attached to

a sturdy board. It is not necessary to have fine motor coordination to indicate the match, therefore the test can be used by children with neurological disabilities.

This test has been used extensively to study normal development in the preschool years in the Cambridge Screening Programme and in clinical assessments of children with neurologic disabilities (Atkinson, Anker, Evans, Hall, & Pimm-Smith, 1988; Atkinson, Anker, Evans, & McIntyre, 1987; Atkinson, Pimm-Smith, Evans, Harding, & Braddick, 1986). Normal preschool children (age 4 years) have the equivalent of 6/9 vision on the CCC, with 6/6 equivalence being reached by 5–6 years.

Isotropic Photorefraction and Videorefraction Photorefraction and videorefraction have been used extensively, both with and without cycloplegia, to measure focusing ability (which can also be used as an indicator of changes in visual attention) and refractive errors. Details of the isotropic technique and the results of its use in screening are described elsewhere (Atkinson & Braddick, 1982b; Atkinson, Braddick, Durden, Watson, & Atkinson, 1984; Atkinson, Braddick, et al., 1987; Braddick & Atkinson, 1984; Braddick, Atkinson, & Wattam-Bell, 1988; Howland, Braddick, Atkinson, & Howland, 1983).

Videorefraction Using Cycloplegia
Screening studies have allowed the course of emmetropization to be studied in children from birth to 5 years. The mean cycloplegic refraction is hyperopic at birth. The mean cycloplegic refraction (of the lower hyperopic meridian) is around one diopter of hyperopia in the majority of children at 9 months of age. Hyperopia under cycloplegia of over 2D, beyond 1 year of age, places the child at risk of strabismus and amblyopia (Atkinson, 1991; Atkinson, in press [b]; Braddick, Atkinson, Wattam-Bell, Anker, & Norris, 1988; Ingram, Traynar, Walker, & Wilson, 1979). In general, emmetropization is rapid over the first 2 years of life with many children reaching adult cycloplegic refractions (having lost their initial astigmatism) by 2 years of age.

Isotropic photorefraction has been used in the Cambridge Infant Screening Programme (Atkinson, in press-b; Atkinson et al., 1987a;

Atkinson & Braddick, 1988) to identify infants at risk of strabismus and amblyopia. In this program, a randomized control trial was conducted in which spectacles were worn in infancy to correct excessive degrees of hypermetropia (long sightedness) and anisometropia (over 1D difference of refraction between the eyes). Without correction, 70% of 4-year-olds who were high hyperopes in infancy showed visual deficits (strabismus and/or amblyopia) compared to 25% of the children with similar degrees of hyperopia in infancy who had worn spectacles partially correcting their refractive errors in infancy. The mechanisms underlying this potentially valuable intervention are not clearly understood; neither conventional models of accommodative strabismus nor uniocular amblyopia fit the data well. It is hypothesized that infant vision screening may identify not only children with refractive errors who are at risk of strabismus and amblyopia, but also a subset of children with mild global developmental delay. If this is the case, it may have implications for understanding the precursors of certain learning disabilities such as dyslexia.

Cycloplegic videorefraction used in clinical assessment enables the tester to gauge whether the refraction of a clinical patient is in line with that of a normal child of the same age. Amblyopia can also be measured in isolation from refractive defocus by measuring acuity with and without spectacles (to correct any refractive errors). If acuity is in the normal range when correcting spectacles are worn, the child can then be said to be non-amblyopic. However, estimates of amblyopia from the forced choice preferential looking method should be viewed with caution, as they often underestimate amblyopia compared to measures of recognition acuity.

Videorefraction Without Cycloplegia

From data in noncycloplegic videorefraction studies, it is known that newborns take up a wide range of focus with the mean tending to be a small degree of myopia. Infants over the first 6 postnatal months improve their ability to change focus and to accommodate accurately to targets at different distances (Braddick, Atkinson, French, & Howland, 1979), although

over 50% of normal infants show some astigmatism (Atkinson, Braddick, et al., 1987; Howland, Atkinson, Braddick, & French, 1978). Infant astigmatism reduces to adult levels of incidence by 2 years of age (Atkinson, Braddick, & French, 1980). By 6–9 months of age, accommodation is reasonably accurate although focusing tends to be slightly myopic on average in dim illumination (dark focus).

Videorefraction can also be used without cycloplegia to monitor switches of visual attention from objects at one distance to another. Normal newborn infants tend to attend visually (and to focus) in relatively nearby space, and do not relax their accommodation sufficiently for targets beyond a meter distance. Infants over 6 months of age can extend their focus to at least 1.5 meters when attending to objects of interest. Many neurological pediatric patients show abnormal patterns of change of visual attention measured in this way (Atkinson, 1989a). For example, many children with cerebral palsy show fixed focus either at near distances (similar to newborns) or at a similar position to their cycloplegic refraction. Some Down syndrome children focus in nearby space in a similar way to normal young infants (although their cycloplegic refraction may be in the normal hyperopic range).

Videorefraction is a very useful technique clinically, in that it is easy to learn and carry out; it compares well with retinoscopy; and it is fast, reliable, safe, and transportable. There is a family of theoretically related photorefractive techniques (Braddick & Atkinson, 1984; Howland, 1991), each of which has certain advantages and disadvantages. Use of a combination of these methods will probably turn out to be an optimal strategy for clinical assessment.

Tests of Cortical Vision

Orientation Discrimination The cortex possesses channels specifically tuned to different orientations (Hubel and Wiesel, 1977). This sensitivity is not found in subcortical systems. A paradigm used to test for the presence of orientation-selective channels has been designed. This consists of analyzing a visual evoked potential (VEP) to a sinusoidal grating pattern, which alternates between two oblique orientations separated by 90 degrees (Atkinson, Hood, & Wattam-Bell, 1987; Atkinson, Hood, Wattam-Bell, Anker, & Tricklebank, 1988; Braddick & Atkinson, 1988; Braddick, Wattam-Bell, & Atkinson, 1986). This paradigm has been used to monitor the development of orientation sensitivity with age. For relatively slow alternation rates (3rps) the orientation response is found shortly after birth, while for more rapid alternation the response emerges around 6 weeks of age. The response is both temporally and spatially tuned (Atkinson, Braddick, Wattam-Bell, Hood, & Weeks, 1989a).

Binocularity—Correlation and Disparity Discrimination The interaction of input from the two eyes is a property of the majority of striate cortical cells but is not found in earlier (subcortical) stages of visual processing. This interaction registers the correspondences between the two images for disparity detection. Stereoscopic vision is absent, or poor, in strabismic individuals, cortical cells becoming dominated in development by input from the nonstrabismic eye.

Two techniques (VEP recordings to random dot correlograms and stereograms and FPL procedures to the same patterns) have been used to assess the development of binocular vision in normal infants (Birch, Shimojo, & Held, 1985; Braddick & Atkinson, 1983b; Braddick et al., 1979; Braddick, Wattam-Bell, Day, & Atkinson, 1983; Fox, 1981). An alternative measure of binocularity is that of the symmetry of monocularly driven optokinetic nystagmus (Atkinson, 1979; Atkinson & Braddick, 1981). In general, the age of onset of the binocular VEP and symmetry of monocular optokinetic nystagmus (MOKN) is similar (Braddick & Atkinson, 1983a), and is around 3–4 months of age post-term.

Shifts of Visual Attention The ability to make rapid saccades to foveate a laterally peripheral target underlies perimetry and field testing. Newborn infants have been found to shift fixation to peripheral targets over a very limited field size (Heersema, Van Hof-van Duin, & Hop, 1989; Mohn & Van Hof-van

Duin, 1986;). They seem to have an additional problem, indicated by a reduction in field size, if a central target remains visible when the peripheral target appears (Atkinson & Braddick, 1985; Atkinson, Braddick, Weeks, & Hood, 1990; Atkinson, Hood, Braddick, & Wattam-Bell, 1988b; Braddick & Atkinson, 1988; Harris & MacFarlane, 1974; MacFarlane, Harris, & Barnes, 1976). Even when the targets are matched across 1- and 3-month-olds for contrast sensitivity (just above contrast threshold), the younger infants show longer latencies to refixate when there is competition between a central and peripheral target.

Mechanisms for shifting visual attention are thought to involve both subcortical (superior colliculus) and cortical (parietal lobes, frontal eye fields) circuitry (Andersen, 1988; Hyvärinen, 1982; Mountcastle, 1978; Posner & Rothbart, 1989; Schiller, 1985). Deficits in selective attention have been found in patients with parietal lobe damage and in primates with damage to the frontal eye fields. For example, patients with Balint syndrome, involving bilateral parietal damage, have great difficulty in disengaging attention from one object of interest in order to attend to another (De Renzi, 1982). This deficit is similar to the behavior in 1-month-olds when viewing competing stimuli. This type of stimulus display, with competing targets, can be used for clinical testing to measure functioning in cortical attentional mechanisms (Hood & Atkinson, 1990).

Current models of human visual development (Atkinson, 1984; Atkinson in press-a; Atkinson & Braddick, 1990) propose different postnatal time-scales for functioning of specific cortical pathways. Each cortical stream processes information for different visual attributes or combinations of attributes. Onset of channels responsible for carrying information on binocularity and orientation discrimination, and attentional shifts necessitate cortical functioning, as subcortical mechanisms cannot underlie these tasks. Using these concepts, a number of "designer" stimuli have been developed to dissociate subcortical from cortical visual systems, and have been used to test specific clinical "at risk" populations.

Studies on three pediatric subgroups are briefly described below to illustrate how these tests of disparity and orientation discrimination can be used to demonstrate cortical function and developmental plasticity. A fourth study describes a preliminary attempt to use tests of attentional shifts to dissociate cortical and sensory visual deficits.

Infants with a First Degree Relative with Strabismus and/or Amblyopia A group of infants at risk of strabismus because of their family history (i.e., infants with at least one first degree relative who had been strabismic and/or amblyopic in childhood) was tested longitudinally to discern the onset of binocularity, as demonstrated by a significant VEP to a correlogram and a symmetrical MOKN response (Wattam-Bell, Braddick, Atkinson, & Day, 1987). Most normal children develop disparity detection at around 4 months postnatally. This was also true for most of the strabismus-history group. The correlation between the age of onset of the correlogram VEP and symmetrical MOKN was significant but weak, and some infants showed early symmetrical MOKN but no binocular VEP. The results suggest that MOKN does not depend on exactly the same neural substrate as the VEP response.

In total, 9.5% of the 105 squint history children became strabismic. One or two infants became strabismic before 4 months and did not show the binocular VEP response (although this could have been due to eye misalignment at the time of testing). Several children in the squint history group developed normal binocularity initially but this became disrupted by later onset strabismus. The results indicate that these strabismic children did not lack the necessary prerequisites for developing this aspect of cortical function early in life, but that some other factor precipitating the strabismus had interfered with the normal course of development. There was a significant increase in ametropia in the cycloplegic refractions of the strabismus history group at 9 months of age compared to the normal population (Anker, Atkinson, Bobier, Tricklebank, & Wattam-Bell, 1991).

Infants with Early Onset Strabismus (Atkin-son et al., 1991; Smith et al., 1989; Smith, Atkinson, Anker, & Moore, 1991) Similar tests to those in the first group have been used to measure binocularity in infants who became strabismic before 6 months postnatally (Atkinson et al., 1991b; Smith et al., 1989, 1991), together with longitudinal monocular acuity testing using FPL, refractive measures using videorefraction, retinoscopy, and standard tests of stereopsis at 4 years of age (Long, Frisby, TNO, and Titmus). In this prospective study, these children were tested before and after surgery to realign the eyes, with surgery taking place before 2 years of age.

Some children demonstrated stereoscopic vision by detecting a relatively large disparity (40 minutes) when tested with FPL stereograms in the months just before and immediately after surgery. There was some overall improvement in binocular status for the entire group after surgery (Figure 1). This result suggests an extraordinary range of cortical plasticity in the first 2 years of life both for developing disparity detectors initially (to accommodate large angles of anomalous correspondence) and for retuning these mechanisms after surgery, when the eyes have been aligned. However, on testing at 4 years of age (2 years after surgery), very few of these same children had any stereoscopic vision, and those who did only responded to relatively coarse disparities on the standard clinical stereo tests (Figure 2). It appears as if their original tenuous stereopsis had been lost (although the surgical realignment was good—within 10 prism diopters). It is possible that better final binocularity would have been obtained if the surgical realignment had been done even earlier, but until control studies are carried out comparing late and early surgery, the answer to this question is not known.

In spite of relatively early surgery, refractive correction, and occlusion therapy prescribed before surgery (and in some cases also after surgery), many of these children showed small degrees of amblyopia when tested at 4 years (acuity being measured with the Cambridge Crowding Cards) (Figure 3). On monocular FPL immediately before and after surgery,

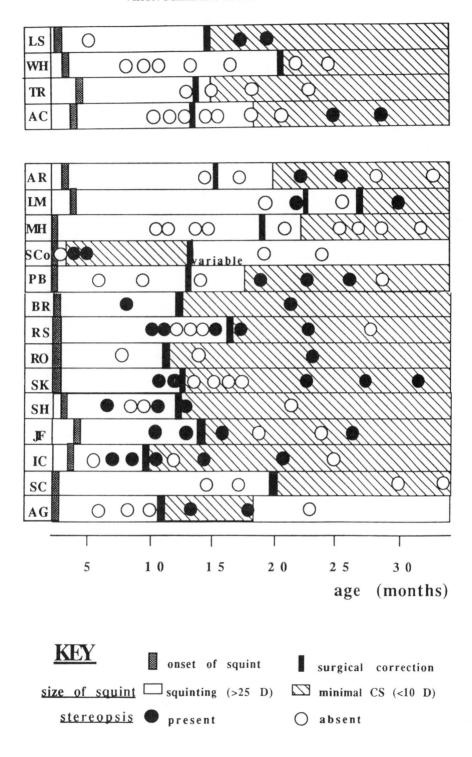

Figure 1. Presence or absence of sensitivity to 2,400 sec disparity target in early onset strabismics before and after surgery. Note that, as a group, there is an increase in the incidence of stereopsis after surgery.

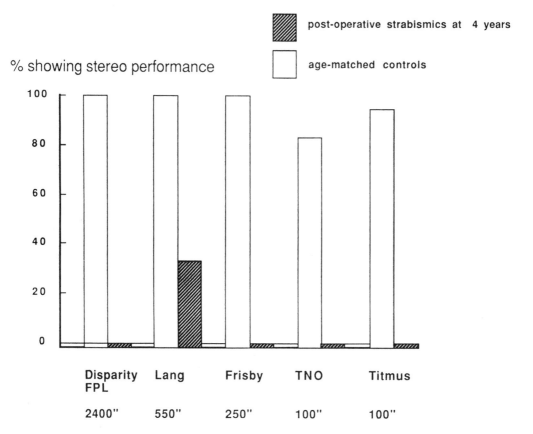

Figure 2.   Poor or absent steropsis at 4 years in the surgically corrected early onset strabismics compared to age matched controls on the same clinical tests.

there was on average an improvement in acuity, with reduced interocular differences following surgery. However, many of the infants showed relatively small or no interocular differences (0.5 octaves or less) even before surgery on FPL. It was also noted that many of these children had abnormal refractions on retinoscopy (moderate to high levels of hyperopia and anisometropia under cycloplegia) through the first 2 years of life.

The results of this study suggest high degrees of plasticity in some individuals in development of binocular systems, allowing development of disparity detectors even though the eyes are not well aligned. The results cast doubt on the belief that good binocularity (normal levels of stereo acuity) can be developed in early onset strabismics following early surgery in the first 2 years of life; any early binocularity seems to be reduced or lost by 4 years. In addi-

Visual acuity: STRABISMICS at 3-4 years

Subject	Cambridge Crowding Cards		Single letters	
	RE	LE	RE	LE
PB	6/12	6/18	6/6	6/9
SC	6/12	6/9	6/6	6/6
IC	np	np	6/18	6/9
SC	6/12	6/12	6/6	6/6
JF	6/9	6/9	6/6	6/6
AG	np	np	6/12	6/9
SH	np	np	6/6	6/6
MH	6/18	6/36	6/9	6/9
SK	6/9	6/12	6/6	6/6
RS	6/9	6/9	6/6	6/6

Cerebral palsy / developmental delay

					FPL (c/deg)	
AC	np	np	6/9	6/9		
WH	np	np	6/9	6/9		
LHS	np	np	np	np	6.5	4
TR	np	np	np	np	6	6
HW	np	np	np	np	10	10

np = not possible

Figure 3.   Acuity in the surgically and refractively corrected early onset strabismics on the single letter matching test and the Cambridge Crowding Cards.

tion, it appears that although dense amblyopia is relatively rare in this group with early intervention, and for the group as a whole, interocular differences were smaller after surgery than before. It is not known from this study whether this would also have been the case with much later surgery. Further studies with both earlier and later surgery, and detailed measures of occlusion compliance, are needed before these questions can be answered.

Very Low Birth Weight (VLBW) Premature Infants As cortical visual function may be a good indicator of the general state of neurological development, the orientation reversal VEP measure (OR-VEP) has been used to investigate development in a "high risk" group—a volunteer cohort of Very Low Birth Weight (VLBW) premature infants (less than 1,500 gms) (Atkinson et al., 1991). This group was matched for gestational age with a group of control infants. Five different tests were compared across the two groups:

1. Orientation reversal (OR) VEP at 5 and 13 weeks post-term
2. Phase reversal (PH) VEP at 5 and 13 weeks post-term
3. Fixation shift test at 4–5 weeks post-term
4. FPL acuity at 12–13 weeks, post-term, and at 28 weeks post-term
5. Cycloplegic videorefraction at 6–8 months post-term

In summary, no difference was found between the groups on acuity estimates from forced-choice preferential looking and accommodative ability measured using videorefraction, nor on any of the VEP measures. However, the VLBW group showed shorter latencies than their post-term age matched controls for re-fixating saccadically a peripheral target. This suggests that the development of control mechanisms for visuomotor tasks of this kind may well be sensitive to the extent of visual experience. Current models of selective attention would suggest that collicular-parietal processing is involved in these responses, whereas acuity and orientation specificity may reflect the maturation of the geniculo-striate pathway. These data may be used to investigate differential critical periods related to different processing streams in human visual development, and to assess neurological delays in at-risk infants.

It is also worth noting that one recent study estimates that only 15% of VLBW infants will develop severe neurological problems (Soual Paediatric and Obstetric Research Unit, University of Glasgow, 1991), and that the Cambridge VLBW group constituted approximately only one third of all VLBW infants born in the Cambridge area within the recruiting period for this study.

Children with Multiple Disabilities: Dissociation of Sensory Visual Loss from Attentional Loss In this study, a group of children with neurological disorders but without gaze apraxia was tested for ability to fixate a target under conditions of competition and non-competition. The children were compared on a fixation shift task with a group of normal 1- and 3-month-olds. Peripheral VEPs were recorded in the same eccentricity and with the same stimuli as used in the fixation shift task (phase reversing at 6 rps, low spatial frequency vertical grating patterns of 50% contrast). Table 1 shows the number of children in each group who showed a significant peripheral VEP and refixated the peripheral target correctly. Nearly all of the 3-months-olds showed both a significant VEP to this pattern in the periphery, and consistently

Table 1. Numbers completing both behavioral and electrophysiological tasks[a]

Group	(a) + BH/ + VEP	(b) + BH/ − VEP	(c) − BH/ + VEP	(d) − BH/ + VEP
1-month-old	4	14	0	0
3-month-olds	12	2	0	0
Clinical	2	5	3	5

+BH/−BH = >8/<8 of 10 correct refixations in NC and C conditions.

+VEP/−VEP = positive/negative VEP signal at first, second, and fourth harmonics.

[a]One 1-month-old, two 3-month-olds, and one in the clinical group failed to complete the behavioral experiments.

refixated the peripheral target in both the competition and noncompetition conditions. Most 1-month-olds showed accurate refixations but did not produce a significant peripheral VEP. Some of the clinical group behaved like the 1-month-olds and some like the 3-month-olds. However, three of the clinical children showed a significant peripheral VEP, indicating that the incoming sensory pathways were intact, but did not actively refixate the target in either the noncompetition or competition conditions. This would indicate a possible dissociation in these children between sensory and attentional mechanisms. Further research using modifications of this type of paradigm may enable us to categorize attentional deficits more finely. However, care will need to be taken regarding spatio-temporal tuning to enable the optimum stimuli to be used.

GENERAL CLINICAL REFERRALS FOR ASSESSMENT

A battery of tests was devised consisting of tests of acuity, binocularity, refraction, focusing ability, and attention. Several other tests were included for assessment of specific subgroups (e.g., field testing in hemiplegics) A summary of the assessment of referrals to the Unit over a 2-year period was published (Atkinson, 1989a). One third of the group of referrals had severe cerebral palsy, and one third showed global developmental delay. Over three quarters of this cohort had one or more visual defects. The most common problems were strabismus, refractive errors, and reduced acuity. A general description of the tests used has already been published together with the results (Atkinson, 1985, 1986, 1989a) and so will not be described in detail here.

A recent summary table of referrals for assessments over the past 2 years is shown in Table 2. A significant point to note is that, in the main, only the severely neurologically impaired group within the total pediatric clinical population is referred for visual assessments to the VDU. Many of these children have common visual problems (strabismus, poor acuity, refractive errors) and many show poor control

Table 2. Clinical referrals to the visual development unit 1989–1991 ($N = 100$) (1989–1991: $N = 504$)

Age range: mainly 0–5 years	
Ophthalmological problem only	11%
Cerebral palsy (CP)	31%
Paediatric neurological disabilities (not CP)	58%
Focal lesions	5%
Outcome of visual assessment	
Abnormal eye movements—strabismus/nystagmus	77%
Reduced acuity	74%
Abnormal cycloplegic refraction	69%
Poor accommodative control on videorefraction	61%
Absence of fine visuomotor coordination	46%
Specific subsets tested on:	
Fields: reduced or asymmetrical	75%
Orientation reversal VEP (cortical): non-sig	83%
Pattern reversal VEP: non-sig	20%
Monocular OKN asymmetry	89%
Fixation shifts: abnormal	40%
Stereopsis: abnormal	85%

of accommodation and fixation shifts, indicating abnormal attentional mechanisms in addition to deficits of sensory and perceptual vision.

THE NEED FOR TESTS OF FUNCTIONAL VISION

From the results of the above assessments, details can be given of the visual, orthoptic, and ophthalmological status of the child. However, one of the major problems with the multiply impaired is understanding their visual defects in terms of implied "disability" and understanding the interactive effects of visual defects with other pediatric problems. What is needed is a functional test of vision which will provide information on which particular everyday tasks will be impeded by the visual defects assessed. At present there are very few pediatric studies which address these problems. In addition, most of the tests described are only concerned with brain mechanisms involved with the initial analysis of visual stimuli into component parts. Perceptual analysis must be used to put these attributes together to recognize objects, to separate them from their background, to categorize objects, and to initiate appropriate actions. This means that tests of perceptuocognitive vision and perceptuomotor vision must be included in visual assessments.

Table 3. Newborn tracking

1. Five trials—separate occasions—within 30 minutes of waking
2. Target—2″ Christmas bauble or other high contrast object—10 deg at 12″ viewing (30 cm)
3. Velocity—5 deg/sec, 10 deg/sec (1″/sec, 2″/sec)
4. Movement from midline, local movement allowed
5. Body support (head/neck) in semi-supine position

Expected result: ⅓ success or ⅔ success with saccadic tracking 15–20 deg from midline
Occasional head movements following eye movements
Long latency for both eye and head movements (several seconds)

As a preliminary attempt to address some of these problems, a battery of tests has been devised called the Atkinson Battery of Child Development for Examining Functional Vision (ABCDEFV) (Atkinson, Gardner, Tricklebank, & Anker, 1989). The battery combines ideas from the present assessments in vision (FPL, videorefraction), established pediatric tests (e.g., Sheridan), and ideas from developmental psychology (Piagetian object permanence tasks, spatial representation, and construction tasks). The battery is divided into seven different age groups between birth and 3 years. Each test will have a defined protocol so that the procedures are standardized across testers. (An example relating to newborn tracking is shown in Table 3.) This is to avoid the obvious problems of misunderstanding, based on clinical procedures such as "fixes and follows," where there is a general notion as to what this phrase means clinically but no easily defined "pass" or "failure" criterion by which to judge an individual child's visual behavior against normal behavior.

The battery is divided into two sections. An outline of part of it is shown in Table 4. On the left are tests which are portable, relate to everyday living, and can be carried out in either the home, community clinic, or clinician's private office. On the right are tasks which require specialist equipment (mainly nonportable) and, in many cases, specialist skills. They are suitable for a specialized unit or hospital clinic. At present the battery is being normalized for each age

Table 4. Atkinson Battery of Child Development for Examining Functional Vision (ABCDEFV)

Community clinic	Assessment unit
A. Newborn (0–1 month) 1. Pupil response 2. Diffuse light reaction 3. Intermittent tracking 4. Videorefraction 5. PL cards	**A. Newborn (0–1 month)** 1. OKN and MOKN 2. VEP (PA and PR) 3. FPL 4. Videorefraction
B. 1–3 months 1. Onset of smiling to face 2. Improved tracking (3/5) 3. Convergence to approach 4. Peripheral refixation in blank field 5. Videorefraction 6. PL cards	**B. 1–3 months** 1. OKN and MOKN 2. VEP (PA and PR) 3. VEP (orientation-cortical) 4. FPL 5. Fixation shifts (attention) 6. Videorefraction
C. 4–6 months 1. Good saccadic tracking (5/5)/some smooth pursuit 2. Batting/protoreach/reach 3. Follows retreat to 3 m. 4. Defensive blink reliable (visual) 3/3 5. Regards hands, then feet 6. Respond to visual peekaboo 7. Peripheral refixation to face 8. No strabismus—corneal reflex test 9. Watches object fall in visual field 10. Retrieves partially covered object 11. Videorefraction 12. PL cards	**C. 4–6 months** 1. FPL acuity 3 c/deg or better 2. VEP (orientation) 3. Videorefraction—focus changes 4. Stereo VEP and FPL 5. MOKN symmetry 6. Fixation shifts and competition

group. There are still many other aspects of functional vision for which assessments methods have to be designed. It is hoped that one endpoint of ABCDEFV will be to define the limits of partial sight and blindness in children of different ages, and to devise more effective treatment, rehabilitation, and educational methods, especially for the multiply-impaired.

REFERENCES

Andersen, R.A. (1988). The neurological basis of spatial cognition: role of the parietal lobe. In J. Stiles-Davis, M. Kritchevsky, & U. Bellugi (Eds.), *Spatial cognition: Brain bases and development* (pp. 57–80). Hillsdale, NJ: Laurence Erlbaum Associates.

Anker, S., Atkinson, J., Bobier, W., Tricklebank, J., & Wattam-Bell, J. (1991). "Infant vision screening programme: can early detection of refractive errors in infants with a family history of strabismus predict later visual problems?" *Abstracts of the 7th International Orthoptic Congress, Nuremberg*, 154.

Atkinson, J. (1979). Development of optokinetic nystagmus in the human infant and monkey infant: An analogue to development in kittens. In R.D. Freeman (Ed.), *NATO advanced study institute series* (pp. 277–288). New York: Plenum Press.

Atkinson, J. (1984). Human visual development over the first six months of life. A review and a hypothesis. *Human Neurobiology, 3*, 61–74.

Atkinson, J. (1985). Assessment of vision in infants and young children. In S. Harel & N.J. Anastasiow (Eds.), *The at-risk infant: psycho/socio/medical aspects* (pp. 341–352). Baltimore: Paul H. Brookes Publishing Co.

Atkinson, J. (1986). Methods of objective assessment of visual functions in subjects with limited communication skills. In D. Ellis (Ed.), *Sensory impairment in mentally handicapped people*. London: Croom Helm Ltd.

Atkinson, J. (1989a). New tests of vision screening and assessment in infants and young children. In J.H. French, S. Harel, & P. Casaer (Eds.), *Child neurology and developmental disabilities* (pp. 219–227). Baltimore: Paul H. Brookes Publishing Co.

Atkinson, J. (1989b). Subcortical or cortical control of newborn vision? A revised model. *Ophthalmic & Physiological Optics, 9*, 469.

Atkinson, J. (1991). Infant vision screening programme. *Transactions of the Boerhaave Commissie voor Postacademisch Onderwijs: Neuro-ophthalmologie IV - Kinderneuro-ophthalmologie*, 17–25.

Atkinson, J. (in press-a). Infant eyes and infant brain: Is newborn vision like 'blind-sight'? In R. Gregory & P. Heard (Eds.), *The artful brain*.

Atkinson, J. (in press-b). The Cambridge infants photorefraction screening programme: Prediction and prevention of strabismus and amblyopia. In K. Simons & D.L. Guyton (Eds.), *Handbook of infant vision: laboratory and clinical research*. New York: Oxford University Press.

Atkinson, J., & Braddick, O.J. (1981). Development of optokinetic nystagmus in infants: An indicator of cortical binocularity? In D.F. Fisher, R.A. Monty, and J.W. Senders (Eds.), *Eye movements: Cognition and visual perception*. Hillsdale, NJ: Lawrence Erlbaum Associates.

Atkinson, J., & Braddick, O.J. (1982a). Assessment of vi-

sual acuity in infancy and early childhood. *Acta Ophthalmologica (Copenhagen) Suppl., 157*, 18–26.

Atkinson, J., & Braddick, O.J. (1982b). The use of isotropic photorefraction for vision screening in infants. *Acta Ophthalmologica (Copenhagen) Suppl., 157*, 36–45.

Atkinson, J., & Braddick, O.J. (1985). Early development of the control of visual attention. *Perception, 14*, A25.

Atkinson, J., & Braddick, O.J. (1988). Infant precursors of later visual disorders: correlation or causality? In A. Yonas (Ed.), *20th Minnesota symposium on child psychology* (pp. 35–65). Hillsdale, NJ: Laurence Erlbaum.

Atkinson, J., Anker, S., Evans, C., Hall, R., & Pimm-Smith, E. (1988). Visual acuity testing of young children with the Cambridge Crowding Cards at 3 and 6 months. *Acta Ophthalmologica, 66*, 505–508.

Atkinson, J., Anker, S., Evans, C., & McIntyre, A. (1987). The Cambridge Crowding Cards for preschool visual acuity testing. *Transactions of the Sixth International Orthoptic Congress*, Harrogate, England.

Atkinson, J., Braddick, O.J., Anker, S., Hood, B., Wattam-Bell, J., Weeks, F., Rennie, J., & Coughtrey, H. (1990). Visual development in the VLBW infant. *Transactions of IVth European Conference on Developmental Psychology*, University of Stirling.

Atkinson, J., Braddick, O.J., Durden, K., Watson, P.G., & Atkinson, S. (1984). Screening for refractive errors in 6–9 months old infants by photorefraction. *British Journal of Ophthalmology, 68*, 105–112.

Atkinson, J. Braddick, O.J., & French, J. (1980). Infant astigmatism: its disappearance with age. *Vision Research, 20*, 891–893.

Atkinson, J., Braddick, O.J., & Moar, K. (1977). Development of contrast sensitivity over the first three months of life in the human infant. *Vision Research, 17*, 1037–1044.

Atkinson, J., Braddick, O.J., & Pimm-Smith, E. (1982). 'Preferential looking' for monocular and binocular acuity testing of infants. *British Journal of Ophthalmology, 66*, 264–268.

Atkinson, J., Braddick, O.J., Wattam-Bell, J., Durden, K., Bobier, W., Pointer, J., & Atkinson, S. (1987a). Photorefractive screening of infants and effects of refractive correction. *Investigative Ophthalmology and Visual Science (Suppl.) 28*, 229.

Atkinson, J., Braddick, O.J., Wattam-Bell, J., Hood, B., & Weeks, F. (1989, October). Temporal frequency and orientation selectivity of young infants' orientation-specific responses. *Ophthalmic and Physiological Optics, 9*.

Atkinson, J., Braddick, O.J., Weeks, F., & Hood, B. (1990). Spatial and temporal tuning of infants' orientation-specific responses. *Perception, 19*(3), 371.

Atkinson, J., Gardner, N., Tricklebank, J., & Anker, S. (1989, October). Atkinson Battery of Child Development for Examining Functional Vision (ABCDEFV). *Ophthalmic and Physiological Optics, 9*, 470.

Atkinson, J., Hood, B., Braddick, O.J., & Wattam-Bell, J.

(1988b). Infants' control of fixation shifts with single and competing targets: mechanisms of shifting attention. *Perception, 17,* 367–368.

Atkinson, J., Hood, B., & Wattam-Bell, J. (1987). Discrimination by infants of orientation in dynamic patterns. *Perception, 16(2),* 232.

Atkinson, J., Hood, B., Wattam-Bell, J., Anker, S., & Tricklebank, J. (1988). Development of orientation discrimination in infancy. *Perception, 17,* 587–595.

Atkinson, J., Pimm-Smith, E., Evans, C., Harding, G., & Braddick, O.J. (1986). Visual crowding in young children. *Documenta Ophthalmologica Proceedings Series, 45,* 201–213.

Atkinson, J., Smith, J., Anker, S., Wattam-Bell, J., Braddick, O.J., & Moore, A.T. (1991). Binocularity and amblyopia before and after early strabismus surgery. *Investigative Ophthalmological and Visual Science, 32(4),* 820.

Atkinson, J., Wattam-Bell, J., Pimm-Smith, E., Evans, C., & Braddick, O.J. (1986). Comparison of rapid procedures in forced choice preferential looking for estimating acuity in infants and young children. *Documenta Ophthalmologica Proceedings Series, 45,* 192–200.

Birch, E.E., Gwiazda, J., & Held, R. (1983). The development of vergence does not account for the development of stereopsis. *Perception, 12,* 331–336.

Birch, E.E., Shimojo, S., & Held, R. (1985). Preferential-looking assessment of fusion and stereopsis in infants aged 1–6 months. *Investigative Ophthalmology and Visual Science, 26,* 366–370.

Braddick, O.J., & Atkinson, J. (1983a). Some recent findings on the development of human binocularity: a review. *Behavioural Brain Research, 10,* 141–150.

Braddick, O.J., & Atkinson, J. (1983b). Stimulus control in VEP and behavioural assessment of infant vision. *Annals of the New York Academy of Sciences, 388,* 642–644.

Braddick, O.J., & Atkinson, J. (1984). Photorefractive techniques: applications in testing infants and young children. *Transactions of the British College of Ophthalmic Opticians (Optometrists) 1st International Congress, 2,* 26–34.

Braddick, O.J., & Atkinson, J. (1988). Sensory selectivity, attentional control, and cross-channel integration in early visual development. In A. Yonas (Ed) *20th Minnesota symposium on child psychology.* Hillsdale, NJ: Lawrence Erlbaum.

Braddick, O.J., Atkinson, J., French, J., & Howland, H.C. (1979). A photo-refractive study of infant accommodation. *Vision Research, 19,* 319–330.

Braddick, O.J., Atkinson, J., Julesz, B., Kropfl, W., Bodis-Wollner, I., & Raab, E. (1980). Cortical binocularity in infants. *Nature, 288,* 363–365.

Braddick, O.J., Atkinson, J., Wattam-Bell, J., Anker, S., & Norris, V. (1988). Videorefractive screening of accommodative performance in infants. *Investigative Ophthalmology and Visual Science (Suppl.), 29,* 60.

Braddick, O.J., Wattam-Bell, J., Day, J., & Atkinson, J. (1983). The onset of binocular function in human infants. *Human Neurobiology, 2,* 65–59.

Braddick, O.J., Wattam-Bell, J., & Atkinson, J. (1986). Orientation-specific cortical responses develop in early infancy. *Nature, 320,* 617–619.

De Renzi, E. (1982). Oculomotor disturbances in hemispheric disease. In C.W. Johnston & F.J. Pirozzolo

(Eds.), *Neuropsychology of eye movements* (pp. 177–200). Hillsdale, NJ: Lawrence Erlbaum Associates.

Dobson, V., & Teller, D.Y. (1978). Visual acuity in human infants: a review and comparison of behavioural and electrophysiological studies. *Vision Research, 18,* 1469–1483.

Fox, R. (1981). Stereopsis in animals and human infants. In R.N. Aslin, J.R. Alberts, & M.R. Petersen (Eds.) *The development of perception: Psychobiological perspectives. Vol. 2: The visual system* (pp. 335–381). New York: Academic Press.

Gwiazda, J., Brill, S., Mohindra, L., & Held, R. (1980). Preferential looking acuity in infants from two to fifty-eight weeks of age. *American Journal of Optometry and Physiological Optics, 57,* 428–432.

Harris, P.L., & MacFarlane, A. (1974). The growth of the effective visual field from birth to seven weeks. *Journal of Experimental Psychology, 18,* 340–384.

Heersema, D.J. (1989). *Perinatale risicofactoren en visuele ontwikkeling bij jonge kinderen* (Perinatal risk factors in the visual development of young children). Thesis, Rotterdam, The Netherlands: Erasmus University.

Heersema, D.J., & Van Hof-van Duin, J. (1990). Age norms for visual acuity in toddlers using the acuity card procedure. *Clinical Vision Sciences, 5,* 167–174.

Heersema, D.J., Van Hof-van Duin, J., & Hop, W.C.J. (1989). Age norms for visual field development in children aged 0 to 4 years using arc perimetry. *Investigative Ophthalmology and Visual Science (Suppl.), 30(3),* 242.

Hood, B., & Atkinson, J. (1990). Sensory visual loss and cognitive deficits in the selective attentional system of normal infants and neurologically impaired children. *Developmental Medicine and Child Neurology, 32,* 1067–1077.

Howland, H.C. (1991). Advances in instrumentation for biometry of infant refractive error. *Investigative Ophthalmology and Visual Science (suppl.), 32(4),* xii.

Howland, H.C., Atkinson, J., Braddick, O.J., & French, J. (1978). Infant astigmatism measured by photorefraction. *Science, 202,* 331–333.

Howland, H.C., Braddick, O.J., Atkinson, J., & Howland, B. (1983). Optics of photorefraction: orthogonal and isotropic methods. *Journal of the Optical Society of America, 73,* 1701–1708.

Hubel, D.R., & Wiesel, T.N. (1977). Functional architecture of macaque monkey visual cortex. *Proceedings of the Royal Society B198,* 1–59.

Hyvärinen, J. (1982). *The parietal cortex of monkey and man.* Berlin: Springer-Verlag.

Ingram, R.M., Traynar, M.J., Walker, C., & Wilson, J.M. (1979). Screening for refractive errors at age 1 year: A pilot study. *British Journal of Ophthalmology, 63,* 243–250.

Lewis, T., & Maurer, D. (1986). Preferential looking as a measure of visual resolution in infants and toddlers: A comparison of psychophysical methods. *Child Development, 57,* 1062–1075.

MacDonald, M.A., Dobson, V., Sebris, S.L., Baith, L., Varner, D., & Teller, D.Y. (1985). The acuity card procedure: a rapid test of infant acuity. *Investigative Ophthalmology and Visual Science, 26,* 1158–1162.

MacFarlane, A., Harris, P., & Barnes, I. (1976). Central and peripheral vision in early infancy. *Journal of Experimental Child Psychology, 21,* 532–538.

Medical Research Council Annual Report. (1988/89), 59.

Miranda, S.B. (1970). Visual abilities and pattern preferences of premature infants and fullterm neonates. *Journal of Experimental Child Psychology, 10*, 189–205.

Mohn, G., & Van Hof-van Duin, J. (1983). Behavioural and electrophysiological measures of visual functions in children with neurological disorders. *Behavioral Brain Research, 10*, 177–189.

Mountcastle, V.B. (1978). Brain mechanisms for directed attention. *Journal of the Royal Society of Medicine, 71*, 14–28.

Posner, M.I., & Rothbart, M.K. (1989). *Attention: Normal and pathological development.* Institute of Cognitive and Decision Sciences, University of Oregon, Eugene.

Royal National Institute for the Blind. (1990). *New directions: Towards a better future for multihandicapped visually impaired children and young people.*

Schiller, P.H. (1985). A model for the generation of visually guided saccadic eye movements. In D. Rose & V.G. Dobson (Eds.), *Models of the visual cortex* (pp. 62–70). Chichester: John Wiley and Sons.

Smith, J.C., Atkinson, J., Anker, S., & Moore, A.T. (1991) A prospective study of binocularity and amblyopia in strabismic infants before and after corrective surgery: implications for the human critical period. *Clincial Vision Science, 6*, 335–355.

Smith, J., Atkinson, J., Braddick, O.J., Wattam-Bell, J., Moore, A.T., & Anker, S. (1989). Stereopsis, visual acuity and optokinetic nystagmus in strabismic infants before and after corrective surgery: implications for the critical period. *Ophthalmic and Physiological Optics, 9*, 466.

Social Paediatric and Obstetric Research Unit, University of Glasgow. (1991). *The Scottish low birthweight study.* Glasgow: Author.

Teller, D.Y., Morse, R., Borton, R., & Regal, D. (1974). Visual acuity for vertical and diagonal gratings in human infants. *Vision Research, 14*, 1433–1439.

Van Hof-van Duin, J., Evenhuis-van Leunen, A., Mohn, G., Baerts, W., & Fetter, W.P.F. (1989). Effects of very low birth weight (VLBW) on visual development during the first year after term. *Early Human Development 20*, 225–266.

Van Hof-van Duin, J., & Mohn, G. (1985). The development of visual functions in preterm infants. In U. Zwiener (Ed.), *Pathogenese, funktionsdiagnostik und therapie gestorter korperfunktionen (Ergebn. exp. Med. 46, Verl. Volk. und Gesundheit)* (pp. 350–362), Berlin.

Van Hof-van Duin, J., & Mohn G. (1986a). The development of visual acuity in normal fullterm and preterm infants. *Vision Research, 26*, 909–916.

Wattam-Bell, J., Braddick, O.J., Atkinson, J., & Day, J. (1987). Measures of infant binocularity in a group at risk for strabismus. *Clinical Vision Sciencesl 4*, 327–336.

Chapter 6

Developmental Vulnerability
New Challenges for Research and Service Delivery

JACK P. SHONKOFF, M.D.
University of Massachusetts Medical School, Worcester

T HE CONCEPT OF EARLY CHILDHOOD INTER-
vention is a phenomenon of modern times.
In past centuries, infants with major congenital
anomalies were viewed as "monsters" and left
alone to die. More recently, many young children who demonstrated significant delays in
their development were labelled "idiots" or
"imbeciles," and segregated in residential institutions where they were left for a life of diminished human interaction and little expectation of individual achievement. It is only since
the late 1960s and the 1970s that a commitment
to the principles and practices of early childhood intervention has gained popular support
(Shonkoff & Meisels, 1990).

The roots of this social revolution can be
found in a variety of domains. As a science, it
draws support from a rapidly growing knowledge base in developmental psychology and
neurobiology. Its theoretical foundation is built
on the work of those who have studied the impact of early experiences on the emergence of
competence, as well as on the empirical investigations of those who have explored the development and plasticity of the immature nervous
system. As a social movement and cultural
phenomenon, early childhood intervention re-

flects a strong moral commitment to the provision of expanded opportunities for those who
are disadvantaged by neurological dysfunction
or by the burdens of poverty and social disorganization. Stated simply, early childhood intervention is a reflection of our compassion for
those who are vulnerable and our willingness
to invest in the best possible future for all young
children.

As we enter the last decade of the twentieth
century, the demand for early intervention services is growing rapidly. The resulting strain
on scarce public resources, however, has inten-
sified the need for an expanded and more
rigorous knowledge base. This chapter examines the current status of early childhood intervention research, offers examples of new directions for empirical study, and reflects on the
service delivery challenges that lie ahead.

A NEW AGENDA FOR
EARLY INTERVENTION RESEARCH

Much has been written about the limitations of
previous empirical research on the development of young children with disabilities and on
the effects of intervention services (Bailey &

Phase I of the Early Intervention Collaborative Study was supported by Grant MCJ-250533 from the Maternal and
Child Health Research Program, Bureau of Maternal and Child Health and Resources Development, DHHS, and a grant
from the Jessie B. Cox Charitable Trust, Boston, MA. The author wishes to acknowledge the contributions of Penny Hauser-
Cram, Ed.D., Marty Krauss, Ph.D., Carole Upshur, Ed.D., Kathy Antaki, M.S., Ann Steele, Ed.M., Helene Fausold,
Ed.M., and Marjorie Erickson, Ph.D.

Bricker, 1984; Dunst, 1986; Dunst & Rhein-grover, 1982; Farran, 1990; Guralnick, 1989; Meisels, 1985; Shonkoff & Hauser-Cram, 1987; Shonkoff, Hauser-Cram, Krauss, & Upshur, 1988). Although a great deal of data have documented the positive impacts of intervention programs on children's short-term performance on standardized cognitive measures, the information needs for contemporary policy making and service planning are more complex. Thus, the research agenda for the 1990s must overcome the critical shortcomings of previous investigations. These include the atheoretical nature of most intervention efficacy studies, the narrow range of outcome measures that have been employed, the disproportionate focus of most investigations on risk factors for poor outcomes, the lack of attention to within-group variability, and the absence of long-term longitudinal data. Each of these issues requires a new research perspective.

A Transactional/Ecological Approach to the Investigation of Service Impacts

The development of children who are at increased risk for disability is a complex process that is influenced by a wide range of variables. Constitutional differences among children, variations in their family circumstances, and selected aspects of the larger social environment in which they live all play a role in determining developmental outcomes. Early intervention service programs represent just one potential influence among many in the lives of young children. Whereas most previous studies have paid relatively little attention to the effects of differences among families and other environmental variables, future efficacy research must generate data that contribute to the building and testing of developmental models that acknowledge the importance of understanding the vulnerable child in context. Indeed, future investigations must seek empirical verification of the transactional/ecological models that guide contemporary thought in normative child development research and that influence decision-making in the arena of early childhood service delivery.

Multidimensional Assessment

The existing database on children who have received early intervention services is burdened by an extraordinarily narrow range of outcomes. Relatively little attention has been paid to the measurement of family adaptation in comparison to the predominant interest in the development of the children. Moreover, assessment of child development has focused primarily on the use of standardized cognitive instruments, with relatively little attention to more ecologically valid domains such as behavior and functional adaptation. Clearly, future research must address a broader and richer outcome variable domain. Equal attention must be paid to both child development and family adaptation. The evaluation of children must move far beyond the traditional reliance on cognition. Family measures must go beyond assessments of parent satisfaction with their service experience. Finally, relationships among young children, parents, and service providers demand careful scrutiny.

Focus on Resilience

Most studies of infants at risk for developmental problems have focused primarily on those factors that predict poor outcomes. Future research must correct this imbalance by identifying sources of resilience and protective factors that increase the likelihood of adaptive outcomes in the face of vulnerability. Much has been learned about the characteristics of children and families who do poorly. Less is known about why some children and families do well despite their designated high risk status. The identification of correlates of successful child and family adaptation can help to inform developmental theory, as well as guide the design of service delivery strategies and decisions regarding resource allocation.

Interest in Variability

Whereas previous research has focused largely on the modal performance of groups, future research must shift the focus toward a greater understanding of human variation. When heterogeneity is substantial, as is found typically within a sample of children with developmental disabilities, mean scores and group averages can be quite misleading. For example, average rates of developmental change for groups that include both children with severe disorders (who change very little) and children with mild delays (who change a great deal) can obscure important subgroup findings. Indeed, it is the differences among the subgroups that constitute the most important findings within a high-risk population. Greater understanding of that within-group variability must be a major priority for future investigation.

The Need for Longitudinal Follow-Up Studies

Most data on early intervention efficacy have come from studies that have assessed children over relatively short periods of time. No previous investigations have followed children and families from their point of entry into an early intervention program through their transition to preschool and beyond. The degree to which short-term change (or its absence) reflects a rate of development that will remain stable over an extended period is essentially unexplored. Similarly, the long-term predictability of early behavioral differences among program participants remains untested. Longitudinal studies are expensive and logistically complex, yet the collection of prospective data is essential if we are to assess the true influence of early life experiences (and early intervention programs, in particular) on the emerging competence of young children and on the ongoing adaptation of their families.

THE EARLY INTERVENTION COLLABORATIVE STUDY: A MODEL FOR EMPIRICAL INVESTIGATION

An ongoing longitudinal investigation that was initiated 7 years ago in 1985 at the University of Massachusetts Medical School provides one example of an attempt to confront the new agenda in early intervention research (Shonkoff, Hauser-Cram, Krauss, & Upshur, 1992). This study was designed to address three primary

goals: 1) to enhance the understanding of variations in the development of young children with disabilities and in the adaptation of their families over time, 2) to evaluate the mediating influences of family ecology and early intervention services, and 3) to generate empirical data to guide the construction of conceptual models of child development and family adaptation in the presence of a disability.

The first phase of this study investigated developmental change in 190 infants (mean age at study entry = 10.6 months) and their families after 1 year of early intervention services. The sample was recruited from 29 community-based service programs in Massachusetts and New Hampshire, and included 54 children with Down syndrome (mean age = 3.4 months; SD = 2.0), 77 children with motor impairment (mean age = 11.5 months; SD = 4.4), and 59 children with developmental delays of uncertain etiology (mean age = 16.0 months; SD = 5.8). Formal child assessments, observations of mother–child interaction, interviews with mothers, and questionnaires completed independently by both parents were collected through two home visits (within 6 weeks of program entry and 12 months later). Subsequent data collection includes a third home visit within 1 month of the child's third birthday, a classroom observation 6 weeks after preschool entry, and a home visit and school observation within 1 month of the child's fifth birthday. Monthly service data were collected for all study participants from the time of their initial assessment until formal discharge from their early intervention program.

This longitudinal investigation employs a nonexperimental design focused on the analysis of within-group differences. Because of ethical and legal restrictions on the identification and long-term follow-up of a true control group for which no services are provided, data analysis for this study did not address questions related to differences between treatment and nontreatment. Rather, analyses focused on differential change in children and families, all of whom received services. Specifically, we investigated which children and families demonstrated greater (or lesser) gains than others (employing standardized residual scores), and tested hypotheses about variables that mediated those gains.

Service Delivery

Analyses of service data revealed considerable variability in the amounts of different services actually received by children and families during their first year of program participation. The average intensity of service delivered was 6.9 hours per month, 3 hours of which involved home visiting, with the remainder divided among center-based activities for children and parents. In addition to services received within their early intervention program, a large percentage of the sample reported involvement in a variety of additional service activities beyond those provided in their core program. These included individual child therapies (e.g., physical therapy, occupational therapy, and speech-language therapy), child support services (e.g., visiting nurse association), and family support services (e.g., respite care and parent counseling). The most striking characteristic of the service experience was its marked variability.

Child Development

Assessment of the emergence of competence in the sample children is based upon a multidimensional approach, focused on two general domains of abilities. The first examines the degree to which the child is able to meet societal expectations. Evaluations within this domain focus on functional behaviors, as measured by the Vineland Adaptive Behavior Scales (Sparrow, Balla, & Cicchetti, 1984), and interactive behaviors, as measured through observation of the child's response to a learning situation with his or her mother, using the Nursing Child Assessment Teaching Scale (Barnard, 1978). The second domain of child competence examines personal development through an assessment of cognitive skills, as measured by the Bayley Scales of Infant Development (Bayley, 1969) or the McCarthy Scales of Children's Abilities (McCarthy, 1972), and through an evaluation of intrinsic motivational behaviors, as mea-

sured through observations of unstructured play (Belsky & Most, 1981).

Analysis of change in child performance over the 12-month study period revealed considerable variability within the sample. On a standardized measure of cognitive skills, the average mental age of the sample increased by 7.9 months. Eleven children (6%), however, showed no change in mental age after 1 year of intervention, whereas 35 children (18.5%) gained 12 months or more over the same time interval. Sample children also showed moderate development of their independent play skills. For the sample as a whole, the average level of play at study entry involved either mouthing or simple manipulation of objects. Twelve months later, the mean level of play involved functional use of objects, with 35 children (18.5%) showing pretense play as a modal level. Analyses of changes in play for the three sample subgroups defined by type of disability (i.e., Down syndrome, motor impairment, and developmental delays of uncertain etiology) revealed expected differences in mean play levels based on differences in chronological age. The rate of change over the 1-year study period, however, was comparable for the three groups, and reflected steady growth between the two data collection points. Observation of spontaneous play was demonstrated to be a useful measure of child competence, demonstrating significant within-group variability and measurable growth over a 12-month period.

Analysis of *differential* change across all child outcomes revealed several consistent findings. Children born prematurely, children with less severe cognitive impairment, and children without seizure disorders demonstrated larger gains in their development than other youngsters. Children with more severe cognitive impairment at study entry changed more slowly than children with milder delays, and children with motor impairment tended to have a lower rate of social development than those in the other two disability groups. Analyses of the service correlates of child change revealed greater gains in cognitive skills associated with more individualized services provided primarily through a single discipline, in comparison to services provided in a group format or through a multidisciplinary team. Of note, however, is the fact that limitations in the research design preclude causal inferences with regard to the correlational findings on service impacts.

Family Adaptation

The assessment of family adaptation and change over time also was conducted through a multidimensional strategy. Aspects of adaptation that were examined during the first phase of the study included: parental locus of control with respect to developmental change in the child, as measured by the Child Improvement Locus of Control Scales (Devillis et al., 1985); size and perceived helpfulness of parental social support networks, as measured by an adaptation of the Parent Support Scale (Dunst, Jenkins, & Trivette, 1984); family functioning, as measured by the Family Adaptability and Cohesion Evaluation Scales (FACES II) (Olson, Bell, & Portner, 1982); parenting stress, as measured by the Parenting Stress Index (Abidin, 1986); and adverse impacts on the family related to rearing a child with disabilities, as measured by the Impact-on-Family Scale (Stein & Reissman, 1980). All data were collected from both mothers and fathers through independent completion of questionnaires.

Analyses of data on parenting stress revealed several interesting findings. In general, most mothers and fathers reported no greater stress related to their parenting role than has been reported, on average, by parents of young children without developmental problems. Moreover, rated levels of parenting stress remained relatively stable over the first 12 months of participation in an early intervention program. Differences were found, however, between mothers and fathers in the relative focus of their stress. Mothers tended to report more stress than did fathers around the personal aspects of parenting, as manifested by perceived difficulties with social isolation, depression, and marital strain. In contrast, fathers were more likely than mothers to report more stress related to their child's temperament and to their own feelings of attachment to their son or

daughter. The implications of such findings for program planning, specifically with respect to the need to target services on the father–infant relationship, are striking.

Despite the finding of a relatively normal level of parenting stress for the study sample as a whole, a subgroup of families generated scores that indicated excessive stress, above the clinical cutoff levels that suggest the need for a mental health referral. Comparisons between these highly stressed families and those demonstrating normative levels of stress revealed several interesting findings. Counter to what might be predicted, there were no significant differences between the highly and normatively stressed families related to the child's type of disability, the severity of the child's cognitive or adaptive impairment, child gender or health status, parent educational levels, family income, or the employment status of the mother or father. Significant differences were found, however, on measures of social support, adverse family impacts, and family functioning. Specifically, highly stressed families were characterized by lower ratings of the helpfulness of their social support networks, higher ratings of negative family impacts on intra- and extra-familial relationships because of the child's disability, and parental perceptions of decreased family adaptability and cohesion. These findings indicate that high levels of parenting stress are not explained by the characteristics of the child but rather by aspects of family function that may very well precede the birth of a child with special needs. Indeed, the data suggest that families with the highest stress levels have underlying dysfunctional features that contribute to stress independent of the child's characteristics.

Analyses of service correlates of family change revealed a number of interesting patterns. On the one hand, more hours of home visiting were associated with greater decreases in maternal stress. On the other hand, more service hours that involved interactions with other parents (i.e., at a center) were associated with greater increases in both the size and the perceived helpfulness of maternal personal support networks. These findings suggest that there may be trade-offs with respect to differential family impacts based on the location and format of service delivery. Data on the family impacts of parent groups indicated a mixed picture. Mothers who attended parent groups more frequently also reported feeling more strain in their personal and family lives compared to mothers who did not attend as frequently. Parent group attendance, on the other hand, was associated with greater increases in the reported size and helpfulness of personal support networks. Interview data confirmed the prevalence of mixed impressions, as some parents characterized such groups as vitally important, while others expressed ambivalence or frank reluctance regarding their participation. In general, the data underline the need for careful delineation of the goals of parent groups and the importance of a thoughtful approach to the selection of participants.

Summary of Study Findings

Three generalizations can be drawn from these data abstracted from the first phase of the Early Intervention Collaborative Study (Shonkoff et al., 1992). First, the receipt of early intervention services implies a multidimensional experience. Moreover, there is considerable variability in the services received by children and families within a 12-month period. Second, the determinants of change in children and families are multivariate and complex. There are no "magic bullets," and significant influences on developmental gains in children and adaptation in their families show marked variability based upon the outcome of interest. Third, subgroups of children and families within an early intervention system demonstrate differential vulnerability and resilience. Thus, a predominant focus on mean group scores obscures within-group differences. Such differential vulnerability has important implications for developmental theory and resource allocation in service programs.

CURRENT SERVICE DELIVERY CHALLENGES

The tasks facing policymakers and service providers in the burgeoning field of early childhood

intervention are staggering. As the demands for resources increase and their availability is more restricted, the need for creative problem-solving is magnified. Three central challenges confront early childhood intervention in the 1990s: 1) the need to rethink disciplinary boundaries, 2) the need to refine intervention goals, and 3) the need to redefine parent–professional relationships.

Rethinking Disciplinary Boundaries

As our service delivery models mature, distinctions among the domains of health, education, and social service become increasingly blurred. Particularly with respect to infants and toddlers, differentiating needs according to traditional disciplinary boundaries is meaningless. The persistence of these barriers is fueled largely by issues related to fiscal accountability. Stated simply, much disciplinary conflict in the field of early childhood intervention has its origin in questions regarding whose budget (health, education, social service, etc.) will pay for needed services. The need for creative strategies for overcoming these dysfunctional bureaucratic barriers represents one of the critical challenges of the coming decade.

Professional identity concerns for early intervention service providers present an additional dimension that influences the conflict over blurred disciplinary boundaries. For many experienced service providers, the growing overlap that characterizes the work of individuals from different disciplines presents an exciting opportunity for professional growth. For others, however, such change and ambiguity is viewed as a threat to one's professional identity. This latter challenge generally is most acute in entry level positions, where young professionals are still in the formative stages of mastering a discrete body of knowledge and developing a professional identity.

Refining Intervention Goals

Efforts to identify the goals of early childhood intervention programs often are deficient in their lack of specificity and their failure to acknowledge the heterogeneity of the service population. For the children enrolled in such programs, for example, realistic long-term achievements may range from the possibility of normal function, to successful adaptation to a permanent disability, or to the prevention of developmental deterioration in the face of a severe handicapping condition.

For many families of children with disabilities, normative levels of stress and well-established informal support networks may indicate the need for relatively modest professional assistance. On the other hand, a subsample of families enrolled in intervention programs experience markedly elevated stress and perceive their existing social networks to be most unhelpful. Under such circumstances, a great deal of professional support may be needed. Thus, intervention goals must be specific, realistic, and individualized. In the absence of refined and individually tailored goals, some families receive services they neither need nor desire, while others do not get enough. When resources are matched to specific child and family service objectives, rather than to arbitrary categories based on the child's diagnosis, their utilization is most efficient.

Redefining Parent–Professional Relationships

Since the early 1980s, increasing numbers of advocacy groups and parent organizations have articulated the need for less hierarchical relationships between parents of children with special needs and professionals. Advocates have underlined the importance of parental autonomy and decision-making, and have decried the traditional paternalism of many professional service providers. This call for a balanced partnership is most appropriate and understandable, and reflects the growing assertiveness of parents of children with disabilities.

Notwithstanding the value of parent–professional collaboration, however, it is clear that relationships are complex and highly variable. The initial formation of a relationship between a parent and a professional is always asymmetric. The rate at which parents demonstrate assertiveness and autonomy within that relationship varies considerably. Some parents move quickly toward independent decision-making and executive functioning; others move slowly or not at all. Moreover, parental independence and autonomy cannot be achieved constructively in the absence of any consideration of the needs of professionals. Developing models of functional partnership between parents and professionals, and understanding the evolution of such alliances, present a crucial challenge for the early intervention efforts of the 1990s.

CONCLUSION

The ultimate challenge for the field of early childhood intervention is to balance the skepticism of the scientist with the faith of the advocate. The Third International Conference on the Infant At Risk embodied the spirit of this mission. Contemporary early childhood intervention draws its energy from the creative thinking of scholars in both human development and neurobiology, from the tireless commitment of service providers and policymakers, and from the passionate investment of parents of young children with disabilities. Together, these forces will shape the direction of our efforts on behalf of vulnerable children and their families well into the 21st century.

REFERENCES

Abidin, R. (1986). *Parenting stress index: Manual* (2nd ed.). Charlottesville, VA: Pediatric Psychology Press.

Bailey, E., & Bricker, D. (1984). The efficacy of early intervention for severely handicapped infants and young children. *Topics in Early Childhood Special Education, 4*, 30–51.

Barnard, K. (1978). *Nursing child assessment teaching scales.* Seattle: University of Washington School of Nursing.

Bayley, N. (1969). *The Scales of Infant Development.* New York: The Psychological Corporation.

Belsky, J., & Most, R. (1981). From exploration to play: A cross-sectional study of infant free play behavior. *Developmental Psychology, 17*, 630–639.

Devillis, R., Devillis, B., Revicki, D., Lurie, S., Runyan, O., & Bristol, M. (1985). Development and validation of the Child Improvement Locus of Control (CILC) Scales. *Journal of Social and Clinical Psychology, 3*, 307–324.

Dunst, C. (1986). Overview of the efficacy of early intervention programs. In L. Bickman & D.L. Weatherford (Eds.), *Evaluating early intervention programs for se-*

54	SHONKOFF

verely handicapped children and their families (pp. 79–147). Austin, TX: PRO-ED.

Dunst, C., Jenkins, V., & Trivette, C. (1984). The Family Support Scale: Reliability and validity. *Journal of Individual, Family, and Community Wellness, 1,* 45–52.

Dunst, C., & Rheingrover, R. (1982). An analysis of the efficacy of infant intervention programs with organically handicapped children. *Evaluation and Program Planning, 4,* 287–383.

Farran, D. (1990). Effects of intervention with disadvantaged and disabled children: A decade review. In S. Meisels & J. Shonkoff (Eds.), *Handbook of early childhood intervention.* (pp. 501–539). New York: Cambridge University Press.

Guralnick, M. (1989). Recent developments in early intervention efficacy research: Implications for family involvement in P.L. 99–457. *Topics in Early Childhood Special Education, 9,* 1–17.

McCarthy, D. (1972). *McCarthy Scales of Children's Abilities.* New York: The Psychological Corporation.

Meisels, S. (1985). The efficacy of early intervention: Why are we still asking this question? *Topics in Early Childhood Special Education, 5,* 1–8.

Olson, D., Bell, R., & Portner, J. (1982). *Family adapt-ability and cohesion evaluation scales (FACES II).* St. Paul, MN: Family Social Science.

Shonkoff, J., & Hauser-Cram, P. (1987). Early intervention for disabled infants and their families: A quantitative analysis. *Pediatrics, 80,* 650–658.

Shonkoff, J., Hauser-Cram, P., Krauss, M., & Upshur, C. (1992). *Infants with disabilities and their families.* Monographs of the Society for Research in Child Development Serial No. 230, Volume 57.

Shonkoff, J., Hauser-Cram, P., Krauss, M., & Upshur, C. (1988). Early intervention efficacy research: What have we learned and where do we go from here? *Topics in Early Childhood Special Education, 8,* 81–93.

Shonkoff, J., & Meisels, S. (1990). Early childhood intervention: The evolution of a concept. In S. Meisels & J. Shonkoff (Eds.), *Handbook of early childhood intervention* (pp. 3–31). New York: Cambridge University Press.

Sparrow, S., Balla, D., & Cicchetti, D. (1984). *Vineland Adaptive Behavior Scales (expanded form manual).* Circle Pines, MN: American Guidance Service.

Stein, R., & Reissman, C. (1980). The development of an Impact-on-Family Scale: Preliminary findings. *Medical Care, 18,* 465–472.

Section II

FAMILIES

Chapter 7

Assessment of the Impact of
Very Low Birth Weight Infants on Families

Carol J. Claflin, Ph.D.
Johnson County Community College, Overland Park, Kansas
Samuel J. Meisels, Ed.D.
University of Michigan, Ann Arbor

The baby in the plastic case lies swathed in a Mickey Mouse blanket whose cartoon characters dwarf him in size. One month after birth, he has already suffered major bleeding in his head, requiring brain surgery, and still needs a respirator to breathe. Born almost four months prematurely, weighing just over a pound, the baby is sustained by a battery of tubes and machines.

His skin is thin as parchment and his eyes are sealed shut, but he is clearly a human child. A minuscule blue and white stocking cap prevents heat loss through his head. . . .

[The doctor] says he has seen infants like his patient become normal children, although he admits the chances that the survivors will be normal are less than 1 in 4.

The remainder suffer brain damage. "Some are handicapped and are a great burden to their families and to society," [he] said, a note of sadness in his voice. It is a price he considers worth paying . . . (Rosenthal, 1991, p. 1)

Most parents consider the survival of their extremely low birth weight infant to be more than worth the "price" in effort, emotion, and sometimes agony that accompanies the early years and subsequent caregiving for their child. But this type of experience takes a toll on parents all the same. Even the birth of a normal, full-term infant can be a significant stressor for family functioning (Bendell, Goldberg, Urbano, Urbano, & Bauer, 1987; Miller & Sollie, 1980). When a baby arrives 2–3 months early, weighing less than half of what newborns usually weigh, families often experience considerably more stress (Crnic, Greenberg, Ragozin, Robinson, & Basham, 1983a). Moreover, the recent decline in mortality of extremely premature very low birth weight (VLBW) infants means that more of these tiny infants are eventually going home with their families. What does this mean for the families of these infants?

Usually, premature labor is unexpected. Parents are unprepared and distressed at the arrival of an infant so different from what was expected (Choi, 1973; Elsas, 1981; Goldberg, 1978). The first time family members see the VLBW infant, they are usually shocked by the baby's unattractive appearance. These infants are small, have little subcutaneous fat, are reddish in color, and are hooked up to a multitude of machines used to assess the infant's status

This work was supported in part by grants to Carol J. Claflin from the National Institutes of Health (NRS Award #1F31 NR06/59-01) and the University of Michigan and to Samuel J. Meisels (Principal Co-Investigator) from the National Institute on Disability and Rehabilitation Research.

and to support life. Concern about whether the infant will survive and the quality of survival is legitimate. Despite improved mortality rates, 27% of VLBW infants in the United States die in the neonatal period (Office of Technology Assessment, 1987). In addition, these infants are known to have higher rates of respiratory morbidity, growth failure, neurological sequelae, developmental delay, and problems in academic achievement than children born at term age (McCormick, 1989; Meisels & Plunkett, 1988).

Social and environmental factors also contribute to the differential family experience of the birth of a VLBW infant. A Neonatal Intensive Care Unit (NICU) is a strange environment in which to become acquainted with a new family member. Surrounded by "high tech" equipment, bombarded by high noise levels, dependent upon experts who know what is "best," looking at the infant through incubator glass—often forbidden to touch their baby for fear of causing stress that the infant cannot tolerate, and required to communicate in a medical language that is distancing and unfamiliar, families have a great deal with which to contend.

Prolonged hospitalization necessitates physical separation. Time, distance, financial, and other obligatory constraints often prevent families from visiting the infant as much as would be liked. In addition, lack of responsibility and involvement in the care of the infant may increase a family's sense of separation (Richards, 1979). Families also face the stress of coming home from the hospital without their baby, and having rituals associated with the birth disrupted or eliminated (e.g., baby showers, birth announcements, formal religious services such as baptisms, circumcisions, naming ceremonies) (Zarling, Hirsch, & Landry, 1988). When preterm infants are well enough to be discharged, they are less alert, responsive, and predictable than full-term infants (Crnic, Greenberg, Ragozin, Robinson, & Basham, 1983b; DiVitto & Goldberg, 1979; Field, 1979; Goldberg, 1978). In addition, preterm infants are less likely to give clear distress signals, and their shrill, high-pitched cry becomes aversive (Goldberg, 1978).

The birth of a VLBW infant confronts fam-
ilies with unexpected financial expenses. Neonatal intensive care is expensive. According to the Office of Technology Assessment (1987), the average hospital cost for VLBW (<1501 grams) infants ranges from $26,740 to $60,015 (all costs are reported in 1984 dollars). However, costs increase with decreasing birth weight. Initial care for infants weighing between 750–1000 grams ranges between $38,750 and $76,390. The smallest infants (500–750 grams) have the highest expenses: $61,700–$149,180. Costs to the family not included in these analyses include expenses for travel, lodging, and meals when visiting the infant; child care for other children at home; and time lost from work. McCormick (1989) also points out that ongoing medical care and intervention services post-discharge can cost "2 to 50 times those of a healthy child through the first three years of life. Despite the availability of private insurance and public programs, a substantial proportion of the burden of providing needed services falls to young families with limited resources and other competing demands" (p. 1771).

Given the additional stressors with which families of VLBW infants may have to contend, it is reasonable to hypothesize that these families are at risk for dysfunction. Yet, one of the most intriguing questions raised from anecdotal reports is how some families manage to continue to function (and function relatively well) when faced with what seem to be overwhelming circumstances. In fact, little is known about the impact on family functioning of the birth and survival of a VLBW infant. Many factors contribute to this dearth of information: 1) until the advent of advanced medical technology beginning in the 1970s, few VLBW infants survived; 2) the primary focus of research has been the outcome of the VLBW infant, rather than the adaptation of the family; and 3) "family functioning" is a complex concept that is difficult to assess. This review is designed to examine theoretical bases for targeting the family as the unit of assessment and to identify and evaluate methods and measures that have been used to assess family functioning in families with preterm infants.

FAMILY FUNCTIONING

Few measures have been developed specifically to evaluate families of premature infants or to be used with VLBW infant/family samples. Thus, in addition to those measures that have been used with VLBW families, this review will also include measures aimed at evaluating family functioning in families with chronically ill children.

Theoretical Perspectives

Recent research has begun to explore "how families cope with and adjust to . . . very difficult situation(s) and at the same time promote the health, well-being, and development of children in the home" (McCubbin et al., 1982, p. 169). This interest is due in part to the recognition of the "interdependence of family members for satisfaction of their biological, psychological, social, and economic needs" (Hymovich, 1974, p. 91). Several theories support the importance of a family-focused approach to studying the impact of a stressful event, such as the birth of an extremely low birth weight infant. These include: General Systems Theory (von Bertalanffy, 1966), Family Systems Theory (Buckley, 1967; Jackson, 1957; Minuchin, 1974), ABC-X Family Crisis Model (Hill, 1949), Double ABC-X Model of Family Functioning (McCubbin & Patterson, 1982), Circumplex Model of Marital and Family Systems (Olson & McCubbin, 1982), Developmental Task Approach (Duvall, 1971; Hymovich, 1974), and the Process Model of Family Functioning (Steinhauer, Santa-Barbara, & Skinner, 1984).

General Systems Theory General Systems Theory (von Bertalanffy, 1966) identifies a system as two or more connected elements that form an organized whole and interact with one another. Although it is suggested that the system is goal-directed and comprised of independent units, there is an interdependence that endures over time. Main components of this theory include: 1) interaction (i.e., the exchange of energy, resources, information; 2) boundary definition (i.e., what is and is not part of the system); 3) flexibility (i.e., a capacity to adapt to internal and/or external changes); and 4) system-relatedness (i.e., the concept that change in any part of the system affects the functioning of the system as a whole).

Family Systems Theory Minuchin (1974) and other family system theorists have adapted General Systems Theory to explain the functioning of a family. Within the context of family systems, the whole is greater than the sum of the parts. It is the structure, role assignment, access to resources, shared and individual histories of members, and dynamics of interaction within the family that contribute to the potential for adaptation in the midst of internal or external stressors (Turk & Kearns, 1985).

ABC-X Family Crisis Model The ABC-X Family Crisis Model states that a stressor event (A) in combination with the family's crisis-meeting resources (B) and the family's definition of the event (C) produce the crisis (X) (Burr, 1973, 1982; Hill, 1958). This model points out that it is not just the event (e.g., the VLBW infant birth), but the family's resources (e.g., the effective communication, social support, financial resources, ability to gain needed resources) and how the family views the event (e.g., extent to which family routine is disrupted, causal attribution to preterm birth, potential for resolution) that determine the crisis (i.e., "amount of crisis") and to some extent, the mobilization of efforts toward "reorganization." Hill also identified several other variables which influence the family's ability to recover from the crisis. These include the suddenness of the event, the kinship/extended family/community ties, the similarity of sentiment in the family, the marital relationship, the type of decision-making utilized within the family, member roles (especially the wife/mother), and successful resolution of previous similar crises. Many of these variables are consistent with characteristics of systems and family systems approaches noted earlier.

Double ABC-X Model of Family Functioning The ABC-X Model was expanded by McCubbin and Patterson (1982) to include adaptation to a crisis over time (post-crisis). Four additional components are included in the revised Double ABC-X Model. Family pile-up of stressors (AA) include unresolved aspects of the original stressor event, "normal" changes within the family that occur over time, role changes as a result of the stressor, and continuing hardships experienced as a result of the event. Unresolved pile-up stressors for families of VLBW infants might include ongoing morbidity of the infant, prolonged separation, and concern regarding the infant's viability and/or "quality" of outcome. Changes over time that may affect families are level of satisfaction of role changes within the family, achievement of developmental tasks of family members (i.e., successful toilet training, beginning of school for siblings), and/or alteration in social support systems resulting from isolation. The BB factor continues to encompass the resources initially available to the family, but now includes strategies for coping that have "strengthened or developed in response to the 'crisis' situation" (McCubbin & Patterson, 1982, p. 45). Families may develop new relationships with care providers and families of other VLBW infants. With time, they may also improve their caretaking skills and learn new methods of managing resources. The family perception of the crisis (CC) involves a redefinition of the situation (i.e., initial event, resources, and response) and attribution of meaning to the situation (which may also include the family's religious beliefs). The XX factor is family crisis and adaptation. "Adaptation involves the processes of stimulus regulation, environmental control, and balancing to achieve a level of functioning, which preserves family unity and enhances the family system and member growth and development" (McCubbin & Patterson, 1982, p. 45). This definition allows for a range of outcomes from negative to positive.

The Circumplex Model of Marital and Family Systems

In an attempt to understand the underlying components of the concepts of family stress theory, Olson and McCubbin (1982) identified two primary dimensions of family behavior—cohesion and adaptability. These dimensions are at the core of The Circumplex Model of Marital and Family Systems which was designed to be used in clinical work with families. Family cohesion is the "emotional bonding that family members have toward one another and the degree of individual autonomy that they experience" (Olson & McCubbin, 1982, p. 49). Family adaptability is "the ability of a marital or family system to change its power structure, role relationships, and relationship rules in response to situational and developmental stress" (p. 51). Four ordinal levels of cohesion and four ordinal levels of adaptation are identified, resulting in 16 possible types of family systems under this model. "Balance" (i.e., cohesion and adaptability at more moderate levels) is postulated to be related to more satisfactory family functioning, while extremes in one or both dimension are associated with greater dysfunction. Also of importance is the agreement/disagreement among family members as to how they see the family dimensions.

Developmental Task Approach

The Developmental Task Approach (Duvall, 1971; Hymovich, 1974) examines the family's ability to facilitate and achieve family, as well as individual, developmental tasks. According to Duvall (1971), there are ten individual tasks and eight family tasks to be accomplished. Specific components and related behaviors for each task are identified for each stage of individual and family development. Hymovich (1974) suggests that stressors the family experiences (i.e., chronic illness or perhaps the birth of a VLBW infant) may have an impact on the family's ability to cope; this can be assessed by monitoring how well the family members, both individually and collectively, master appropriate developmental tasks.

Related to this approach, Strauss (1975) suggests that families dealing with chronic illness have specific tasks that are superimposed over the normal developmental tasks of individuals and families. These include: 1) preventing medical crises, 2) controlling symptoms, 3) carrying out prescribed regimes, 4) preventing social isolation, 5) attempting to normalize developmentally appropriate interactions with others, 6) adjusting to changes in the course of the illness, and 7) assuring adequate finances. These tasks may also be relevant for the families who deal with ongoing sequelae that are sometimes associated with VLBW infants.

Process Model of Family Functioning   The Process Model of Family Functioning (Steinhauer et al., 1984) evaluates the interaction between the individuals in the family and the family as a whole. "The overriding goals of the family are to provide for the biological, psychological and social development and maintenance of family members" (p. 78). These goals are influenced by society, stage of family life, and the values and norms of the family, and are accomplished by a variety of tasks. Components of the model that contribute to family functioning are: 1) the values and norms held by the family, 2) control and management issues, 3) affective involvement of members, 4) effectiveness and style of communication, 5) performance of prescribed familial role, and 6) task accomplishment. This model specifically tries to focus upon family process instead of structure.

These models reflect the complexity of the phenomena embedded in "family functioning." Early attempts to analyze the impact of stress associated with childhood illness upon the family were relatively simplistic, due to their limited focus on one aspect of the family, namely, the child. Criticisms such as these have encouraged family-oriented research. However, this multidimensional focus raises other concerns. Can complex theoretical models be operationalized and applied usefully in research and clinical settings? As one researchers laments, "Nobody knows how to measure a family because it is a dynamic and ever-growing unit" (Klein, 1974, p. 187).

METHODS OF ASSESSMENT: MEASURES AND INSTRUMENTS

Instruments that are used to assess functioning (or a component of family functioning) in families with chronically ill children or premature infants are discussed in this section. The instruments and measures have been grouped according to the dimension of family functioning addressed (i.e., family dynamics, stressors and stress, resources, and parental attitudes).

Family Dynamics

The interaction and interdependence of family members are among the key concepts identified in the theoretical models of family functioning. The changing structures, role assignments, values, control mechanisms, communication patterns, affective affiliations, facilitation of developmental task achievement, and responses to challenging situations within a family do not occur spontaneously, but by a continuous give-and-take within family members, between family members, and with the greater societal environment. In an attempt to better understand this dynamic system, researchers have begun to develop instruments specifically designed to assess the interactive and interdependent qualities of families. Table 1 describes eight such instruments (seven family measures and one dyadic measure) identified from the review.

One aspect of the family dynamic measures that is encouraging is that they can be administered to all family members capable of understanding them. The Family Assessment Measure (FAM) (Skinner, Steinhauer, & Santa-Barbara, 1983) has been used with children 7 years and older and The Children's Version of the Family Environment Scale (CVFES) (Moos, 1974) is designed for children ages 5–12 years of age. While studies involving FAM and The Family Adaptability and Cohesion Evaluation Scales (FACES) (Olson, Bell, & Portner, 1978) strive to include all appropriate family members in the assessment, these are exceptions. In most cases, the mother is the primary, if not the sole source of information regarding family functioning. Since families are comprised of more than one individual, it seems essential to have the perspective of more than one person, if the goal is to understand the family. The degree of consensus and/or discrepancy among family members is also important, and may be related to the level of stress experienced within the family (Olson & McCubbin, 1982; Spanier, 1976; Steinhauer, 1984). Measures that provide a means for evaluating similarities and differences have an advantage over those which do not.

Although a case can be made for some link

Table 1. Measures of family functioning

Measure	Authors	Description	Concept or factors measured	Scoring	Internal reliability
Family Adaptability and Cohesion Evaluation Scales (FACES)	Olson, Bell, and Portner (1978)	111 self-report items: 6 items for each of the 16 variables from the Cir- cumplex Model; 15-item social desirability scale	1. Family cohesion 2. Family adaptability 3. Social desir- ability	4-point Likert rat- ing of "how true" the statement is for their own family; scores computed for: 1. Cohesion 2. Adaptability 3. Social desirability Sample item: Family members are concerned with each other's welfare.	Cohesion: .83 Adaptability: .75 Social desir- ability: not reported
Family Assessment Measure (FAM)	Skinner, Steinhauer, and Santa- Barbara (1983)	134 self-report items based on Process Model: 50-item General scale, 42-item Dyadic Relation- ship, 42-item Self-rating scale	1. Task accom- plishment 2. Role per- formance 3. Communi- cation 4. Affective involvement 5. Control 6. Values and norms	Not available	General scale: .90 adult, .93 child; Dyadic scale: .94 adult, .93 child; Self- rating scale: .90 adult, .87 child
Family Concept Q-sort (FCQS)	Novak and Van der Veen (1970)	80 cards de- scribing family unit, sorted twice: "as your family is now," "as you would ideally like your family to be"	1. Family adjustment 2. Family satisfaction 3. Family congruence	10-point Likert rating; cards sorted by piles from "least like my family" to "most like my family" 1. Family adjustment = compari- son of per- son's real family to pre-existing sort of the "ideal fam- ily" by men- tal health professionals 2. Family satis- faction = comparison of person's real and ideal family concepts 3. Family con- gruence = agreement of family	Not reported

(continued)

Table 1. (continued)

Measure	Authors	Description	Concept or factors measured	Scoring	Internal reliability
				concepts between mother and father Method of computing comparisons not described Sample items: We cannot tell each other our real feelings. We forgive each other easily.	
Family Effectiveness Test (FET)	Novak and Van der Veen (1970)	48 self-report items	Social and emotional aspects of family	9-point Likert rating of "how like" the statement is of the family; rating of >4 = positive; total number of positive items = degree of family adjustment; total range = 0–48; 35 or more = good adjustment; less than 30 = poor adjustment	Not reported
Family Environment Scale (FES)	Moos (1974)	90 self-report items, 10 subscales	Social climate: 1. Cohesion 2. Expressiveness 3. Conflict 4. Independence 5. Active recreation orientation 6. Moral-religious emphasis 7. Organization 8. Control 9. Achievement orientation 10. Intellectual-cultural orientation	True/false statements; statements can be grouped into sets of relationships, personal growth, and system maintenance; scales can also be administered three times to evaluate "real" vs. "ideal" family and "expectancies" for change Sample items: Family members really help and support one another. Activities in our family are carefully planned.	Subscales: .67–.78

(continued)

Table 1. (continued)

Measure	Authors	Description	Concept or factors measured	Scoring	Internal reliability
Family Environment Scale—Children's Version (CVFES)	Moos (1974)	30 items presented by examiner, 3 pictures for each item; pictures include mother, father, and child and "situation varied along the dimension"	Same as above	Child's description of family elicited by "Which looks like your family?" *Some pictures have captions at the 3rd grade reading level.	Not reported
Family Relations Test (FRT)	Bene and Anthony (1957)	Figures representing family members matched with cards that have a single emotion, attitude, or statement	"Affective relationship" with individual family members For adults/teens: early memories of family and current family relations For children: "perception of interpersonal relationships"	Counting of number of affective items from each "attitudinal area" matched for each family figure; conceptualized to represent the psychological importance of each family member and the positive, negative, and/or ambivalent feelings associated with the family member	Not reported
Dyadic Adjustment Scale	Spanier (1976)	32 self-report items; factor analyzed into 4 subscales	1. Dyadic satisfaction 2. Dyadic consensus 3. Dyadic cohesion 4. Affectional expression	5- and 6-point Likert ratings of "how much agreement you and your partner have" (always agree to always disagree) or "how often you and your partner encounter some event" (all the time to never). Sample items: agreement on handling finances; how often you or your partner leave the house after an argument	Satisfaction: .94, consensus: .90, cohesion: .86, affective expression: .73, total: .96

to a theoretical base in all of these measures, only two (FACES and FAM) are explicitly theory-based. Theoretically-based models begin to shed some light on how families function, not only that families differ. Both FAM and FACES have been useful in guiding the development of therapeutic goals to maintain and improve individual and familial functioning, and in the assessment of response to intervention (Olson & McCubbin, 1982; Steinhauer, 1984). In addition, FAM is an aid in the education of students and therapists (Steinhauer, 1984).

The measures of family functioning presented in Table 1 are not free from criticism. It can be argued that some do not measure functioning, but level of satisfaction (Family Concept Q-sort) (FCQS) (Novak & Van deer Veen, 1970), attitude toward other family members (Family Relations Test) (Bene & Anthony, 1957), or "good" or "bad" outcome (Family Effectiveness Test) (FET) (Novak & Van der Veen, 1970). Similarly, the validity of these measures is not well established. In addition, measures that lack evaluation of internal consistency, and/or vary considerably within and between subscales, make interpretation difficult, as items may have little empirical relationship to one another. Finally, it is recognized that when the number of family members increases, it becomes more difficult to agree upon the functioning dynamics of the family unit (Olson & McCubbin, 1982).

Stressors and Stress

Families are confronted by a variety of stressful events. These events differ between families according to the type (normative or non-normative; daily hassle or life event); overall number, frequency, and timing; and interpretation (Burr, 1982; Kanner, Coyne, Schaefer, & Lazarus, 1981; McCubbin & Patterson, 1982; McCubbin et al., 1980). It follows, therefore, that the same event (stressor) experienced by several families could have several different effects (stress) that range in quality as well as intensity; conversely, it is possible that exposure to different stressors could result in similar effects (stress). The measures presented in Table 2 are designed to examine the familial experience of stressors and stress.

Once again, it is important to consider each family member's perspective in an assessment of the family's experience of events. Two of the measures, the Family Inventory of Life Events and Changes (FILE) (McCubbin, Patterson, & Wilson, 1983) and the Daily Hassles Scale

(Kanner et al., 1981) are designed so that the responses of family members can be compared. However, these measures are limited by the lack of consideration for developmental, age-appropriate events. Therefore, even if these measures were administered to children capable of completing the measure, they may not reflect their experience. Most of the measures are designed for adult or parent use only.

Three measures take into account the individual's evaluation of the effect of the stressor (Daily Hassles; FILE; Life Experiences Survey [LES] [Sarason, Johnson, & Siegel, 1978]). Although these are an improvement over early checklist approaches to the experience of stressors, they still do not take into account what factors influence the perceived stressfulness of the event.

The Impact on Family Scale (Stein & Riessman, 1980) and the Problem Inventory (Tavormina, Boll, Dunn, Luscomb, & Taylor, 1981) focus on areas that may be related specifically to the parent's experience of caring for an ill child. These measures are not designed for sibling evaluations of the experience. In addition, it is possible that the age of the ill child may affect the validity of these measures (e.g., even a healthy toddler may place extra demands on time and energy compared to children of other ages). Used in isolation, these measures do not take into account non–illness-related stressors. Similarly, the general stress measures may not be specific enough to assess many of the issues that are associated with the care and emotional aspects of having an ill child.

Finally, the psychometric characteristics of these instruments should be considered. Reliability measures of subscales, when available, vary considerably on some instruments. The validity of the Parenting Stress Index (PSI) (Abidin, 1983) is questionable. Although it is aimed at "parenting" stress, it is heavily influenced by infant temperament and maternal anxiety/depression measures; it may be identifying difficult babies or depressed mothers. In contrast, the Daily Hassles Scale has demonstrated validity in the prediction of psychological symptoms and adaptational outcomes (Kanner et al., 1981).

Table 2.   Measures that assess the type, area, and/or amount of stress experienced by families

Measure	Authors	Description	Concept or factors measured	Scoring	Internal reliability
Daily Hassles Scale	Kanner, Coyne, Schaefer, and Lazarus (1981)	117 self-report items	Daily hassles: "irritative, frustrating, and distressing demands that to some degree characterize everyday transactions with environment"; 7 areas of hassle: work, health, family, friends, environment, practical considerations, and chance occurrences	3-point Likert rating of "severity of hassle" from "mild" to "severe." Three scores: 1. Frequency of hassles = count of items experienced 2. Cumulated severity = sum of severity points 3. Average intensity of hassles = total of severity points divided by number of hassles experienced Sample items: Misplacing or losing things; problems with your children	Not reported
Family Inventory of Life Events and Changes (FILE)	McCubbin, Patterson, and Wilson (1983)	71 self-report items based upon Double ABC-X Model; 9 subscales	1. Level of stress experienced with normative and non-normative events 2. "Pile-up" of stressors 3. Perceived strain in 9 areas: intrafamily, marital, childbearing, finances/ business, work–family transitions, losses, illness and family care, general transitions, and legal violations	9-point Likert rating of severity Total stress = number of events experienced times a standard weight per item (derived from sample of 75 families assessing how the "average" family would view the event) Total demand = number of events experienced times the family's perception of severity Sample item: A member gave birth or adopted a child.	Total: .72

(continued)

Table 2. *(continued)*

Measure	Authors	Description	Concept or factors measured	Scoring	Internal reliability
Impact on Family Scale	Stein and Riessman (1980)	24 self-report items	Effect of child illness on family system in four areas: 1. Financial impact 2. Social/family impact 3. Personal strain 4. Mastery	4-point Likert rating of agreement with statement from "strongly agree" to "strongly disagree" Score is the sum of rating points Total possible range = 24–96 Standardized on a sample of 100 mothers of chronically ill children: range 24–76, mean = 48.0, standard deviation = 8.2 Sample item: Additional income is needed in order to cover medical expenses.	Financial: .72, Social/family: .86, Personal: .81, Mastery: .60, Total: .88
Life Experiences Survey (LES)	Sarason, Johnson, and Siegel (1978) (adapted by Crnic, Greenberg, & Slough, 1986, for use with mothers of newborn infants)	46 self-report items	"Negative" life stress: 1. Occurrence 2. Evaluation (good/bad) 3. Degree of effect	4-point Likert rating of degree of effect from "none" to "great"; sum of the degree of effect of all occurring items conceptualized as index of negative life stress Sample item: Major change in sleeping habits	Not applicable
Parenting Stress Index (PSI)	Abidin (1983)	101 self-report items	"Stress" in parent-child relationship Child characteristics: adaptability, acceptability, demandingness, mood, distractability/hyperactivity, reinforces parent Parent characteristics: depression, attachment,	5-point Likert rating from "strongly agree" to "strongly disagree" Sample item: My child's sleeping or eating schedule was much harder to establish than I expected.	Child subscales: .62–.70, Parent subscales: .55–.80, Total scale: .95

(continued)

Table 2. *(continued)*

Measure	Authors	Description	Concept or factors measured	Scoring	Internal reliability
			restriction of role, sense of competence, social isolation, spousal relationship, health Situational/ demographic information		
Problem Inventory	Tavormina, Boll, Dunn, Luscomb, and Taylor (1981)	10 self-report items	"Difficulties" related to the care of a child who is ill or has a disability	5-point Likert rating of frequency of occurrence from "never" to "always"; score is sum of ratings Sample items: Extra demands on time and energy; life centered around the child's needs; decreased social life with spouse.	Not reported

Resources

A family's resources to respond to an event may be material, social, emotional, and/or mental. Family resources also vary in availability, accessibility, utilizability, and manageability. How individual members within the family use resources may be complementary, contradictory, and/or detrimental to the family as a unit. Table 3 presents measures that address familial resources.

Two of the measures are explicitly based upon the Double ABC-X Family Crisis Model (McCubbin & Patterson, 1982): the Family Inventory of Resources for Management (FIRM) (McCubbin, Comeau, & Harkins, 1981) and the Coping Health Inventory for Parents (CHIP) (McCubbin, McCubbin, & Cauble, 1979). The CHIP focuses on parental coping strategies only, but does allow for interparental comparisons. The advantage of the FIRM is that it is a measure designed for all family members and focuses on a wider domain. Its disadvantage is that it does not address the specifics of potential "extra" resources needed for life with an ill child.

The Home Observation for Measurement of the Environment (HOME) (Caldwell & Bradley, 1984) and questionnaire adaptation are intended to address the resources available to children younger than 6 years of age. There are concerns, however, regarding this measure. Although a resource must be available to be taken advantage of, availability alone does not imply that it will be or can be used. The scale also contains biases related to the number of children in the home; there are probably more toys and more toys of varying developmental levels when there are more children in the home. Socioeconomic factors may also influence the scoring of the HOME. General household items converted into "toys" (e.g., pots, spoons, shoe boxes, milk cartons, clothespins) may not count as toys (i.e., "three or more puzzles"). The time of year the observation takes place may also influence the scoring. In harsh winter weather, the infant may not be taken out of the home enough to get credit for the item. However, in the spring, summer, or fall, credit would be received. In addition, the child who "goes out" to daycare is scored for an outing.

Table 3. Measures of family resources

Measure	Authors	Description	Concept or factors measured	Scoring	Internal reliability
Coping Health Inventory for Parents (CHIP)	McCubbin, McCubbin, and Cauble (1979)	80 self-report items based on Double ABC-X Model; 3 strategies from factor analysis	Strategies used to manage life with a chronically ill child (designed for cystic fibrosis) Strategy 1: Maintenance of family integration, cooperation, and optimistic definition of situation Strategy 2: Maintenance of social support, self-esteem, and psychological stability Strategy 3: Understanding medical situation through communication with others	4-point Likert rating of "how helpful" strategy is in managing stress Score is the sum of rating points. Sample items: Believing that my child is getting the best possible medical care; talking with other parents in the same situation	Strategy 1: .79, Strategy 2: .79, Strategy 3: .71
Family Inventory of Resources for Management (FIRM)	McCubbin, Comeau, and Harkins (1981)	69 self-report items based on Double ABC-X Model	Family availability of and management of resources 1. Esteem & Communication: esteem, communication, mutual assistance, optimism, problem solving, autonomy 2. Mastery & Health: mastery-mutuality, physical/ emotional health 3. Extended Family Support: giving/ receiving help, material help, supportive communication 4. Financial Well-Being: ability to meet commitments, adequacy of resources, ability to help others, optim-	4-point Likert rating of "how well" the statement describes the family situation from "not at all" to "very well" Score is the sum of rating points. Sample item: Our family is under a lot of emotional stress.	Esteem: .85, Mastery/ Health: .85, Extended Family: .62, Finances: .85, Resource Strain: .86

(continued)

Table 3. (continued)

Measure	Authors	Description	Concept or factors measured	Scoring	Internal reliability
			ism, management practices 5. Resource Strains: Difficulty in acquiring/ maintaining resources		
Home Observation for Measurement of the Environment	Caldwell and Bradley (1984)	55 items (observation and interview); 8 subscales	"Quality and quantity of social, emotional, and cognitive supports" available to preschoolers (3–6 years) Subscales: Stimulation through toys, etc.; language stimulation; physical environment; pride, affection, warmth; stimulation of academic behavior; modeling and encouragement	Yes/No scoring of items Scoring is based upon the sum of the items with "yes" observations and/or responses Sample items: Three or more puzzles; mother uses correct grammar. Mother kisses/cuddles child at least once during visit.	Subscales: .53–.83, Total: .93
Questionnaire adaptation of Home Observation for Measurement of the Environment	Elardo, Bradley, and Caldwell (1977)	45 self-report items	"Quality and quantity of social, emotional, and cognitive support" available to infants (0–3 years) Subscales: Maternal/family style; emotional/ verbal responsiveness; avoidance of restriction/ punishment; organization; provision of appropriate toys; maternal involvement; variety	Yes/No scoring of items	Subscales: .44–.89, Total: .89

(continued)

Table 3. *(continued)*

Measure	Authors	Description	Concept or factors measured	Scoring	Internal reliability
Social Support Measure (Adaptation of scale developed by Henderson, Byrne, & Duncan-Jones, 1981)	Crnic, Greenberg, Ragozin, Robinson, and Basham (1983), Crnic, Greenberg, and Slough (1986)	9 self-report items; 3 sub-scales by factor analysis	Availability and satisfaction of social support: 1. Intimate support 2. Friendships 3. Neighborhood/community	4-point Likert rating of satisfaction from "very satisfied" to "very dissatisfied" Sums for subscales and total scores	Intimate: .69, Friendship: .65, Neighborhood: .50

The HOME does, however, have an advantage, in that it involves direct observation and is not totally self-report like the other measures. It also attempts to address the resources that are available for young children, while the other measures do not do this.

Parental Attitudes

"How parents treat children is presumably determined in part by what parents believe about children, both children in general and their own children in particular (Miller, 1988, p. 259). It follows, therefore, that parental attitudes are often considered as possible contributors to the parent-child interaction dimension of family dynamics. Measures of parental attitudes are described in Table 4.

These scales vary as to what they measure. The Hereford Parent Attitude Survey (Hereford, 1963) suggests components that contribute to a parent's overall comfort level of parenting, while the Mother-Child Relationship Evaluation (MCRE) (Roth, 1980) is more reflective of how the mother would be likely to interact with the child. The Satisfaction with Parenting Scale (SWPS) (Ragozin, Basham, Crnic, Greenberg, & Robinson, 1982) attempts to assess satisfaction. The remaining three instruments (Vulnerable Child Scale [VCS] [Perrin, West, & Culley, 1989], and the two Your Baby and Average Baby Perception Inventories [Broussard & Hartner, 1970; Danko, Nagy, & Holmes, 1982]) examine how parents view their child in comparison with the "average" child. These measures invite the interesting question as to whether they reflect the "true picture" of a child, or a self-fulfilling prophecy.

Summary of Strengths and Weaknesses

Instruments used to assess family functioning offer the advantage of producing a continuous or categorical value that can be used in statistical analyses. In addition, use of the same measure by various researchers facilitates the comparison of results. Practical advantages also follow from the use of the measures presented: they are predominantly paper and pencil measures that can be completed in a relatively short time; they can be mailed to subjects; and they are often less threatening than face-to-face encounters.

However, there are concerns about the measures cited. The reliability and validity of most of the instruments are not clearly documented. In addition, socioeconomic and cultural biases are likely inherent given the practice of development and/or standardization on predominantly white middle-class samples.

Methods of assessment used by researchers to assess family functioning in response to a stressor event (e.g., the birth of an extremely premature infant or life with a chronically ill child) lag behind the available theoretical conceptualizations. Although theories have expanded to include many aspects of family functioning, most measures examine only a limited number of components. Whether this is sufficient depends upon the specific aim of the study. Is the goal to classify families according to certain dimensions, or to create a typology?

Table 4. Measures of parental attitudes

Measure	Authors	Description	Concept or factors measured	Scoring	Internal reliability
Hereford Parent Attitude Survey	Hereford (1963)	75 items; 5 subscales with 15 items each	Parental attitudes: 1. Confidence in parental role 2. Causation of child's behavior 3. Acceptance of child 4. Mutual understanding (reciprocity of feelings) 5. Mutual trust (confidence in each other)	5-point Likert rating of agreement; summary measures for subscales and total Sample item: I feel I am faced with more problems than most parents.	Confidence: .78, Causation: .77, Acceptance: .68, Understanding: .86, Trust: .84
Mother-Child Relationship Evaluation (MCRE)	Roth (1980)	48 items; 4 categories with 12 items each	Measuring maternal attitudes of child: acceptance, overprotection, overindulgence, rejection	5-point Likert rating of agreement from "strongly agree" to "strongly disagree" Subscale and total scores are the sums of ratings.	Acceptance: .57, Overprotection: .53, Overindulgence: .41, Rejection: .47
Satisfaction with Parenting Scale (SWPS)	Ragozin, Basham, Crnic, Greenberg, and Robinson (1982)	12 items; 2 subscales	Maternal satisfaction with: 1. Infant (child care chores, doubts about maternal confidence, irritation with baby, overall feeling toward baby) 2. Role (satisfied with amount of infant care responsibility, household responsibility, time for self, social time away from baby, nonprofessional advice, people with whom to	Method of scoring not available Sample item: Do you ever find your baby irritating?	Satisfaction with baby: .48, Role satisfaction: .61, Total: .67

(continued)

Table 4. (*continued*)

Measure	Authors	Description	Concept or factors measured	Scoring	Internal reliability
			discuss negative feelings regarding baby)		
Vulnerable Child Scale (VCS)	Perrin, West, and Culley (1989)	16 items	Maternal perception of child's vulnerability	4-point Likert rating of "trueness" of statement to child Summary scores Sample items: I often think about calling the doctor about "name."	Not reported
Your Baby and Average Baby Perception Inventories	Broussard and Hartner (1970)	6 items	Evaluation of infant behavior: crying, spitting, feeding, elimination, sleeping, and predictability	5-point Likert rating of occurrence from "a great deal" to "none." Summary scores of ratings for own baby and "average" baby	Not reported
Your Baby and Average Baby Perception Inventories Modified	Danko, Nagy, and Holmes (1982)	10 items	Infant behavior	7-point Likert rating of bipolar behavioral characteristics Sample item: eats well/eats poorly	Not reported

Is the interest to identify a level of stress that is different from families that do not experience the stressor? Or, is there an attempt to understand how families function? Is the aim of assessment to develop and guide interventions to facilitate family adaptation? In contrast, it appears that a combination of measures could be used to examine several dimensions of family functioning: family dynamics, family stress, family resource management, developmental task achievement, parental attitudes, and individual functioning.

Another area of concern with assessment of family functioning is the common practice of obtaining only one perspective of family functioning—that of the mother. Although this is most likely due to convenience sampling, this practice does not promote a thorough understanding of a dynamic system in which the intricacies of the interdependence and interaction of all family members have been emphasized repeatedly in theory. A mother is not a family; ideally, all family members, individually and collectively, should be included in assessments of family functioning.

IMPACT OF VLBW INFANTS ON FAMILY FUNCTIONING

A summary and critique of the limited number of studies that have considered the impact of VLBW infants on family life are provided in this section. A brief description of the available studies is presented, followed by a report of the variables found to be associated with family functioning in samples of preterm infants.

Little research has addressed how families respond and adapt to the birth of a VLBW infant. Eleven studies were identified that could be considered in some sense to include a component of family functioning. These few studies examined limited component aspects of family functioning and are presented from the mother's point of view. Ten of the research teams used measures of family functioning completed by the mother that addressed the following areas: social support, attitudes toward the child (including a sense of vulnerability), and type of impact. The remaining study (Rivers, Caron, & Hack, 1987) reported that families were interviewed about "the effect the child's premature birth and neurologic outcomes has had upon the family" (p. 224). However, the interview questions were parent-focused and there was no mention in the results about sibling appraisal of the impact of the VLBW infant or any viewpoint other than that of the "parent." In addition, the infants varied in birth weight; some were <1,800 grams and/ or of <37 weeks gestational age with no birth weight reported, and the large multi-center study also included infants of birth weights <2,500 grams.

Several of the studies examined differences between groups of mothers of preterm and full term infants to assess component aspects of family functioning. These studies primarily assessed differences in social support and maternal attitudes; they will be presented first. Following this, the factors associated with maternal reports of the level of impact that a VLBW infant has upon family functioning are addressed.

Social Support

The amount and quality of social support does not appear to differ between groups of preterm and full term mothers (Crnic et al., 1983a; Zarling et al., 1988). Within groups of mothers, greater social support relates to greater maternal satisfaction with parenting and general life satisfaction. In addition, the quality of intimate (i.e., spousal) support appears more important than the mere availability of this type of support. Crnic, Greenberg, and Slough (1986)

demonstrated a relationship between preterm mother report of social support (intimate, friend, and community support) and positive mother-infant interaction. Zarling et al. (1988) examined the boundary densities in social support networks (i.e., "the extent to which ties are believed to exist between members of different segments of an individual's network" [p. 179]). As hypothesized, higher boundary density (i.e., more individuals and increased contact with those people in the social network) in the premature infant–mother group was associated with less maternal sensitivity to the infant. Zarling et al. speculate that increased attention to topics centered on the VLBW infant may lead mothers to "experience anxiety and self-doubt, which may inhibit their ability to attend fully to their infant" (p. 179).

Maternal Attitude

It has been suggested that a life-threatening illness in infancy can disrupt the parent-child relationship because parents come to view their children as "vulnerable" even beyond the resolution of the acute threat (Green & Solnit, cited in Perrin et al., 1989). Mothers of preterm infants were found to have a higher sense of vulnerability than mothers of full term infants (Perrin et al., 1989). In a large multi-center sample consisting primarily of infants with birth weights <2,500 grams (McCormick, Shapiro, & Starfield, 1982), 72% of children functioning at an appropriate developmental level were rated as "slow" or lagging in development by their mothers. Infant variables associated with inappropriately low maternal assessment of abilities were low birth weight, hospitalization, congenital anomalies, physician visits, and male gender. These findings are consistent with the "vulnerable child" approach. A sense of vulnerability may elicit a tendency for mothers to be overprotective and/or overindulgent. O'Mara and Johnston (1989) examined this hypothesis. Although they did not measure maternal sense of vulnerability, preterm infants were assumed to be more "vulnerable." In comparing mothers of preterm and full term infants, they did not find any difference in overprotectiveness. The difference found in tendency for overindulgence was accounted for by respiratory morbidity status of the infant.

As is implied from the studies above, the primary assumption in "vulnerability" is that beliefs in higher infant risk on the mother's part translate into lower (i.e., below average) expectations. Yet, contrary to many vulnerability studies, when mothers were asked to rate their infant's behavior compared to "the average infant," no differences in overall ratings were found between mothers of preterm and full term infants (Danko et al., 1982). Interestingly, all mothers rated their infants favorably and were more positive about them than the "average" infant.

Factors Associated with the Level of Impact

Contributing factors to maternal perception of the impact of a VLBW infant on the family were examined by McCormick, Stemmler, Bernbaum, and Farran (1986). Although mothers rated their infant's health as "good," high levels of impact (as measured by Stein & Riessman's Impact on Family Scale [1980]) were found to be related to the child's level of limitation in activities of daily living and the lack of resources (especially financial) to meet the increased service requirements related to the medical/developmental needs of the child. Additionally, socioeconomic factors of marital status other than married, lower educational level, and more than two children in the family contributed to higher perceived impact.

Tobey and Schraeder (1990) examined maternal stress as measured by The Daily Hassles Scale. They concluded that mothers of 5-year-old VLBW children reported a higher intensity of daily stress than a comparison standard. However, the standard was based on adult norms (which included non-parents) and a sample of mothers of 6- to 9-year-olds who had been full term at birth. Both of these comparisons are inappropriate. Mothers are likely to experience qualitatively different stressors and perhaps a different quantity of stressors than male and female non-parents. Thus, the inclusion of non-parents of both sexes and fathers as well as mothers in the comparison group may

account for the variation in stress intensity. Similarly, mothers of full term 6-year-olds have children who may have different developmental abilities than 5-year-old VLBW children. In addition, these older, full term children may be in school, whereas 5-year-old VLBW children may not yet be in school or may be first adjusting to that major change in their life. These potential differences in developmental abilities, coupled with differences in the amount of time the children may spend with their mothers, may account for the discrepancy in stress intensity.

Rivers et al. (1987) assessed the quality of life for families of surviving VLBW infants by interview when the child was a mean age of 4.3 years (range 3–7 years). Their sample was stratified by neurological status of the infant (abnormal vs. normal). The most frequent concern of parents from their recall of the neonatal period focused on interactions with health care providers. Specifically, their concerns fell into three areas: communication, attitude toward parents, and lack of knowledge about later infant development. Parents in both groups identified the following as stressful: not being informed about their infant's status, not having medical procedures explained, and having their concerns regarding later outcome dismissed. In addition, several families (especially of the abnormal neurologic group) had ongoing financial problems related to initial hospitalization and subsequent rehospitalization costs. On the positive side, many parents stressed the importance of social support and, through it all, the majority of parents felt that the experience had brought them closer together as a spousal unit and as a family.

Summary

Though limited in their scope, these research studies suggest that social support, health status or perceived health status of the infant, and interaction with the health care system (i.e., communication with medical personnel and financial burdens imposed by medical care) influence how mothers view components of the family experience of life with a VLBW infant. Three interesting findings emerge regarding social support: 1) mothers of preterm infants do not differ from mothers of full term infants; 2) in both groups of mothers, it seems that satisfaction with, or the "quality" of the social support, is more important than mere availability or "quantity" of social support; and 3) support is associated with positive mother-infant interaction in groups of preterm dyads as long as the social network is not "too dense." Concerning maternal attitude, mothers of preterms often appraise their infants as more "vulnerable" than do mothers of full term infants. Whether this difference is meaningful is unclear, since both groups rate their respective infants as "above average." Maternal reports of the level of impact that a VLBW infant has upon family functioning were associated with the child's limitation in daily activities (which may reflect increased physical, emotional, time, and/or financial demands). Lack of financial resources is repeatedly documented in maternal reports of familial stressors. Finally, even after an average of 4 years, many parents recall interactions with health care providers as a stressful part of the experience of having a VLBW infant.

DISCUSSION

The birth and early experience of a very low birth weight infant is qualitatively different from that of a full term infant. Similarly, the experience that surrounds the birth of a VLBW infant is very different for the family than what was hoped for or expected. Families may find that their "survival" through the hospitalization experience (seeing the VLBW infant dependent on highly technical medical treatment, worrying about infant survival and outcome, communicating with medical personnel, parenting in a strange environment, experiencing extended separation, and accumulating financial expenditures) is as challenging as the infant's adjustment to extrauterine life. Even when the infant is deemed likely to survive, families often face uncertainty in terms of the infant's risk for and potential development of sequelae. Surprisingly, many families function well despite these seemingly overwhelming circumstances.

Theories of family functioning provide a framework to evaluate the birth of a VLBW infant's impact upon family functioning and how families respond to this "crisis." The interaction and interdependence of family members are key concepts that are identified in models of family functioning. Although the impact of the family on the infant is not a focus of this chapter, it should be noted that "infants . . . are inextricably embedded within their families" (Krauss & Jacobs, 1990, p. 303). Recognition of this bidirectional relationship has been influential in the emergence of intervention programs and legislative mandates (e.g., PL 99-457) to require family assessments and parental involvement in the education of children with disabilities or those who are at-risk developmentally (Krauss & Jacobs, 1990; Meisels & Shonkoff, 1990).

It is not surprising that living with children who require alterations in the activities of daily living is associated with maternal reports of increased family impact. This suggests that VLBW infants who demonstrate ongoing morbidity, developmental delay, or neurologic sequelae may have a greater impact on family functioning than "healthy" VLBW infants. However, the studies reviewed did not assess or take into account social support. Does social support moderate this effect of the child's functional ability?

In addition, financial burden (which often accompanies VLBW infant birth) and non-VLBW financially-related variables (i.e., non-married, low educational level, and two or more children) are related to higher levels of impact. Since the initial, follow-up, and hidden costs (i.e., travel, meals, child care) related to VLBW are likely to increase the longer the infant is hospitalized, it is likely that the impact will be greater for families of more severely ill infants. How much do financial aspects of life contribute to mothers' overall view of impact? Will impact be reduced if financial aid meets the identified needs of the family? Are families able to recover from the potential financial avalanche that accompanies the birth of an extremely preterm infant? These questions remain unanswered.

Parents report that one of the most stressful aspects of having a VLBW infant is the contact that is required with health care providers. Parents were distressed by the lack of communication, lack of knowledge of later infant development, and dismissive attitudes they encountered from hospital staff. These findings suggest that parents who have to contend with longer hospitalizations may report higher levels of impact due to the stressful nature of ongoing interactions with medical personnel. Once again, social support was not assessed; would social support in the form of a parent support group or a patient advocate have diminished this stressor?

These findings lead to speculation that the health status of the infant affects the level of impact on family functioning. Increased cost, increased contact with caregivers, and increased risk of sequelae are all likely to be associated with extended hospital stay which is required until the VLBW infant is well enough to go home.

In essence, how families respond and change over time to the impact of the birth of a VLBW infant has not yet been assessed systematically. In addition, the influence and fluctuation of social support as it relates to impact over time has not been addressed. Longitudinal study designs are needed to address these issues. As we learn more about them, hopefully our interventions will alter so that the impact is buffered and the outcomes for children and families are improved.

REFERENCES

Abidin, R. (1983). *Parenting Stress Index: Manual.* Charlottesville, VA: Pediatric Psychology Press.

Bendell, D., Goldberg, M., Urbano, M., Urbano, R., & Bauer, C. (1987). Differential impact of parenting sick infants. *Infant Mental Health Journal, 8,* 28–37.

Bene, E., & Anthony, J. (1957). *Manual for the Family Relations Test.* London: National Foundation for Educational Research in England and Wales.

Broussard, E., & Hartner, M. (1970). Maternal perception of the neonate as related to development. *Child Psychiatry and Human Development, 1,* 16–25.

Buckley, W. (1967). *Sociology and modern systems theory.* Englewood Cliffs, NJ: Prentice-Hall.

Burr, W. (1973). *Theory construction and the sociology of the family.* New York: Wiley.

Burr, W. (1982). Families under stress. In H. McCubbin, A. Cauble, & J. Patterson (Eds.), *Family stress, coping, and social support* (pp. 5–25). Springfield, IL: Charles C Thomas.

Caldwell, B., & Bradley, R. (1984). *Manual for the Home Observation of the Environment* (HOME; rev. ed.). Little Rock: University of Arkansas.

Choi, M. (1973). A comparison of maternal psychological reactions to premature and full-size newborns. *Maternal and Child Nursing, 2,* 1–13.

Crnic, K., Greenberg, M., Ragozin, A., Robinson, N., & Basham, R. (1983a). Effects of stress and social support on mothers and premature and full-term infants. *Child Development, 54,* 209–217.

Crnic, K., Greenberg, M., Ragozin, A., Robinson, N., & Basham, R. (1983b). Social interaction and developmental competence of preterm and full-term infants during the first year of life. *Child Development, 54,* 1199–1210.

Crnic, K., Greenberg, M., & Slough, N. (1986). Early stress and social support influences on mothers' and high risk infants' functioning in late infancy. *Infant Mental Health Journal, 7,* 19–32.

Danko, M., Nagy, J., & Holmes, D. (1982, May). *The effect of prematurity and illness on parents' perceptions of their infants.* Paper presented at the 44th Annual Meeting of the Midwestern Psychological Association, Minneapolis, MN.

DiVitto, B., & Goldberg, S. (1979). The effects of newborn medical status on early parent-infant interaction. In T.M. Field, A.M. Stostek, S. Goldberg, & H.H. Shuman (Eds.), *Infants born at risk: Behavior and development* (pp. 311–323). New York: Spectrum.

Duvall, E. (1971). *Family development* (4th ed.). Philadelphia: J.B. Lippincott.

Elardo, R., Bradley, R., & Caldwell, B. (1977). A longitudinal study of the relation of infants' home environment to language development at age three. *Child Development, 48,* 595–603.

Elsas, T. (1981). Family mental health care in the neonatal intensive care unit. *Journal of Obstetric and Gynecological Nursing, 10,* 204–206.

Field, T.M. (1979). Interaction patterns of pre-term and term infants. In T.M. Field, A.M. Stostek, S. Goldberg, & H.H. Shuman (Eds.), *Infants born at risk: Behavior and development* (pp. 333–356). New York: Spectrum.

Goldberg, S. (1978). Prematurity: Effects on parent-infant interaction. *Journal of Pediatric Psychology, 3,* 137–144.

Henderson, S., Byrne, D., & Duncan-Jones, P. (1981). *Neuroses in the social environment.* New York: Academic Press.

Hereford, C. (1963). *Changing parental attitude through group discussion.* Austin: University of Texas Press.

Hill, R. (1949). *Families under stress.* New York: Harper & Row.

Hill, R. (1958). Generic features of families under stress. *Social Casework, 49,* 139–150.

Hymovich, D. (1974). A framework for measuring outcomes of intervention with the chronically ill child and his family. In G. Graves & I. Pless (Eds.), *Chronic childhood illness: Assessment of outcome* (DHEW Publication No. NIH 76-877). Bethesda, MD: National Institutes of Health.

Jackson, D. (1957). The question of family homeostasis. *Psychiatric Quarterly, 31,* 79–90.

Kanner, A., Coyne, J., Schaefer, C., & Lazarus, R. (1981). Comparison of two modes of stress measurement: Daily hassles and uplifts versus major life events. *Journal of Behaviorial Medicine, 4,* 1–39.

Klein, S. (1974). Measuring the outcome of the impact of chronic childhood illness on the family. In G. Graves & I. Pless (Eds.), *Chronic childhood illness: assessment of outcome* (DHEW Publication No. NIH 76-877). Bethesda, MD: National Institutes of Health.

Krauss, M.W., & Jacobs, F. (1990). Family Assessment: Purposes and techniques. In S.J. Meisels & J.P. Shonkoff (Eds.), *Handbook of early childhood intervention* (pp. 303–325). New York: Cambridge University Press.

McCormick, M. (1989). Long-term follow-up of infants discharged from neonatal intensive care units. *Journal of American Medical Association, 261*(12), 1767–1772.

McCormick, M., Shapiro, S., & Starfield, B. (1982). Factors associated with maternal opinion of infant development—clues of the vulnerable child? *Pediatrics, 69*(5), 537–543.

McCormick, M., Stemmler, M., Bernbaum, J., & Farran, A. (1986), The very low birth weight transport goes home: Impact on the family. *Developmental and Behavioral Pediatrics, 7*(4), 217–223.

McCubbin, H., Comeau, J., & Harkins, J. (1981). *FIRM: Family inventory of resources for management.* Madison, WI: University of Wisconsin.

McCubbin, H., Joy, C., Cauble, A., Comeau, J., Patterson, J., & Needle, R. (1980). Family stress and coping: A decade review. *Journal of Marriage and the Family, 11,* 855–871.

McCubbin, H., McCubbin, M., & Cauble, E. (1979). *CHIP: Coping health inventory for parents.* St. Paul, MN: University of Minnesota.

McCubbin, H., Nevin, R., Cauble, A., Lorsen, A., Comeau, J., & Patterson, J. (1982). Family coping with chronic illness: The case of cerebral palsy. In H. McCubbin, A. Cauble, & J. Patterson (Eds.), *Family stress, coping, and social support* (pp. 169–188). Springfield, IL: Charles C. Thomas.

McCubbin, H., & Patterson, J. (1982). Family adaptation to crisis. In H. McCubbin, A. Cauble, & J. Patterson (Eds.), *Family stress, coping, and social support* (pp. 26–47). Springfield, IL: Charles C Thomas.

McCubbin, H., Patterson, J., & Wilson, L. (1983). *FILE: Family inventory of life events and changes.* Madison: University of Wisconsin.

Meisels, S.J., & Plunkett, J.W. (1988). Developmental consequences of preterm birth: Are there long-term effects? In P.B. Baltes, D.P. Featherman, & R.L. Lerner (Eds.), *Life-span development and behavior* (Vol. 9, pp. 87–128). Hillsdale, NJ: Lawrence Erlbaum.

Meisels, S.J., & Shonkoff, J.P. (Eds.) (1990). *Handbook of early childhood.* New York: Cambridge University Press.

Miller, B., & Sollie, D. (1980). Normal stress during the transition to parenthood. *Family Relations, 29,* 459–465.

Miller, S. (1988). Parents' beliefs about their children's cognitive development. *Child Development, 59,* 239–286.

Minuchin, S. (1974). *Families and family therapy.* Cambridge: Harvard University Press.

Moos, R. (1974). *Family environment scale and preliminary manual.* Palo Alto, CA: Consulting Psychologists Press.

Novak, A., & Van der Veen, F. (1970). Family concepts and emotional disturbance in the families of disturbed adolescents with normal siblings. *Family Process, 9,* 157–171.

Office of Technology Assessment. (1987). *Neonatal intensive care for low birthweight infants: Costs and effectiveness* (Health Technology Case Study 38). Washington, DC: Congress of the United States.

Olson, D., Bell, R., & Portner, J. (1978). *FACES: Family adaptability and cohesion evaluation scales.* St. Paul, MN: Family Social Science.

Olson, D., & McCubbin, H. (1982). Circumplex model of marital and family systems V: Applications to family stress and crisis intervention. In H. McCubbin, A. Cauble, & J. Patterson (Eds.), *Family stress, coping, and social support* (pp. 48–68). Springfield, IL: Charles C Thomas.

O'Mara, L., & Johnston, C. (1989). Mothers' attitudes and their children's behaviors in 3-year-olds born prematurely and at term. *Developmental and Behavioral Pediatrics, 10,* 192–197.

Perrin, E., West, P., & Culley, B. (1989). Is my child normal yet? Correlates of vulnerability. *Pediatrics, 83*(3), 355–363.

Ragozin, A., Bashan, R., Crnic, K., Greenberg, M., & Robinson, N. (1982). Effects of maternal age on parenting role. *Developmental Psychology, 18,* 627–634.

Richards, M.P.M. (1979). Effects on development of medical interventions and the separation of newborns from their parents. In D. Shaffer & J. Dunn (Eds.), *The first year of life* (pp. 37–54). New York: Wiley.

Rivers, A., Caron, B., & Hack, M. (1987). Experience of families with very low birthweight children with neurologic sequelae. *Clinical Pediatrics, 26,* 223–230.

Rosenthal, E. (1991, 29 Sept.). As more tiny infants live, choices & burdens grow. *The New York Times,* pp. 1A, 16A.

Roth, R. (1980). *The Mother-Child Relationship Evaluation.* Los Angeles, CA: Western Psychological Services.

Sarason, I., Johnson, J., & Siegel, J. (1978). Assessing the impact of life changes: Development of the Life Experiences Survey. *Journal of Consulting and Clinical Psychology, 46,* 932–946.

Skinner, H., Steinhauer, P., & Santa-Barbara, J. (1983). The family assessment measure. *Canadian Journal of Community Mental Health, 2,* 91.

Spanier, G. (1976). Measuring dyadic adjustment: New scales for assessing the quality of marriage and similar dyads. *Journal of Marriage and the Family, 38,* 15–28.

Stein, R., & Riessman, C. (1980). The development of an impact-on-family scale: Preliminary findings. *Medical Care, 18,* 465–472.

Steinhauer, P. (1984). Clinical applications of the process model of family functioning. *Canadian Journal of Psychiatry, 29,* 98–111.

Steinhauer, P., Santa-Barbara, J., & Skinner, H. (1984). The process model of family functioning. *Canadian Journal of Psychiatry, 29,* 77–88.

Strauss, A. (1975). *Chronic illness and the quality of life.* St. Louis, MO: C.V. Mosby.

Tavormina, J., Boll, T., Dunn, N., Luscomb, R., & Taylor, J. (1981). Psychosocial effects on parents of raising a physically handicapped child. *Journal of Abnormal Child Psychology, 9,* 121–131.

Tobey, G., & Schraeder, B. (1990). Impact of caretaker stress on behavioral adjustment of very low birth weight preschool children. *Nursing Research, 39,* 84–89.

Turk, D., & Kearns, R. (1985). The family in health and illness. In D. Turk & R. Kearns (Eds.), *Health, illness and families: A life-span perspective* (pp. 1–22). New York: Wiley.

von Bertalanffy, L. (1966). General systems theory and psychiatry. In S. Arieti (Ed.), *American handbook of psychiatry* (Vol 3.) (pp. 705–721). New York: Basic Books.

Zarling, C., Hirsch, B., & Landry, S. (1988). Maternal social networks and mother-infant interactions in full-term and very low birthweight infants. *Child Development, 59,* 178–185.

Chapter 8

Enhancing Parent Sensitivity

TIFFANY FIELD, PH.D.
University of Miami, Florida

INFANCY RESEARCHERS HAVE BEEN EXPLOR-ing techniques for enhancing parent sensitivity to their infants. Some examples of these techniques are: 1) teaching infant massage, 2) demonstrating newborn assessments, and 3) interaction coaching. Some of the work in these areas will be reviewed.

INFANT MASSAGE

Until recently, massaging healthy babies was virtually unknown in western countries. In contrast, infant massage is a common childcare practice in many parts of Africa and Asia. For example, infants are massaged for the first several months of life in Nigeria, Uganda, India, Bali, Fiji, New Guinea, New Zealand (the Malori), Venezuela, and the former Soviet Union (Auckett, 1981). In most of these countries the infant is massaged with oil following the daily bath and prior to sleeping. The western world has only recently discovered this practice and begun researching its effects. In the United States, for example, infant massage schools have been established to train infant masseuses in the art of teaching infant massage to parents. Their techniques are based on the teachings of two individuals who trained in India (Auckett, 1981; McClure, 1989). Although infant massage training groups are now located in most parts of the United States, very little research has been conducted on the use of infant massage with healthy infants. Nonetheless, anec-dotal reports from the infant massage training groups suggest that massage: 1) helps the bonding process and the development of a warm, positive parent-child relationship; 2) reduces stress; 3) reduces colic; 4) reduces pain associated with teething and constipation; 5) helps induce sleep; and 6) makes the parent masseuse "feel good." They also offer several examples of different infants with special needs benefiting from infant massage, such as blind and deaf infants (becoming more aware of their bodies), quadriplegics, cerebral palsied infants, and preterm infants.

The data on the positive effects of infant massage come primarily from studies on premature infants. Since the 1970s several investigators have studied the effects of massage (tactile/kinesthetic stimulation) on the preterm newborn (Barnard & Bee, 1983; Rausch, 1981; Rice, 1977; Solkoff & Matuszak, 1975; White & LaBarba, 1976). Generally, the results reported by all of these investigators have been positive. A recent meta-analysis of 19 of these stimulation studies estimated that 72% of infants receiving some form of tactile stimulation were positively affected (Ottenbacher et al., 1987). Most of these investigators reported weight gain and better performance on developmental tests.

In 1984 a study was conducted in which 40 preterm neonates were given 45 minutes of massage per day for 10 days (Field et al., 1986). The infants averaged 31 weeks gestational age,

1280 grams birthweight, and 20 days intensive care. They entered into this study when they graduated to the "grower" nursery. The massage sessions were composed of three 5-minute phases. During the first and third phases, tactile stimulation was given. During these phases the newborn was placed in a prone position and given body stroking of the head and face region, neck and shoulders, back, legs, and arms for five 1-minute segments. This Swedish-like massage was given because the infants preferred some degree of pressure as opposed to light stroking; light stroking is too much like a tickle stimulus, which infants do not like. The middle phase (kinesthetic phase) involved general flexing of the infant's limbs while the infant was lying on its back, much like bicycling motions. The results of this study suggested that: 1) the massaged infants gained 47% more weight, even though the groups did not differ on calorie intake; 2) the massaged infants were awake and active a greater percentage of the observation time; 3) the massaged infants showed better performance on the Brazelton Scale on habituation, orientation, motor activity, and range of state behaviors; and 4) the massaged infants were hospitalized 6 days less than the control infants, yielding a hospital cost savings of approximately $3,000 per infant.

In 1987, the same study was repeated and basically replicated the data. In this sample the stimulated infants showed a 21% greater daily weight gain, were discharged 5 days earlier, showed superior performance on the Brazelton habituation items, fewer stress behaviors (mouthing, grimacing, and clenched fists), and their vagal activity and catecholamines increased (norepinephrine and epinephrine) (Scafidi et al., 1990). It is now believed that one of the reasons massage leads to weight gain is that the increase in vagal tone and catecholamine activity associated with stimulation contributes to the release of gastrointestinal food absorption hormones such as gastrin and insulin. Thus, the study is being repeated again to examine this hypothesis. Similar effects have also begun to show with cocaine addicted infants, namely, a reduction in irritability, an increase in performance on the Brazelton ha-bituation items, and increased weight gain. Finally, an assessment on the effects of parents administering this kind of massage with their infants will be examined. Thus far, preliminary data suggest that the infants whose parents are taught to massage them and who continue to massage them after they are discharged from the hospital show superior weight gain and performance on the Bayley Developmental Assessments at 8 months. It can be speculated that these long-term effects were not necessarily the direct results of massage, but are mediated by the improved relationship between the parents and infants. The infants are more like Gerber babies; for example, they weigh more and are more responsive to social stimulation items on the Brazelton. Because of this, they elicit more sensitive and contingent responses from their parents, which in turn contribute to improved development.

DEMONSTRATIONS OF THE BRAZELTON SCALE

One of the most effective ways of enhancing parental sensitivity to infant behavior is to make the parents aware of the newborn's capabilities. Since newborn assessments such as the Brazelton Neonatal Behavioral Assessment Scale are increasingly used during the neonatal period, they can just as easily be demonstrated to parents as an educational tool. Brazelton and others have argued that demonstrations of these assessments to new parents may not only improve their knowledge but also enhance mother– and father–infant interactions (Nugent & Brazelton, 1989).

In 1978, a Brazelton demonstration study was conducted with teenage mothers of preterm infants (Widmayer & Field, 1980, 1981). In this study, 30 healthy preterm infants were randomly assigned either to a control group or to one of two experimental groups. In the first experimental group the mothers were given a demonstration of the Brazelton Neonatal Behavior Assessment Scale (BNBAS) and were asked to complete the Mother's Assessment of the Behavior of Her Infant (MABI) at birth and weekly for 4 weeks after the discharge of their infants. The MABI was a scale that was adapted from the Brazelton; mainly, a simplified scale so it could be completed by mothers (Field, Hallock, Dempsey, & Shuman, 1978). It differs from the Brazelton by the exclusion of reflex items and the pinprick habituation items and features an easier-to-score 4-point scale rather than the Brazelton 9-point rating scale. The score on the MABI can then be converted to Brazelton equivalent scores so that comparisons can be made between mothers' ratings and examiners' ratings. In the second experimental group the mothers were not given a demonstration of the Brazelton but were asked to complete the MABI scale at birth and weekly for the first month after discharge. Finally, the mothers in the control group did not observe the Brazelton or complete the MABI scale but were instead asked to complete a questionnaire on the developmental milestones of their infants. The mothers and infants were then visited in their homes at 1, 4, and 12 months.

At 1 month, the experimental groups performed more optimally on the Brazelton scale interactive process items. These infants also received superior ratings on videotaped feeding and face-to-face play sequences. By 4 months the groups performed in a stepwise fashion with the Brazelton group doing better than the MABI group, in turn doing better than the control group on developmental assessments and face-to-face interactions. These advantages for the experimental groups persisted at 1 year on the Bayley Developmental Scales. Seemingly, the mother, via her observation of the Brazelton Scale or her own assessment using the MABI scale, may have become more sensitized to the unique skills of her infant, more interested in observing the infant's development, and more active in providing appropriate stimulation to facilitate development. The Brazelton demonstration mothers frequently expressed amazement that their newborns were capable of following moving faces, looking in the direction of sound, and being so aware of their environment. Having seen this demonstrated by the examiner, they reported feeling encouraged to try it themselves on the MABI scale. Presumably the mothers of the Brazelton and MABI groups continued to perceive their infants as more receptive to stimulation and continued to provide more optimal levels of stimulation. As in the transactional model suggested by Sameroff and Chandler (1975), the mothers may have discovered the amazing skills of the newborns, which in turn affected their early interaction behaviors, and these in turn affected their infants' later cognitive skills. Given that this is a routinely administered scale the demonstration for the mother is a cost-effective intervention.

Several other investigators have explored the use of Brazelton demonstrations with other populations (Anderson, 1981; Dolby, English, & Warren, 1982; Olsen, Olsen, Pernice, & Bloom, 1981; Worobey & Belsky, 1982). Worobey and Belsky (1982), for example, used a similar approach with middle class mothers of healthy term infants. One of their groups received a verbal description of their newborn's performance on the BNBAS, another group watched the examiner administer the BNBAS, and a third group was guided through an interaction with their newborns in which they administered the BNBAS items themselves. A month later each mother-infant dyad was observed for 1 hour at their home for baseline and bathing sessions. The mothers who were guided through the interactive situation of administering the items themselves were noted to engage in more contingent interactions during the bath times and more "embellished involvement" during the unstructured period prior to the bath session. While the differences between the experimental groups were not very great, the demonstration of the Brazelton, nonetheless, had positive effects on the mothers' behavior. The authors attributed these effects to the mothers' enhanced awareness of the newborns' capabilities.

In an extension of this paradigm to fathers, Dolby et al. (1982) studied Brazelton demonstrations in both preterm and full-term infants. Dolby et al.'s Australian parents were both invited to assess their infants' responses using the parent version of the Brazelton Scale, the MABI (Field et al., 1978). The examiner's assessment of the infant was videotaped. Following the assessment, the parents' observations and the videotape were discussed with each family to highlight the infant's responses to the handling. The authors particularly focused on the infant's responses to social stimulation since this appeared to be more rewarding to the parents. At 6 months the parents were visited in the home where they were given the home scale and a modified form of Field's Interaction Rating Scales (Field, 1980). The infants were also assessed on the Bayley Scales. The mothers who assessed their infants on the MABI received more optimal ratings on their play interactions, and the fathers who were part of the Brazelton assessment group received higher scores on the home scale. Specifically, they were more proud of their baby and more responsive to their infant's vocalizations. The authors suggested that these positive findings were related to the parents' gaining confidence in their parenting skills and learning how to expand on their infant's efforts to solve problems.

These are just some examples of studies that demonstrate how parents' sensitivity can be increased by simply showing them their infants' skills. Since developmental assessments such as the Brazelton Scale and the later Bayley Scales of Infant Development are frequently used in research projects, the parents participating in these assessments could be given these cost-effective demonstrations. It would seem, as Goldberg has suggested (Goldberg, 1979) that research assessments often indirectly serve as interventions.

Although some recent skepticism was raised by Belsky (1986), Worobey and Brazelton (1986) rightfully point out that there are simply too many studies that have documented positive effects to question the value of this intervention. Positive effects have been reported for mothers and fathers (e.g., Beal, 1984; Davidson, 1979), for adolescent and adult parents (e.g., Anderson & Sawin, 1983; Widmayer & Field, 1980), lower and middle class parents (e.g., Liptak, Keller, Feldman, & Chamberlain, 1983; Olsen, Olsen, Pernice, & Bloom, 1981; Worobey & Belsky, 1982) and for fullterm and preterm newborns (e.g., Clarke & Tesh, 1980; Peters-Martin, 1985). In addition,

Worobey and Brazelton (1986) cite the possibility that there may be sleeper effects. At least some investigators have already reported long-term follow-up effects, including Widmayer and Field (1981), who noted positive effects on Bayley scores at 1 year of age, and Rauh, Achenbach, Nurcombe, Howell, and Titi (1988), who noted superior performance on developmental assessments at 3 and 4 years of age for those infants whose parents received Brazelton demonstrations.

In a review of the most recent data on Brazelton demonstrations, Nugent and Brazelton (1989) suggest that the long-term effects of Brazelton demonstrations are not direct longterm effects. Rather, short-term changes in parental attitude and behavior in response to the BNBAS demonstration seem to initiate positive cycles of interactions between parents and infants that then have long-term consequences. They speculate about several possible reasons for the effectiveness of the BNBAS demonstration, including that the parents learn new information about their newborn's capabilities, which then enables them to respond more sensitively to their infant's communication signals. They also suggest a potential social learning model in which parents effectively learn handling and interaction techniques from the clinician as the Brazelton is being demonstrated. Finally, they suggest that parents may unlearn unrealistic perceptions of their infants, or negative attributions that come from conflicts about their own earlier relationships. They cite the works of Stern (1985) and Cramer (1987) on the psychoanalytic approach to misrepresentations of infants. Whatever the underlying process may be, the Brazelton demonstration appears to be a powerful intervention for enhancing parental sensitivity to infant behavior.

INTERACTION COACHING

Interaction coaching is a term coined for attempts to help improve early interactions (Field, 1978). To do this, a number of manipulations were designed that seemed to enhance behaviors often seen in more harmonious interactions. For example, face-to-face play interactions typically feature mothers or fathers taking turns, or not interrupting, respecting the infant's occasional breaks from the conversation, infantizing or slowing down their behaviors, exaggerating and repeating their behaviors, and contingently responding by imitating or highlighting the infant's behaviors. In contrast, the atypical or disturbed face-to-face interaction features an overactive, intrusive, controlling parent and a gaze averting, fussing infant. Our attempts to improve interactions have typically focused on the parent's behaviors since they are more amenable to change than are the infant's behaviors.

Manipulations of interactions vary in their effectiveness. Nonetheless, they seem to reduce distress vocalizations and squirming on the part of the infant, and the infants engage in longer periods of eye contact with their parents. Our most effective manipulations have been asking mothers to count slowly as they interact, to imitate all of their infant's behaviors, to repeat their words slowly, and to be silent during their infant's sucking or looking away periods (Field, 1977; 1983). Other forms of interaction coaching include teaching the mother age-appropriate games, coaching her through an interaction by an earpiece microphone, and replaying videotapes and viewing them either with or without the investigator's running commentary (Clark & Seifer, 1983; Field, 1978, 1983). Most parents experiencing difficult interactions are willing to try anything. Although we still know very little about harmonious interactions, and even less about disturbed interactions and intervention techniques, these interaction coaching techniques seem to help.

Another more recent technique developed in France and Switzerland (Cramer & Stern, 1988; Stern-Bruschweiler & Stern, 1989) is called representation-oriented psychotherapy. This form of intervention is directed more at the mother's representations of early interactions rather than at her behaviors. The actual intervention is based on confrontation and interpretation. The therapist does not tell the mother how to change her behavior (as in interaction coaching). According to the three psychiatrists who are studying this form of therapy (Cramer,

Stern, & Stern-Bruschweiler), the procedure is comprised of three processes: 1) the mother describes her infant's symptoms and what they mean to her, and the therapist gradually perceives a pattern of the mother's related conflicts and anxieties; 2) this pattern is then related to the mother's past and current history; and 3) when the mother is able to separate her own mental representation of her infant from the representations of her own history (that are interfering), then the mother's and infant's interaction can improve. This too is an increasingly popular method for improving parent–infant interactions.

Videotaped Feedback

Videotaped feedback is a type of interaction coaching that has been investigated by Clark and Seifer (1983, 1985). In the Clark and Seifer program (1983) videotapes are made of the mothers and infants engaging in spontaneous play. A speech pathologist then views the videotapes and determines which dyads could improve their interactions. During the feedback sessions the mother is shown the videotapes of their free play and is reinforced for those behaviors that seem to be contributing to a good interaction. The therapist then focuses on the behaviors that could be modified and asks permission of the parent to try making some changes that might improve the interaction. The therapist then makes specific suggestions about modifications that the parent can make while the interaction is actually being videotaped. After the videotaping, the tape that has been made with feedback from the therapist is reviewed and ideas on how to maintain that behavior in the natural settings are reviewed. Several viewings are usually necessary for the mother to become accustomed to seeing herself on video and to concentrate on the behaviors. Clark and Seifer (1983) have reported that both providing video feedback and coaching directly from the sidelines have been effective in modifying interaction behavior.

A similar videofeedback technique has been used to alter depressed mothers' negative attributions about their infants, themselves, and their interactions. When the tape is replayed, the mother and examiner simultaneously code the mother's behavior (e.g., negative, neutral, or positive affect) on separate lap top computers (on the second run they simultaneously code the infant's behavior). Whenever the mother codes more negatively than the examiner, a buzzer sounds to make her aware of her negative attribution.

Specific Interaction Coaching Techniques

Some of the most effective interaction coaching techniques have included asking the mother to count slowly to herself as she interacts (Tronick, Als, Adamson, Wise, & Brazelton, 1978), asking the mother to repeat her words slowly (Field, 1977; Stern, Beebe, Jaffe, & Bennett, 1977), asking her to imitate all of her behaviors (Field, 1977), or to be silent during her infant's looking away periods (Fields, 1977, 1978). All of these techniques seem to result in longer periods of eye contact, fewer distress vocalizations, and less squirming on the part of the infant (Field, 1981).

Techniques used to simplify and "slow down" the interactive behavior of mothers include silencing when infants look away, repeating the infant's verbal expressions, and imitations. All of these "slowing down" techniques were studied with mothers of preterm infants who tend to be overstimulating (Field, 1983). When mothers were asked to remain silent during their infant's pauses, they increased their silence during pauses from 65% of the infant gaze aversion time to 90% of the infant gaze aversion time. In turn, the infants reduced the amount of infant gaze aversion from approximately 60% to 30% of their interaction time (Field, 1983).

Repetition of phrases has been noted in spontaneous interactions by Fogel (1977) and Stern et al. (1977). In one study (Field, 1983), repetition of phrases accounted for approximately 64% of the mother's phrases. As expected, the amount of repetition increased when the mother was invited to repeat her phrases (from approximately 40% of her phrases to approximately 78% of her phrases). Again, this technique was shown to be effective by an increase in infant gaze from approxi-

mately 42% to approximately 58% of the interaction time. Although very little is known about the infant's information processing of interaction behaviors, the repetition of phrases would presumably make it easier for the infant to process intonation quality and emotional expressions. Infants seem to look away or gaze avert when there is excessive stimulation or the infant is unable to process the information and modulate arousal. If the task is made easier for the infant by the mother repeating phrases, it is not surprising that the infant looks for longer periods at the mother.

One of the most effective interaction coaching techniques is imitation. Mothers of young infants imitate their infants' behaviors quite frequently (Pawlby, 1977; Trevarthen, 1974). For the imitation interaction coaching, the mothers are simply asked to imitate everything the baby does. Although mothers sometimes feel a bit silly imitating behaviors such as crying and hiccuping, they usually perform this task quite effectively. Imitations in this case are taken to be behaviors that have similar form and the same modality and occur within 3 seconds of the infant's behavior. When asked to imitate their infants, mothers' imitative behavior increased from a level of about 38% during spontaneous interactions to a level of 82% during the coaching sessions. Again, the infant's gaze at the mother increased from a level of approximately 40%–62%, suggesting that this coaching technique was effective. Like the repetition of phrases, imitative behaviors are perhaps easier to process because they are similar to the infant's own behaviors. Many of the mother's imitations turned into chains of behavior, with the mother imitating the infant's behavior and the infant then imitating the mother's behavior (or repeating his own behavior), as in an infant game.

For mothers whose interaction behavior is depressed (e.g., depressed mothers), maternal activity was increased by giving them attention-getting and game-playing techniques. Usually asking mothers to keep their infant's attention results in increases in infant gaze aversion (Field, 1977). However, in the case of depressed mothers who are "understimulating," the infants' gaze aversion may be related to the aversiveness of receiving very little stimulation. When mothers are simply asked to keep their infants looking at them, most of them immediately begin talking, making funny sounds, making exaggerated facial expressions, waving their hands about, and placing their face in front of the infant's face whenever the infant gaze averts. In this case the situation is a "stimulus overload." However, in the presence of depressed mothers, infant's activity levels increased (from approximately 38% to 59%) and infant gaze increased (from 22% to 43%), as if the infant was becoming more interested in the interaction when the mother became more active.

Similarly, when this group of depressed mothers was invited to play infant games, in this case, "I'm gonna get you," the incidence of game playing increased from a low 12% to 38% of the interaction time and infant gaze in turn increased from approximately 18% of the time to 42% of the time. Other games that occur quite frequently between parents and infants include "pat-a-cake," "peek-a-boo," "walking fingers," or "creepy crawlies" (a game that is characterized by fingers crawling spider-like up the torso of the infant), and "so big" (a game in which the parent "tries to make the infant taller" by extending his or her arms upward and saying "so big"), as well as "tell me a story" (which consists of the parent asking the infant to tell a story, the infant making vocalizations, and the parent supplying the words for both the story and their reactions to the story).

Other games that are frequently played by American mothers are "itsy bitsy spider," "hickory dickory dock," "peas porridge hot," and "this little piggy went to market" (Field, 1979).

Mothers (and fathers) who are experiencing difficult interactions with their infants are typically aware of the difficulties they are having and are concerned about them. Usually, they are willing to try anything. The techniques we use in interaction coaching sessions have been extremely effective and very well received by parents. However, it is not clear whether there is any carryover between the positive effects seen in the laboratory situation and their interactions at home. Nonetheless, these interaction coaching data suggest that parents and infants can easily be taught other ways to interact.

SUMMARY

Parents can be taught a number of different techniques to enhance their sensitivity to their infants and thereby improve their relationship. Learning to massage their infants helps parents to be aware of body signals, such as muscle tension, and enhances physical intimacy. Observing developmental assessments increases awareness of infants' motor and communication skills. Interaction coaching teaches parents strategies for improving their interactions, such as contingently responding and paying attention to infants' turn-taking signals. These are some examples of ways parents can be taught to increase their sensitivity to their infants' behaviors.

REFERENCES

Anderson, C.J. (1981). Enhancing reciprocity between mother and neonate. *Nursing Research, 30,* 89–93.

Anderson, C.J., & Sawin, D.B. (1983). Enhancing responsiveness in mother–infant interaction. *Infant Behavior and Development, 6,* 361–368.

Auckett, A.D. (1981). *Baby massage.* New York: Newmarket Press.

Barnard, K.E., & Bee, H.L. (1983). The impact of temporally patterned stimulation on the development of preterm infants. *Child Development, 54,* 1156–1167.

Beal, J.A. (1984). *The effect of demonstration of the Brazelton Neonatal Assessment Scale on the father–infant relationship.* Paper presented at the Fourth Annual International Conference on Infant Studies, New York.

Belsky, J. (1986). A tale of two variances: Between and within. *Child Development, 57,* 1301–1305.

Clark, G.N., & Seifer, R. (1983). Facilitating mother-infant communication: A treatment model for high-risk and developmentally delayed infants. *Infant Mental Health Journal, 4,* 67–82.

Clark, G.N., & Seifer, R. (1985). Assessment of parents' interactions with their developmentally-delayed infants. *Infant Mental Health Journal, 6,* 214–225.

Clarke, B.A., & Tesh, E. (1980). *Promoting development in infants of teenage mothers.* Paper presented at the third annual symposium of the Robert Wood Johnson Nurse Faculty Fellow in Primary Care, Nashville.

Cramer, B. (1987). Objective and subjective aspects of

parent-infant relations. In J. Osofsky (Ed.), *The handbook of infant development* (2nd ed., pp. 1037–1059). New York: Wiley.

Cramer, B., & Stern, D.N. (1988). Evaluation of changes in mother-infant brief psychotherapy. *Infant Mental Health Journal, 9,* 20–45.

Davidson, S.M. (1979). *An experiment in teaching parenting skills.* Paper presented at the biennial meeting of the Society for Research in Child Development, San Francisco.

Dolby, R., English, B., & Warren, B. (1982). *Brazelton demonstrations for mothers and fathers: Impact on the developing parent–child relationship.* Paper presented at the International Conference on Infant Studies, Austin, TX.

Field, T. (1977). Effects of early separation, interactive deficits, and experimental manipulation on infant-mother face-to-face interaction. *Child Development, 48,* 763–771.

Field, T. (1978). The three Rs of infant-adult interactions: Rhythms, repertoires, and responsivity. *Journal of Pediatric Psychology, 3,* 131–136.

Field, T. (1979). Games parents play with normal and high-risk infants. *Child Psychiatry and Human Development, 10,* 41–48.

Field, T. (1980). Interactions of preterm and term infants with their lower- and middle-class teenage and adult mothers. In T. Field, S. Goldberg, D. Stern, & A. Sostek (Eds.), *High-risk infants and children: Adult and peer interactions.* New York: Academic Press.

Field, T. (1981). Infant gaze aversion and heart rate during face-to-face interactions. *Infant Behavior and Development, 4,* 307–316.

Field, T. (1983). Early interactions and interaction coaching of high-risk infants and parents. In M. Perlmutter (Ed.), *Minnesota symposium on child psychology.* Hillsdale, NJ: Lawrence Erlbaum Associates.

Field, T., Hallock, N., Dempsey, J., & Shuman, H.H. (1978). Mothers' assessments of term and preterm infants with Respiratory Distress Syndrome: Reliability and predictive validity. *Child Psychiatry and Human Development, 9,* 75–85.

Field, T., Schanberg, S., Scafidi, F., Bauer, C., Vega-Lahr, N., Garcia, R., Nystrom, J., & Kuhn, C.M. (1986). Tactile/kinesthetic stimulation effects on preterm neonates. *Pediatrics, 77*(5), 654–658.

Fogel, A. (1977). The role of repetition in the mother-infant face-to-face interaction. In H.R. Schaffer (Ed.), *Studies in mother–infant interaction.* London: Academic Press.

Goldberg, S. (1979). The pragmatics and problems of longitudinal research with high-risk infants. In T.M. Field, A.M. Sostek, S. Goldberg, & H.H. Shuman (Eds.), *Infants born at risk* (pp. 427–442). New York: Spectrum.

Liptak, G.S., Keller, B.B., Feldman, A.W., & Chamberlain, R.W. (1983). Enhancing infant development and parent-practitioner interaction with the Brazelton Neonatal Assessment Scale. *Pediatrics, 72,* 71–78.

McClure, V.S. (1989). *Infant massage.* New York: Bantam.

Nugent, J.K., & Brazelton, T.B. (1989). Preventive intervention with infants and families: The NBAS model. *Infant Mental Health Journal, 10,* 84–99.

Olsen, R., Olsen, F., Pernice, J., & Bloom, K. (1981). *The use of Brazelton assessment as an intervention with high risk mothers.* Paper presented at the annual meeting of the Ambulatory Pediatric Association, San Francisco.

Ottenbacher, K.J., Muller, L., Brandt, D., Heintzelman, A., Hojem, P., & Sharpe, P. (1987). The effectiveness of tactile stimulation as a form of early intervention: A quantitative evaluation. *Journal of Developmental and Behavioral Pediatrics, 8,* 68–76.

Pawlby, S. (1977). Imitative interaction. In H.R. Schaffer (Ed.) *Studies in mother-infant interaction* (pp. 203–226). London: Academic Press.

Peters-Martin, P. (1985). *Hospital-based intervention with mothers of preterms.* Paper presented at the biennial meeting of the Society for Research in Child Development, Toronto.

Rauh, V.A., Achenbach, T.M., Nurcombe, B., Howell, C.T., & Titi, D.M. (1988). Minimizing adverse effects of low birthweight: Four-year results of an early intervention program. *Child Development, 59,* 544–553.

Rausch, P.B. (1981). The effects of tactile and kinesthetic stimulation on premature infants. *Journal of Obstetric, Gynecological and Neonatal Nursing, 10,* 34–37.

Rice, R.D. (1977). Neurophysiological development in premature infants following stimulation. *Developmental Psychology, 13,* 69–76.

Sameroff, A., & Chandler, M. (1975). Reproductive risk and the continuum of caretaking casualty. In F. Horowitz (Ed.) *Review of child development research* (Vol. 4, pp. 187–249). Chicago: University of Chicago Press.

Scafidi, F., Field, T., Schanberg, S., Bauer, C., Tucci, K., Roberts, J., Morrow, C., & Kuhn, C.M. (1990). Massage stimulates growth in preterm infants: A replication. *Infant Behavior and Development, 13,* 167–188.

Solkoff, N., & Matuszak, D. (1975). Tactile stimulation and behavioral development among low-birthweight infants. *Child Psychiatry and Human Development, 6,* 33–37.

Stern, D.N. (1985). *The interpersonal world of the infant.* New York: Basic.

Stern, D., Beebe, B., Jaffe, J., & Bennett, S.L. (Eds.) (1977). The infant's stimulus world during social interaction: A study of caregiver behaviors with particular reference to repetition and timing. In H.R. Schaffer (Ed.), *Studies in mother–infant interaction* (pp. 177–202). New York: Academic Press.

Stern-Bruschweiler, N., & Stern, D.N. (1989). A model for conceptualizing the role of the mother's representational world in various mother-infant therapies. *Infant Mental Health Journal, 10,* 142–156.

Trevarthen, C. (1974). Conversations with a 2-month-old. *New Scientist, 22,* 230–235.

Tronick, E., Als, H., Adamson, L., Wise, S., & Brazelton, T.B. (1978). The infant's response to entrapment between contradictory messages in face-to-face interaction. *Journal of Child Psychiatry, 17,* 1–13.

White, J.L., & LaBarba, R.C. (1976). The effects of tactile and kinesthetic stimulation on neonatal development in the premature infant. *Developmental Psychobiology, 6,* 569–577.

Widmayer, S.M., & Field, T.M. (1980). Effects of Brazelton demonstrations on early interactions of preterm infants and their teenage mothers. *Infant Behavior and Development, 3,* 79–89.

Widmayer, S.M., & Field, T.M. (1981). Effects of Brazelton demonstrations for mothers on the development of preterm infants. *Pediatrics, 67,* 711–714.

Worobey, J., & Belsky, J. (1982). Employing the Brazelton Scale to influence mothering: An experimental comparison of three strategies. *Developmental Psychology, 18,* 736–743.

Worobey, J., & Brazelton, B. (1986). Experimenting with the family in the newborn period: A commentary. *Child Development, 57,* 1298–1300.

Chapter 9

Factors Affecting
the Efficacy of
Early Family Intervention

CHRISTOPH M. HEINICKE, PH.D.
University of California at Los Angeles

IT IS NOW WIDELY BELIEVED THAT EFFECtive early family intervention is a powerful tool in preventing later family and child pathology, and that such intervention provides an efficient setting for the study of treatment process and outcome.

In this chapter, the following questions and issues will be addressed:

1. Do families experiencing early family and child-focused intervention show more positive changes than their non-intervention controls?
2. What characteristics of the defined intervention are associated with more significant and long-lasting changes in family and child development?
3. The factors of duration-intensity, and the comprehensiveness of the intervention will be discussed, as well as the variations in the amenability to intervention of the families involved.
4. What areas of family and related child functioning (outcome) are more likely to respond significantly to a relationship intervention?
5. The family and relationship context of the development of the following components

of the self will be focused on: the competent self, the secure self, and the separate self.
6. Within a relationship intervention approach to family functioning, how do we conceptualize the process and define the various intervenor roles?
7. The profile of intervention roles that have been used as part of the UCLA Family Development Project will be discussed.

IS EARLY FAMILY
INTERVENTION EFFECTIVE?

How effective is early family intervention? Three recent reviews (Heinicke, 1991; Heinicke, Beckwith, & Thompson, 1988; Olds & Kitzman, 1990) have established that families experiencing intervention show a more positive development than their nonintervention controls on all of three outcome criteria:

1. One as opposed to no significant effects
2. Three or more significant effects
3. Three or more significant effects in different domains of family functioning

A total of 24 studies is included in two of these reviews (Heinicke, 1991; Heinicke et al.,

The author wishes to acknowledge the generous financial support of the Lawrence Welk Foundation. The research is being continued with support from the National Institute of Mental Health, Grant No. MH 45722-01A2.

1988). In each instance, intervention began in the period from pregnancy to the first 3 months and included samples of premature children; but for the purpose of these reviews, disabled children, or those who were born to seriously mentally disturbed parents, were not included. Intervention studies have been done with these populations but are best reviewed separately because of the striking differences in the defining characteristics of the sample. The application of the three different outcome criteria indicates that 19 out of 24 studies showed one significant effect, 14 out of 24 studies showed three or more significant effects, and 13 out of 24 studies showed three or more significant effects in different domains of family functioning.

FACTORS AFFECTING THE EFFICACY OF EARLY FAMILY INTERVENTION

As is the case in the history of various treatment approaches, once the answer to the question of, "Is it effective?" has been established, the next set of questions has to do with determining the factors which maximize that effectiveness. In developing a strategy of research in the early family intervention domain, experience in doing parent and child psychotherapy research with school-age children became particularly helpful. Thus, after the initial questions as to, "Does psychotherapy work?", the field turned to defining the parameters that made that particular treatment experience more effective. In fact, recent documentation supporting generic principles governing the process and outcome of parent and child psychotherapy can be generated as well from preventive early family intervention studies (Heinicke, 1990). In that article it was shown that the factors of intensity/duration, comprehensiveness, and the amenability to treatment of the family are parameters that signicantly affect the process and outcome of both parent and child psychotherapy with school-age children and early family intervention.

Turning to the factors in the early family intervention setting, the above reviews first of all demonstrated that the more pervasive outcome was a function of the duration/intensity of the interventions. A more successful outcome was associated with at least a dozen contacts in the period from birth to 3 months. This finding suggested that there is a threshold phenomenon in terms of duration-intensity, which has to be reached in order to have any significant, especially more pervasive, effect. To explore what length of intervention and/or intensity as well as comprehensiveness of service and type of family served was likely to lead to both a pervasive and sustained effect, studies were chosen from the pool of 24 that had the following characteristics: 1) there were at least 12 contacts over the first 3 months of life, 2) a pervasive effect was obtained during the intervention, and 3) these results were sustained by at least one follow-up evaluation. A total of nine studies met these requirements. The questions then became "How lengthy was the intervention in these successful interventions?", "How comprehensive was it?", and "What initial characteristics of the families made them more or less amenable to intervention?" (Cowan & Cowan, 1987; Garber & Heber, 1981; Gross 1990; Gutelius, Kirsch, MacDonald, Brooks, & McErlean, 1977; Lally, Mangione, & Honig, 1988; Minde, Shosenberg, & Thompson, 1983; Nurcombe et al., 1984; Olds, Henderson, Tatelbaum, & Chamberlin, 1986; Seitz, Rosenbaum, & Apfel, 1985). It is important to stress that examination of the characteristics of these successful studies can only lead to hypotheses which then guide future systematic study of the impact of these factors.

Duration-Intensity

The most striking feature characterizing the duration and number of contacts of these successful studies is their great variation. Thus, the months of contact range from 3 to 72; 24 months is the median value. As for the number of contacts, these range from the minimum by definition, namely, 11, to approximately 1,250. The median value for the number of contacts is approximately 50. In terms of intensity, one can divide the number of contacts by the number of months that the family was being served and get some indication of the frequency of contacts per month. This ranges from 4 to, in some cases, 20. For those characterized by the index of 20, this involved both attendance at a daycare center, home-visiting, and sometimes group participation as well. In conclusion, while no particular duration or intensity characterizes these successful studies, the evidence does suggest that a minimum of 11 contacts, starting either shortly before or after birth and extending through the first 3 months of life, as well as the characteristic of at least four contacts per month, are perhaps the minimal conditions necessary for a successful outcome as defined in this chapter. Once these minimal conditions of an early family intervention are met, then a great deal of variation can be found. It is recognized of course that these variations may be correlated with a great number of different parameters that hold for a particular study.

The Comprehensiveness of the Intervention

The comprehensiveness of a particular family intervention approach will be defined by the articulated effort to attempt to intervene in various aspects of family functioning rather than a single aspect. That is, it appears most fruitful to conceptualize the comprehensiveness in terms of the articulated efforts rather than simply counting the number of different services given to the family. A framework has previously been provided to abstract these different aspects of family functioning (Heinicke et al., 1988), but for purposes of this review, the mother's experienced support system is focused on: 1) extended family, friends, and community resources; 2) the experienced relationship to a partner; 3) the nature of her own adaptive functioning; 4) the interaction with the child; and 5) aspects of the child's functioning. The question then becomes: How many of these five aspects of family functioning are explicitly addressed in the articulation and delivery of the intervention? Given the above defined five domains, the number can range from one to five. Here, again, the range was considerable, going in fact from two to five. The median value was three. It should be stressed again that the investigators' specifically articulated goal is being used as the guide. What may have occurred in addition to what is articulated is very difficult to determine. What is notable is that in each of the nine interventions, the adaptive capacities of the mother were specifically targeted. Not surprisingly, in eight of these family oriented interventions, the parent–child interaction was also an explicit target of intervention. If then, successful early family intervention studies deal with several domains of that family functioning, but particularly the adaptive capacities of the mother and the caregiver–child interaction, it is not that surprising but nevertheless significant that the major mode of delivery in relation to these domains of family functioning is the relationship to the intervenor. In eight of the nine studies, a home visitor provided that relationship which then served as the entry point to other services. In one study, the contact consisted of a couple group which was held for a 6-month period. In conclusion, without suggesting a particular definition of comprehensiveness, it may well be that early family intervention directed to at least the adaptive functioning of the primary caregiver and his or her interaction with the child, and delivered through the primary entry point of the relationship to the intervenor, is an important minimal characteristic of successful intervention.

Amenability to Intervention

Focusing again on the nine studies that meet certain minimal criteria, it should first of all be noted that in all of these intervention projects, the families cooperated with the intervention (i.e., the intervention for a particular population was not court-ordered, but rather entered into by the family on a voluntary basis). This is of course a very important characteristic of amenability.

Another feature of eight of these nine studies should be noted, namely, that the populations either involved premature infants or poverty status, or a combination of both. Therefore, these are families who can be defined at risk in terms of certain obvious criteria, and who are likely to be experiencing some conscious need to receive help.

It is also clear that the issue of amenability to help needs to be examined in relation to whether the initial characteristics of the family permit the formation and development of a working relationship.

Analysis of the factors affecting the outcome in five current intervention studies (Barnard et al., 1988; Beckwith, 1988; Lieberman, Weston, & Pawl, 1989; Lyons-Ruth, Coll, Connell, & Odom, 1987; Osofsky, Culp, & Ware, 1988) showed that whether or not the mothers developed a working relationship with the intervenor clearly affected the outcome. Thus, the amenability to or "taking" of the treatment was a function of the differential initial characteristics of the mothers. In a study by Lieberman et al. (1989), a home visitor made herself emotionally available to mothers in order to enhance their availability to their child, and thus affect the security of their attachments. In the initial comparison of the intervention and control groups at 2 years of age, the intervention, having started at 1 year of age, showed no difference on the Waters and Deane (1986) Q-sort security measure. However, when those rated as developing a working relationship with the intervenor were compared with the control group, significant differences in the security of attachment in the children did emerge.

Lyons-Ruth et al. (1987) also found positive changes in childrens' 18-month attachment behavior as a function of an extensive relationship-focused home-intervention with high-risk families. Several comparisons of high-risk treated and untreated (control) infants are presented and show a significantly higher proportion of secure attachments in the treated group. Most relevant to the present article is the finding that a sample of mothers, all of whom reported being depressed and some of whom also had maltreated their children or had been hospitalized for psychiatric reasons, responded less to treatment than a group of mothers who reported depression but did not show evidence of the additional risk characteristics. Thus, for the first group showing the highest risk, the proportion of secure children was 61% for the treated and 35% for the untreated children, a difference of 26%. The percentages for the sample excluding the maltreating and hospitalized mothers (depressed only) were, respectively, 73% and 25%. That is, families with the greater number of maternal risk criteria responded less to treatment.

Systematic Comparison of Factors Affecting Efficacy of Early Family Intervention

In examining the factors associated with the efficacy of early intervention, characteristics of the more successful studies have been studied thus far. What evidence is there as to the efficacy of these factors as determined by systematic comparison or variation of the parameters?

In regard to duration-intensity, Powell and Grantham-McGregor (1989) compared the impact of once-a-week, bi-weekly, and once-a-month home visiting on poor urban children in Jamaica. Using the Griffith Mental Development Scales as outcome measures, these authors concluded that in the population they served, at least weekly visiting is necessary to make a substantial impact on the children's development. There are no other known studies that systematically compare intensity and/or duration as a factor affecting the outcome of home visiting. Taken together with the observations made in the above paragraphs, it would seem that the once-a-week home visiting intervention lasting at least 3 months, and going on as long as 1 or 2 years, may be necessary to make a substantial impact on family development. This type of intensity and duration is likely to be called for in dealing with families from a poverty or premature infant background.

The next consideration is one of comprehensiveness. A study by Wasik, Ramey, Bryant, and Sparling (1990) systematically compares the impact on three samples. One sample received both a family home-based education program and a center-based educational daycare program, one received only the family education program, and both of these were compared with a matched control group which received neither of these. The HOME inventory (Caldwell & Bradley, 1976), was administered when the children were 6, 12, 18, 30, 42, and 54 months old. The three samples did not differ on this outcome measure at any of the assessment points. However, using the Bayley Mental Development Index (Bayley, 1969), it was found that the children experiencing the most comprehensive program, namely, the child development center plus the family education group, differed significantly from both the family education and control groups at 12 and 18 months of age. On the Stanford Binet Intelligence Test (Terman & Merrill, 1973) at 24, 36, and 48 months, and the McCarthy Scales (McCarthy, 1972) at 30, 42, and 54 months, differences were again found between the sample experiencing both the child development center and the family education experience and those experiencing only the family education experience. A concept of greater comprehensiveness is again supported. Interestingly, there was no difference between the more comprehensive program group and the control group. This was discussed as possibly due to the fact that the control group in fact attended some form of center program in many instances.

Aside from the possible lack of difference between the program groups and the control group, because the control group was in fact getting many of the program experiences, one can also raise the question of why the family education group did not differ from the control group and was in fact much less effective in its results than either of the two groups. The authors suggest that since, in fact, the families in the family education group were visited only on a bi-weekly basis, this intensity may not be sufficient to make a significant impact. However, at least two further questions should be raised, namely: Are cognitive measures the most relevant in terms of the possible outcome of a family-based relationship invervention? and, Do we not need to examine what is meant by a family intervention and what profile of interventions is most effective with defined populations?

Now turn to the question of what aspect of family development is likely to be most responsive to an environmentally based relationship intervention.

Finally, the issue of variations in the family intervention strategy itself will be addressed by discussing the profile of intervention role used in the UCLA Family Development Project.

THE NATURE OF THE OUTCOME MEASURES

In order to assess the efficacy of early family intervention, it is important to conceptualize what types of measures might be most appropriately used for that assessment. Given a family systems relationship perspective, and given the predominance of a relationship type of intervention used in the home setting, it is important to go beyond measures of the cognitive functioning of the child and to include other areas of child and family development. Like other researchers (Stern, 1985), it has been found useful to focus conceptualization on definitions of the components of the self. These are seen as emerging from the interaction of early infant characteristics and the qualities of the caretaking relationship. The self is seen as an organization which integrates the infant adaptation and the accompanying feelings and thoughts. Development of the components of the self can then be related to the quality and goals of the relationship. These relationships in turn need to be put in the context of family system functioning, and the larger ecological setting. Justice can not be done to all these issues, but a basis should be provided for choosing among various outcome measures. First of all, the competent self which is associated with a sense of being an agent, goal orientation, sustained attention, and the capacity for self-regulation should be focused on. It emerges out of and continues in the context of the type of parental responsiveness that exposes and teaches the child new cognitive experiences. Measures of the construct of the competent self are very likely to be correlated with measures of the IQ or general mental development of the child (Heinicke & Lampl, 1988).

A second component of the self has been called "the secure self." As a construct, it is further defined by measures of the inner expectation of being cared for, the sense of self as worthy, and the ability to modulate aggression in the first 2 years of life. Most importantly, it has been extensively documented that the development of a secure self emerges out of and continues in a relationship that is characterized by the parents' or caregiver's responsiveness to the needs of the infant (Heinicke & Guthrie, 1992).

The third component of the self, called, "the separate self," includes a subjective awareness of the self and other as separate, and the child's capacity for autonomous initiative. It is seen as emerging out of and continuing in a relationship to a caregiver that prepares for and promotes autonomy, as well as providing control (i.e., limits, for that expansion) (Heinicke & Guthrie, 1992).

It must be stressed again that each of these constructs can be anchored in a variety of measures of the infant transacting with the caregiver in the first 2 years of life. Furthermore, these transactions can in turn be linked to characteristics of the personality of the parents or caregivers, and the nature of the partnership involvement of these caregivers. Using path analysis models, these links have been documented in a number of longitudinal studies (Heinicke, Diskin, Ramsey-Klee, & Oates, 1986; Heinicke & Guthrie, 1992).

What then is the relevance of these conceptualizations to the choice of outcome measures? Insofar as the variations and the development of the competent self are governed by genetic variations in IQ, outcome indices related to the developing competent self may actually be less responsive to a relationship intervention than indices related to the concepts of secure and separate self. Paradoxically, a great number of the early intervention studies have focused on changes in IQ and parental educational stimulation. The findings of these studies suggested that initial gains could be made but then tended to "wash out" in the early school years. More recent studies (Gross, 1990; Wasick et al., 1990) do indicate that family/cognitively oriented interventions produce significant gains when involving the premature or less educated child and family, who in the normal course of development, have not been exposed to certain minimal levels of cognitive stimulation.

Since, however, there is considerable evidence that measures related to the secure and separate self are less likely to be determined to a significant extent by genetic predispositions, these indices are therefore also likely to be more promising in the sense of responding to a relationship intervention that is directed at the marital partner characteristics of the family system, the personality characteristics of the caregivers, and the relationship components of these aspects of the developing self. It is a sequence of measures going from the experienced support of the caregivers, the nature of the partnership of the caregivers themselves, the personality characteristics of these caregivers, the quality of the relationship to the child, and especially their responsiveness to the needs of the infant and their encouragement of autonomy that are promising indices of outcome in the study of an early family intervention.

DEFINING THE PROFILE OF INTERVENTION ROLES

Just as it has been attempted to document that the choice of outcome measures must be conceptually framed in relation to the rationale and technique of intervention, so it follows that the definition of the home-visiting relationship intervention also needs to be conceptually articulated and related to the form and rationale of the overall family intervention. To illustrate this, the various intervention roles used in the UCLA Family Development Service need to be defined (see Heinicke, 1991 and UCLA Family Development Project, 1991, for description of sample and procedures). These roles have been organized in terms of four major domains:

1. Consolidating the helping, working relationship
2. Enhancing communication and personal adaptation
3. Enhancing alternate approaches to parent-child interaction
4. Providing direct support

To promote the working relationship, the intervenor takes steps to consolidate the real helping relationship and to understand and respond to the emerging transference, counter-transference, and counter-feeling reactions. Consolidation of the real relationship involves becoming *aware* of what aspects of a relationship are operating and *explaining* the nature of that relationship. The help offered is explained as addressing those areas of coping that are associated with becoming a first time parent: Issues of personal and partner adaptation, issues of interacting with their infant, and issues of obtaining support. The expectable conditions for delivering the help are assured through defining the length of the weekly home visit (about 1 hour), fixing a regular appointment time, and defining the duration of the intervention (usually 2 years).

In addition to awareness of and explanations relating to the real relationship, both intervenor and mother also *act* to increase their positive mutality (see Figure 1 for specific categories describing these interactions).

If the above characteristics define the real relationship, the repetition in relation to the interviewer of unresolved past relationships (transference) and the reactions to these, both conscious (counter-feeling) and unconscious (countertransference), must be understood and discussed if the parent is to trust the continuity of the help and allow the exploration of sensitive and intimate issues. The nature of the parent's relationship to the intervenor becomes a powerful tool for assessing the parent's specific expectations regarding work and relationships, and most importantly, the sense of self-efficacy (Bandura, 1986) in adapting successfully in these domains. For Gill (1982), the core of the continuing working relationship is the realistic mutuality. To maintain the helping process, one must be aware of the transference and countertransference phenomena that intrude into and impair that mutuality. Luborsky, Crits-Christoph, Mintz, and Auerbach (1988) have shown that it is the strength of the working relationship that predicts success in adult psychotherapy.

Specific intervention roles in regard to awareness, verbalization, and action in the transference have been defined and are listed in Figure 1.

The second major domain is enhancing the communication and personal adaptation of the parent. The primary task of the intervenor in this regard is to listen and to formulate the understanding of the antecedents, corollaries, and consequences of the defined difficulty. Following this initial formulation of the links to the perceived difficulties, one of two major directions should be taken. The first of these directions has been heavily influenced by cognitive behavioral and social cognitive theories (Bandura, 1986; Meichenbaum, 1979). The primary role is to articulate alternate perceptions of the difficulties, articulate various options for action in relation to these perceptions, and finally, to evaluate these actions after they have occurred. The emphasis is on enhancing the parents' ability to autonomously cope with their own issues, including of course the issue of parenting. In that sense, self-efficacy is a key goal.

The intervenor, in articulating and understanding the difficulties, may, in contrast, focus more on reflecting and clarifying thoughts and feelings, and in certain cases make psychodynamically based interpretations that relate the conflict of feelings to current as well as past situations. Experience has shown that this approach is not inconsistent with those other moments when a cognitive–behavioral approach is more appropriate for enhancing the effectiveness of the parents. (See Figure 1 for a listing of specific intervention roles.)

A theoretically similar approach, including the various steps outlined above, is used to help the parent enhance the effectiveness of their interaction with the infant. Of course, important additions arise in this situation since intervenor and parent, first of all, observe the infant, often share developmental information, and finally, whatever approaches are articulated and used can be modelled by the intervenor.

In regard to the fourth major domain, providing direct affirmation and support, following Barkley (1981), both general positive reinforcement techniques, as well as more specific types of behavior, positive reinforcement of parental behavioral have been articulated and consistently used. The activities in this domain are not, however, confined to reinforcement techniques. They include advocacy of specific instrumental steps, such as helping the parent to deal with the health system, and do include direct assistance to the parent in terms of going to an agency to help the parents buy

Date of visit: _____

Family name: _____

Intervenor: _____ Length of visit: _____ (Total mins.)

Frequency
(No, one, or two
checks)

A. **Consolidation of the helping, working relationship**

     1. Intervenor *Aware* of helping aspects of relationship   ___
         a. Aware what aspects of real relationship help   ___
         b. Aware what aspects of real relationship mother seeks   ___
     2. Intervenor *Explains* nature of helping relationship   ___
         a. What intervenor (project) offers to mother   ___
         b. What mother offers to project   ___
     3. Intervenor and mother *Act* to confirm positive mutuality   ___
         a. Intervenor and mother share enjoyment   ___
             i. Of infant   ___
             ii. Of other things (e.g., food)   ___
         b. Intervenor and mother take steps to be with each other   ___
             i. Ensure continuity of meeting; make up missed meetings   ___
             ii. Try to lengthen contact   ___
         c. Intervenor and mother express feelings about relationship   ___
             i. Direct positive or negative affect   ___
             ii. Appreciate affirmation by other; appreciate relationship   ___
     4. Intervenor *Aware* of transference/counter transference and/or
        own feeling reactions to mother   ___
         a. Resistance of mother related to above   ___
     5. Intervenor *Discusses* or *Verbalizes* aspects of transference, etc.   ___
         a. *Reflection* of feelings and thoughts   ___
         b. *Clarification* of feelings and thoughts   ___
             i. Clarify phenomena   ___
             ii. Show conflict of feelings related to transference, etc.   ___
         c. *Interpretation* of feelings and thoughts in transference, etc.   ___
             i. Linking current feelings and thoughts to transference   ___
             ii. Same as i but include reference to past   ___

B. **Enhancing communication and personal adaptation**

     1. Listening to formulate concerns   ___
     2. Clarifying the antecedents, correlaries, and consequences of
        perceived difficulties   ___
     3. Articulating alternate perceptions of the difficulties   ___
     4. Articulating alternate solutions to the difficulties   ___
     5. Evaluating the consequences of the solutions   ___
     6. Empathic reflection of feelings and thoughts   ___
     7. Clarification of feelings and thoughts   ___
         a. Clarify sets of feelings and thoughts: This like that   ___
         b. Show conflict of feelings and thoughts   ___
     8. Interpretation of causal connections   ___
         a. Linking current feelings, thoughts, and conflicts to similar ones   ___
         b. Same as above but includes past thoughts, feelings, and conflicts   ___
         c. Interpret resistance-defense of mother   ___

C. **Enhancing alternate approaches to parent–child interaction**

     1. Listening to formulate concerns   ___
     2. Clarifying the antecedents, correlaries, and consequences of the
        difficulties   ___
     3. Observing the behavioral sequence   ___
     4. Articulating alternate perceptions of the difficulties
     5. Providing development information in relation to concerns   ___
     6. Articulating alternate solutions to the difficulty   ___
     7. Modelling alternate solutions to the difficulty   ___
     8. Evaluating the consequences of the solution   ___

(continued)

Figure 1. UCLA family development project intervention roles.

		Frequency (No, one, or two checks)

9. Empathic reflection of feelings and thoughts ____
10. Clarification of feelings and thoughts ____
  a. Clarify sets of feelings and thoughts: This like that ____
  b. Show conflict of feelings and thoughts ____
11. Interpretation of causal connections ____
  a. Linking current feelings, thoughts, and conflicts to similar ones ____
  b. Same as above, but include past thoughts, feelings, and conflicts ____
  c. Interpret resistance-defense of mother ____

D. **Providing direct affirmation and support**
  1. General positive reinforcement of the parent's adaptation & parenting ____
  2. Positive reinforcement of specific responses ____
  3. Advocacy of specific instrumental steps
  4. Direct assistance in pursuing goal ____

Figure 1. (continued)

food stamps, or in certain instances, purchasing something like a car seat or toy that is seen as ultimately facilitating the efficacy and autonomy of the parent. The above techniques of advocacy and direct assistance are consistent with techniques outlined by Polansky (1981) in his book on damaged parents.

SUMMARY

Focus on nine early family intervention outcome studies, which included comparison with a control group and follow-up evaluation, revealed that this type of intervention does promote family development and that duration/intensity, comprehensiveness, and the amenability to intervention are likely to impact the extent and nature of that outcome. Given the choice of a relationship intervention, it was argued that outcome variables associated with the development of the child's secure and separate self are more likely to respond to such a home visiting intervention than such cognitive measures as IQ. It was further argued that as part of a strategy to define how process relates to outcome, the various intervention roles used must be defined both theoretically and operationally.

REFERENCES

Bandura, A. (1986). *Social foundation of thought and action: A social cognitive theory.* Englewood Cliffs. NJ: Prentice Hall.

Barkley, R.A. (1981). *Hyperactive children.* New York: Guiford Press.

Barnard, K.E., Magyary, D., Sumner, G., Booth, C.L., Mitchell, S.K., & Spieker, S. (1988). Prevention of parenting alterations for women with low social support. *Psychiatry, 51,* 248–253.

Bayley, N. (1969). *Bayley Scales of Infant Development.* New York: The Psychological Corporation.

Beckwith, L. (1988). Interrention with disadvantaged parents of sick, pre-term infants. *Psychiatry, 51,* 242–247.

Caldwell, B., & Bradley, R. (1976). *Home Observation for Measurement of the Environment.* Unpublished manuscript. University of Arkansas.

Cowan, C.P., & Cowan, P.A. (1987). A preventive intervention for couples becoming parents. In C.F.Z. Boukydis (Ed.), *Research on support for parents and infants in the post-natal period* (pp. 225–251). Norwood, NJ: Ablex.

Garber, H., & Heber, R. (1981). The efficacy of early intervention with family rehabilitation. In M.J. Regab, H.C. Haywood, & H.L. Garber (Eds.), *Psychosocial influences in retarded performance, Vol. 2. Strategies for improving competence* (pp. 71–88). Baltimore: University Park Press.

Gill, M.M. (1982) *Analysis of transference* (Vol. 1). New York: International Universities Press.

Gross, R. (1990). Enhancing the outcomes of low-birth weight, premature infants: A multisite, randomized trial. *The Journal of the American Medical Association, 263,* 3035–3042.

Gutelius, M.F., Kirsch, A.D., MacDonald, S., Brooks, M.R., & McErlean, T. (1977). Controlled study of child health supervision: Behavioral results. *Pediatrics, 60,* 294–304.

Heinicke, C.M. (1990). Toward generic principles of treating parents and children: Integrating psychotherapy with the school-aged child and early family intervention. *Journal of Consulting and Clinical Psychology, 38,* 6, 713–719.

Heinicke, C.M. (1991). Early family intervention: Focusing on the mother's adaptation-competence and quality of partnership. *Prevention in Human Services, 9*, 127–142.

Heinicke, C.M., Beckwith, L., & Thompson, A. (1988). Early intervention in the family system: A framework and review. *Infant Mental Health Journal, 9*, 111–141.

Heinicke, C.M., Diskin, S.D., Ramsey-Klee, D.M., & Oates, D.S. (1986). Pre and postbirth antecedents of 2-year-old attention, capacity for relationships, and verbal expressiveness. *Developmental Psychology, 22*, 777–787.

Heinicke, C.M., & Guthrie, D. (1992). Stability and change in husband-wife adaptation and the development of the positive parent-child relationship. *Infant Behavior and Development, 58*, 713–719.

Heinicke, C.M, & Lampl, E. (1988). Pre and post birth antecedents of three and four year old attention, IQ, verbal expressiveness, task orientation, and capacity for relationships. *Infant Behavior and Development, 11*, 381–410.

Lally, J.R., Mangione, P.L., & Honig, A.S. (1988). The Syracuse University Family Development Research Program: Long-range impact of an early intervention with low-income children and their families. In D.R. Powell (Ed.), *Parent education as early childhood intervention* (pp. 79–104). Norwood, NJ: Ablex.

Lieberman, A.F., Weston, D., & Pawl, J.H. (1989). *Preventive intervention with anxiously attached dyads* [Abstract]. Abstracts, Bi-annual Meeting, Society for Research in Child Development, 7, 175.

Luborsky, L., Crits-Christoph, P., Mintz, J., & Auerbach, A. (1988). *Who will benefit from psychotherapy?* New York: Basic Books.

Lyons-Ruth, K., Coll, D., Connell, D.B., & Odom, R. (1987). *Maternal depression as mediator of the effects of home-based intervention services* [Abstract]. Abstracts, Bi-annual meeting, Society for Reseach in Child Development, 7, 189.

McCarthy, D. (1972). *Manual for the McCarthy Scales of Children's Abilities*. New York: The Psychological Corporation.

Meichenbaum, D. (1979). *Cognitive behavior modification*. New York: Plenum Press.

Minde, K., Shosenberg, N., & Thompson, J. (1983). Self-help groups in a premature nursery, infant behavior and parental competence one year later. In E. Galenson &

J. Call (Eds.). *Frontiers of infant psychiatry* (pp. 264–271). New York: Basic Books.

Nurcombe, B., Howell, D.C., Rauh, V.A., Teti, D.M., Ruoff, P., Brennan, J., & Murphy, B. (1984). An intervention program for mothers of low birth-weight infants: Preliminary results. *Journal of the American Academy of Child Psychiatry, 23*, 319–325.

Olds, D., Henderson, C., Tatelbaum, R., & Chamberlin, R. (1986). Preventing child abuse and neglect: A randomized trial of nurse home visitation. *Pediatrics, 78*, 65–78.

Olds, D.L., & Kitzman, H. (1990). Can home visitation improve the health of women and children at environmental risk? *Pediatrics, 86*, 108–116.

Osofsky, J.D., Culp, A.M., & Ware, L.N. (1988). Intervention challenges with adolescent mothers and their infants, *Psychiatry, 51*, 236–241.

Polansky, N.A. (1981). *Damaged parents*. Chicago: University of Chicago Press.

Powell, C., & Grantham-McGregor, S. (1989). Home visiting of varying frequency and child development. *Pediatrics, 84*, 157–164.

Seitz, V., Rosenbaum, L.K., & Apfel, N.H. (1985). Effects of family support intervention: A ten-year follow-up. *Child Development, 56*, 376–391.

Terman, L.M., & Merrill, M.A. (1973). *Stanford-Binet Intelligence Scale*. Boston: Houghton Mifflin.

UCLA Family Development Project. (1991). *Operational manuals for preventive intervention plan*. Los Angeles: University of California, Department of Psychiatry and Biobehavioral Sciences (The three operation manuals are available from Christoph M. Heinicke, Department of Psychiatry and Biobehavioral Sciences, University of California, Los Angeles, 760 Westwood Plaza, Los Angeles, California 90024-1759.)

Wasik, B.H., Ramey, C.T., Bryant, D.M., & Sparling, J.J. (1990). A longitudinal study of two early intervention strategies: Project CARE, *Child Development, 61*, 1682–1696.

Waters, F., & Deane, K.F. (1986). Defining and assessing individual differences in attachment relationships: Q-methodology and the organization of behavior in infancy and early childhood. In I. Bretherton & E. Waters (Eds.), *Growing points of attachment theory and research. Monographs of the Society for Research in Child Development, 50* (Serial No. 209), 41–65.

Chapter 10

Family Issues of Children with Disabilities
How Research and Theory Have Modified Practices in Intervention

GLORIA L. HARBIN, PH.D.
The University of North Carolina at Chapel Hill

SINCE THE 1970S, EARLY INTERVENTION IN the United States "has been transformed from an emerging service with a primitive empirical base, scant funding, and virtually no public mandate to a robust area of theory, research and practice" (Meisels & Shonkoff, 1990, p. xv).

The professionals working with children with disabilities have drastically changed their view of intervention with children, as well as their families (Simeonsson & Bailey, 1990). Ideas and practices that were once regarded as "facts" are now seen as misguided and incorrect. The view that autism was the result of a "refrigerator mother" is just such an example. For many years, professionals believed that the behaviors of an autistic child were caused by an emotionally "cold" mother, who did not have enough affection to facilitate the development of a loving bond with her child (Bettelheim, 1967). Currently, however, professionals have a better understanding of the complexities of autism and no longer blame the mother (Bristol & Shopler, 1989; Gallagher and Bristol, 1987). These fundamental changes in beliefs and approaches to intervention not only with regard to autism, but also concerning children with disabilities in general, have occurred as a result of the complex interactions of four broad factors: 1) the conceptual contributions of scholars and theorists, 2) the innovative ideas and concepts

of skilled and experienced clinicians, 3) research studies from a variety of disciplines and philosophical approaches, and 4) a host of social and political factors.

The purpose of this chapter is to synthesize the information from these four broad factors and to describe how they have shaped the parents' role in intervention since 1960. It is from an understanding of this historical background that a more systematic and comprehensive set of guidelines for policy and practice can be developed with regard to the role of families in early intervention for infants with disabilities and those at risk of developing disabilities. The second section of this chapter will address the need for a more comprehensive conceptual framework for those interventionists from diverse disciplines who are currently struggling to integrate and operationalize the many theories and models into a more cohesive whole. The final section will focus on some promising approaches which have been developed to operationalize some aspects of the currently accepted assumptions regarding the parents' role in early intervention.

HISTORICAL OVERVIEW

The shifts in the attitudes and expectations of professionals regarding families of children with developmental delays and disabilities

The author wishes to thank Melva Covington and Beverly Paige for their assistance in the preparation of this chapter.

have been dramatic (Dunst & Trivette, 1990; Gallagher, 1990; Kraus & Jacobs, 1990; Simeonsson & Bailey, 1990; Winton, 1986). The role of the parents of children with disabilities has essentially evolved through five major and qualitatively different stages. Each of these stages can be characterized by distinct roles assumed by both the families of infants with disabilities as well as the professionals working with these children. The stages presented here, with the corresponding role of the families, are based upon the four forms of family involvement described by Simeonsson and Bailey (1990). Each of these historical stages will be described in terms of the primary role of the family in intervention as seen by professionals. The interaction of the primary conceptual, empirical, social, and political forces interacting to shape the interventionists' view of the family will also be addressed briefly in each stage. There is always the danger, when selecting major forces, that some important force will be omitted, or because of the brevity and limits of the presentation, reality will be distorted. It is hoped that this does not occur, or at least is minimized in this brief overview of several decades. Table 1 presents a list of the five major stages, including the general historical period in which they occurred.

Stage One: Parents Relinquish Child to Care of Institution

During the first half of this century (1900–1950s), physicians routinely recommended that developmentally delayed children be institutionalized. The prevailing view of society concerning the disabled was that not only were these individuals incapable of learning, but also that they were potentially a public menace as well (Mercer & Richardson, 1975). During this time, the energies of society seemed to be focused on the involvement in two World Wars, the armed conflict in Korea, as well as a devastating economic depression. Thus, individuals, as well as society as a whole, had limited energies and resources to invest in children, let alone children with disabilities. Parents were encouraged to *relinquish* their caregiving or

Table 1. Stages of family involvement in intervention for infants with disabilities

Stages number	Date	Stage title
I	1900–1950s	Parents relinquished care of child to institution
II	1950s and 1960s	Parents as bystanders and observers of professionals
III	Early 1970s	Parents encouraged to become involved in intervention
IV	Mid-1970s	Parents as teachers and educational decision-makers
V	1980s	Families as planners and recipients of services

parenting role for their disabled child to the institution. The predominant view of the time was that parents should allow their child to be placed in an institution immediately after birth or immediately after diagnosis, if this occurred at a later date. It was thought that this was emotionally best for the parent, since the child would be taken before the parents developed emotional ties to their child. In addition, some physicians recommended that once the child was institutionalized parents should not visit their child. In some instances, parents were also counseled that it was best if the other children in the family were spared knowing about the existence of a disabled sibling. Hence, in some families, it was not until they reached adulthood that other children in the family learned of their sibling with disabilities, whom they had never seen, since he or she had spent his or her life in an institution. Professionals felt that this was the most humane approach, since little or nothing could be done to enable the disabled infant to become a self-sufficient and contributing member of society. Thus, institutionalization would allow parents to expend their limited energy and resources in areas where change and progress could be made, such as in work and in the rearing of other children.

Stage Two: Parents as Bystanders and Observers of Professionals

During the 1960s, child development researchers became aware of evidence indicating that children with developmental delays or disabilities could learn if they were provided with a stimulating environment (Kirk, 1958; Skeels & Dye, 1939; Skinner, 1938). While the work of Skeels and Dye (1939) and Skinner (1938) were completed in the 1930s, it was not until the late 1950s and early 1960s that their work gained prominence. Other investigators discussed the importance of early development in shaping later developmental outcome (Bloom, 1964; Hunt, 1961). As a result of these conceptual contributions, professionals encouraged parents to care for their disabled child at home.

Also in full swing were a variety of rich social factors, such as the civil rights movement and the movement focusing on normalizing the life experiences of individuals with disabilities by removing them from institutions and placing them in "homelike" settings. Professionals capitalized on these movements and studies, espousing the philosophy that individuals with disabilities could learn and contribute, and hence, deserved the right to an education. Thus, many professionals and parents began to demand that children residing in the institutions be returned to the home and be cared for by their parents, as well as professionals within the community (Rhodes, 1977). The development of early intervention for the poor, created by the Head Start program, also provided further impetus to the development of early intervention programs for young children with disabilities.

The earliest form of intervention often consisted of general sensory stimulation for these young children (Stedman & Eichorn, 1964). The early intervention programs were based upon the assumption that such stimulation could improve the child's development, as well as prevent the onset of secondary disabling conditions. While parents often attended intervention or therapy sessions, which in some instances occurred in their own homes, they were most often considered to be *bystanders* or *observers* of the intervention activities conducted by professionals (Simeonsson & Bailey, 1990). Since parents were encouraged to care for their infant with disabilities at home, one of the purposes of early intervention programs was to make the tasks of caring for their child at home easier (Wiegerink & Posante, 1977). While the child was the primary focus of formal intervention, professionals also believed that parents should be helped to deal effectively with their feelings of grief that resulted from having a child with disabilities.

As a result of the prevailing attitudes among professionals and policy makers regarding the importance of early intervention, Congress, in 1968, established the Handicapped Children's Early Education Program (HCEEP). The purpose of this monumental federal program was to develop innovative models of early intervention and to increase the availability of service programs across the country. Parent involvement was a requirement for receiving one of these innovative federal grants. The assumption of this requirement was that the involvement of the parent in the child's intervention program was likely to improve the child's development. Parental involvement was seen as important because their influence would last throughout the child's life, while the influence of teachers and therapists would be transient. In this instance, federal policy preceded the widespread practice of parent involvement in intervention. The policy set forth by HCEEP established programs which laid the foundation for the emergence of the next stage.

Stage Three: Parents' Involvement in Intervention Encouraged

In this stage, the recognition of the importance of *parent involvement* in their child's intervention program became widely accepted (Winton & Turnbull, 1981). However, the type and amount of parent involvement varied from program to program (Simeonsson, Cooper, & Scheiner, 1982). Based upon meager empirical evidence, but strong theoretical assumptions, many early interventionists felt that all parents needed information about their child's handicapping or disabling condition, as well as emotional support, to better accept and cope with the demands of their child's disability. To that end, many of the early intervention programs contained a formal parent involvement component. Parents were encouraged in some programs, and required in others, to attend meetings designed to meet parental needs, as identified by professionals. Professionals determined that parents needed to be involved in group meetings in order to receive emotional support and information from the program staff, as well as from the other parents of children with disabilities.

The importance of parent involvement was given even greater prominence and acceptance as a result of Bronfenbrenner's (1974) review of the effectiveness of early intervention programs. In this review, Bronfenbrenner concluded that early intervention was effective, with parent involvement emerging as the most salient factor across studies associated with improvement in the child's development. These results provided the impetus for a new stage with regard to the interventionists' view of families.

Stage Four: Parents as Teachers and Educational Decision-Makers

Bronfenbrenner's (1974) review of program effectiveness encouraged a proliferation of *parent training* programs. As a result, parents became more formally involved in their child's intervention (Simeonsson & Bailey, 1990). Parents, and in some instances, other family members, were encouraged or required to carry out the intervention activities designed by professionals. In order to be able to perform the role of "teacher" or "therapist," parents received instruction from a variety of professionals who were involved with their child. Hence, the term *parent training* emerged.

During the early and mid 1970s, the parents of school-age children were advocating for a more official and formalized participation in the educational planning process and the right to be considered a member of their child's intervention team. This movement of parents as educational decision-makers, which built upon the Head Start program emphasizing parent empowerment and decision-making, culminated with the passage of PL 94-142 (the Education for All Handicapped Children Act of 1975). This law has recently become reauthorized as Part B of the Individuals with Disabilities Education Act (1990). This monumental federal policy (PL 94-142) created an important and fundamental shift in the interventionists' view of the family. Previously, professionals were in control of educational planning and decision-making. Now, control, or power, was to be "shared" with the parents.

Stage Five: Families as Planners and Recipients of Services

In the mid to late 1970s, two conceptual contributions emerged that have shaped the research agenda and the view of interventionists concerning the role of the families of children with disabilities for over a decade and a half. Just about the time of the passage of PL 94-142 (now referred to as Part B of IDEA), the concept of the transactional model of child development was presented by Sameroff and Chandler (1975). In this model of human development, both the child and the caregiver were seen as influencing the interactions or transactions taking place between them, and hence, influencing the behaviors or development of each. Previously, child development had been viewed as a uni-directional construct, where the child's development and behavior were influenced by the parents. Sameroff and Chandler's bi-directional model contended that each party influenced and shaped the behavior of the other.

The second conceptual contribution was presented by Bronfenbrenner (1979) in which he urged researchers to consider the ecological context in which an individual develops, and which, in turn, mediates an individual's behavior. Bronfenbrenner conceptualized the individual as residing within a nested arrangement of ecostructures, each contained within the next, and each influencing the other in an interdependent fashion. These ecostructures consisted of the family in which the child resides, the subculture and community, and the broader environment of society.

As a result of the conceptual contributions of Sameroff and Chandler (1975), Bronfenbrenner (1977, 1979) and several investigators became interested in addressing the broad complexities of working with the families of young disabled children. These individuals turned to the conceptual contributions and research of investigators from different, but relevant, professional disciplines for enlightenment (Kraus & Jacobs, 1990). These professional disciplines provided different lenses for conceptualizing and understanding family functioning. From the area of family sociology, the work of Moos and Moos (1976) identified three broad areas in which families differed: relationships, personal growth, and system maintenance. An additional sociological perspective, presented by Olson and colleagues in 1979 and updated in 1983, focused on three concepts that they viewed as central to family processes: adaptability, cohesion, and communication. From the area of family systems, early intervention researchers utilized the theoretical work of Minuchin (1974) among others and the principles delineated by Walsh (1980). A third lens from which to view family functioning was provided by the work of McCubbin and his colleagues related to family stress theory (1980, 1981, 1982, and 1983).

Several investigators utilized these theoretical frameworks, as they undertook a variety of studies addressing different areas that related to families of young children with disabilities. Among these pioneers in early intervention family research were: Dunst and his colleagues at the Western Carolina Center; Drs. Bailey, Bristol, Gallagher, and Simeonsson at the Frank Porter Graham Child Development Center at the University of North Carolina at Chapel Hill; Turnbull and her colleagues from both the University of North Carolina at Chapel Hill and the University of Kansas; Vincent and her colleagues at the University of Wisconsin; and Fewell and her colleagues at the University of Washington. As a result, there was a dramatic increase in family-focused research. Studies conducted in the 1970s and 1980s have provided us with rich information about the families of various types of disabled and at-risk children, as well as the differing characteristics of those families.

PROLIFERATION OF FAMILY-FOCUSED RESEARCH

Review of relevant research indicates that many parent variables have been correlated with both positive and negative child outcome. These include such characteristics as the socioeconomic status of the parent (Braswell, 1977; Dumas & Wahler, 1983; McMahon, Forehand, Griest, & Wells, 1981); level of education of the parents (Braswell, 1977; Sharav, Collins, & Shlomo, 1985); home environment (Best & Roberts, 1976; Piper & Ramsay, 1980); maternal locus of control (Maistro & German, 1981); and parental adjustment, marital difficulties, and dysfunctional family interactions (Griest & Forehand, 1982).

A variety of studies have examined the effects of parents as the primary teacher or therapist for their child. Some studies reported that parents were able to: be successful language teachers (Lombardino & Mangan, 1983); improve motor development through the use of physical therapy techniques (Gross, Eudy, & Drabman, 1982); and manage and modify the behaviors of their child through the use of behavior modification techniques (Bidder, Bryant, & Gray, 1975). However, other studies indicated several drawbacks of the parents playing the role of the teacher. These drawbacks include: some parents preferred not to serve as their child's teacher (Winton & Turnbull, 1981); a high attrition rate in many parent involvement programs (Stile, Cole, & Garner, 1979); many mothers generalized and used structured teaching techniques in situations (e.g., play) that did not warrant such didactic techniques (Mash, 1984).

Another group of studies has examined aspects of mother–child interaction. Various characteristics of the child, such as delayed social and communication skills, limited mobility, and temperament have been reported to affect both the quality of interaction and the development of maternal attachment (Blacher & Meyers, 1983; Kelly, 1982; Stoneman, Brody,

& Abbott, 1983). Frodi (1981) reported that child abuse was disproportionately high among developmentally delayed children. Beckman-Bell (1981) reported that the nature of the caregiving demands of the young child seemed to affect the level of stress experienced by the mother.

In their review of the literature, Dunst and Trivette (1990) contend that there is a growing body of evidence indicating that stress and social support directly and indirectly affect both child and family functioning in several important ways: they enhance parent and family well-being (Patterson & McCubbin, 1983); they decrease time demands placed on the family by the child with a disability; they promote positive caregiver interactive styles, while decreasing negative or interfering styles of interaction (Trivette & Dunst, in preparation); and they enhance the positive perceptions of the parents regarding child functioning (Colletta, 1981). Conversely, Dumas and Wahler (1983) reported that the insularity, or social isolation, of mothers is negatively related to treatment outcome. Dunst and Trivette (1990) also contend that results of their own studies indicate that the provision of social support is particularly successful when the assistance provided matches family identified needs.

NEW ASSUMPTIONS REGARDING FAMILIES IN INTERVENTION

All of these studies, in combination with numerous others related to families of young children, reveal the complex needs and characteristics of families. No longer can interventionists design a parent component where parents are seen as a homogeneous group, receiving identical training and services. The proliferation of family research in the late 1970s and early 1980s has given birth to a new set of assumptions concerning the view of the family in the process of early intervention. These assumptions include:

1. Parenting a child with disabilities is a persistent and ever-changing source of stress which affects the entire family. It is not a single occurrence of the passage through the four discrete stages of grief, as once thought.
2. Intervention efforts with families should be broader in focus, recognizing the importance of broader ecological contexts and helping families cope with the variety of associated stresses of rearing a child with disabilities.
3. Parents play a multiplicity of roles with respect to their child. Education is only one of nine functions (Turnbull, Brotherson, & Summers, 1985), thus, all parental roles should be recognized and supported.
4. Families are unique, possessing individual strengths and needs. The work of Werner (1990) and others related to "protective" factors and "resiliency," as well as "risk" factors, has been useful in recognizing that each family possesses its own combination of protective factors (strengths) and risks (needs).

The acceptance of these assumptions by both researchers and advocates helped to shape the contents of Part H of PL 99-457 (The Education of the Handicapped Act Amendments of 1986 and recently reauthorized as the Individuals with Disabilities Education Act). These federal policies required that early interventionists from all disciplines view families as *planners* and *recipients* of services (Simeonsson & Bailey, 1990). The law also required the individualization of services to infants and toddlers with developmental delays and their families. The parents' role as the decision-maker concerning various aspects of their child's intervention was even more firmly embedded in Part H of PL 99-457. Not only are families eligible to receive services such as family counseling, but they are also the ones who decide, if they wish, on the nature of and types of services their child will receive. This federal support for services to families represents a significant shift in public policy for families of young children with disabilities. In the previous stages, "parents" (usually the mother) were seen as secondary targets of intervention. Part H of IDEA (formerly PL 99-457) uses the term *family* instead of parents, which is an important distinction and shift, and certainly in keeping with a more ecological approach to intervention. Once again, however, practice is being prodded by policy. Table 2 presents a comparison of the most salient characteristics of each of the five stages previously described.

NEED FOR CONCEPTUAL FRAMEWORK

Despite the mandates of Part H of IDEA, a clear conceptual framework for integrating all of the elements of family research into a comprehensive and systematic view of family intervention is lacking (Sameroff & Friese, 1990; Simeonsson & Bailey, 1990; Winton, 1986). Currently, early interventionists are struggling

with the complexities of operationalizing a more ecologically based, individualized intervention program for families that varies by type of strategy and activity (Sameroff & Friese, 1990) and by level of involvement in intervention (Simeonsson & Bailey, 1990).

What is needed to facilitate the development of this comprehensive and cohesive conceptual framework is the development and utilization of research methodologies that can address the complex interactions of variables within individual families, as well as the broader ecological systems within which families operate (Gallagher, 1990; Sameroff & Friese, 1990; Winton, 1986). Indeed, Gallagher (1990) ques-

Table 2. Comparison of selected characteristics of stages of family involvement

Stages	Role of parent	Focus of intervention	Conceptual contributions	Research	Social and policy factors
I	Relinquished role to institutions	Institutionalization of child			World wars Armed conflict Economic depression
II	Bystanders or observers	Home care Sensory stimulation Professionals were experts Cope with grief and caregiving demands	Bloom Hunt Skinner* Skeels and Dye* Kirk		Sputnik* Civil rights movement Normalization/deinstitutionalization Head start
III	Parent involvement	Focus on child Parents encouraged to be involved, but not systematically Provide parents information and emotional support			HCEEP*
IV	Teachers and educational decision-makers	Parent Training Program		Bronfenbrenner—review of literature*	PL 94-142 Parent advocacy—civil rights for people with disabilities
V	Families as planners and recipients of services	Individualized	Sameroff and Chandler* Bronfenbrenner* Moos and Moos* Olson, Russell, and Sprenkle Minuchin* McCubbin and Patterson	• Dunst • Bailey and Simeonsson • Bristol and Gallagher • Turnbull, Brotherson, and Summers • Vincent	PL 99-457 Parent and professional advocacy

Note: Asterisks indicate contributions or research that actually occurred chronologically in an earlier stage, but its influence is experienced in this stage.

tions the limited usefulness of the standard experimental-control design when he states:

> If we have reason to believe, as we do, that there are multiple interactive factors determining outcomes for different families, then combining such data in group analyses may have the effect of obscuring such idiosyncratic interactions—the very discovery we are seeking—that explain success for a particular family. (p. 556)

PROMISING APPROACHES: DEVELOPMENT OF CONCEPTUAL FRAMEWORKS

The conceptual contributions and research of several investigators included in this edited volume, as well as many others from special education, psychology, nursing, and medicine show much promise for developing a comprehensive conceptual framework related to families of infants with disabilities. A few of these promising approaches will be described briefly. The reader is encouraged to examine the original and more extensive presentation of each of these approaches. First, Winton (1986) has developed a conceptual framework which utilizes six concepts organized in a topological arrangement similar to Bronfenbrenner's ecological model (1976, 1977). This topology contains three ecological contexts: intrafamily variables, formal and informal supports, and the socio-historical context. Figure 1 depicts Winton's conceptual framework for assessing the major variables related to families of chil-

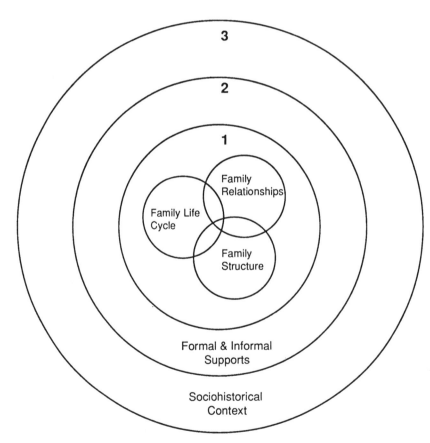

Figure 1. Model illustrating intrafamily (Circle 1) and extrafamily (Circles 2 and 3) variables important in assessing impact of developmentally delayed child on the family. (From Winton, P. [1986]. *Advances in special education* [Vol. 5, p. 226]. Greenwich, CT: JAI Press. Copyright 1986 by JAI Press, Inc. Reprinted by permission.)

dren with disabilities. In her description of the conceptual framework, Winton (1986) discusses the major factors that are contained in each of the three ecological contexts. Table 3 presents the major factors discussed by Winton.

Secondly, there are at least five innovative approaches for the individualization of intervention with families of young children with disabilities. Bailey and Simeonsson (1988) have developed a tool which is based upon a functional approach to assessing the needs of families in order to provide individualized services. The Family Needs Survey (Bailey & Simeonsson, 1988) contains 35 items designed to document the family's identification of needs for the purpose of planning family-focused early intervention. The survey consists of six scales: 1) needs for information, 2) needs for support, 3) explaining to others, 4) community services, 5) financial needs, and 6) family functioning. Simeonsson and Bailey (1990) have developed a continuum of levels of family involvement. At the lower end of this continuum, family involvement is nonexistent because families choose not to participate in early intervention. At the upper end of the continuum, families are actively involved in early intervention. For each of the six levels or dimensions of family involvement, Simeonsson and Bailey (1990) describe both the roles of the family and the interventionist. Dunst and Triv-

Table 3. Concepts included in Winton's ecological model

Intrafamily variables
  Family relationships
  Family structure/membership
  Family life cycle
  Cultural style—ideological style

Formal and informal supports
  Agencies
  Service providers
  Friends
  Relatives
  Neighbors
  Co-workers

Sociohistorical context
  Political climate
  Attitudes of the public
  Cultural expectations

ette (1990) describe a model for assessing the social supports available to families, in order to match the intervention with family identified needs. Their model contains four components: 1) identification of family concerns, issues, and priorities using needs-based assessment procedures and strategies; 2) identification of family strengths and capabilities emphasizing those areas in which the family is doing well, and to identify those intra-family resources that increase their ability to use extrafamilial resources to meet their needs; 3) "mapping" the family's personal and social network in terms of support and resources, including potential untapped sources of aid; and 4) use of different types of assistance that enable the family to mobilize and use resources in order to meet family needs and goals (Dunst & Trivette, 1990).

An additional promising approach for individualizing intervention has been developed by Sameroff and Friese (1990). They present an approach designed to target three types of intervention strategies more appropriately, based upon multiple determinants or areas of need. These strategies include: 1) remediation, focusing on changing the child with eventual changes occurring in the parent; 2) redefinition, focusing primarily upon the facilitation of more optimal parenting behaviors and interactions; and 3) reeducation, teaching the parents appropriate child rearing techniques. Three different levels of regulation (micro, mini, and macro) are included for each of the three types of strategies as well. The transactional model of development is used as a framework for determining both the areas where intervention is needed, as well as the strategies to be utilized (Sameroff, 1983, 1987; Sameroff & Chandler, 1975). The work by Heinicke and his colleagues (chap. 9, this volume) also seems to address the use of multiple areas of intervention with children and their families.

Dokecki and Heflinger (1989) developed a values-based framework for the development of policies for services to young children with disabilities and their families. This framework seeks to ensure that public policies are respectful and responsive to families. Kaiser and Hayden (1984) have applied the framework developed by Dokecki and Heflinger to intervention with families.

Finally, Dunst, Trivette, Alexander, Gatens, Parkey, and Mankinen (in preparation) have developed an innovative approach for documenting the benefits of intervention with young children with severe disabilities and their families. A social systems framework was used to demonstrate and document the various systems' influences of intervention.

SUMMARY

Since the 1950s, the interventionists' view of the family has evolved through five qualitatively different stages, each building upon the previous stage and influencing the next stage. This evolution has been influenced by the interaction of conceptual, empirical, social, and political factors. The role of the family, which was once viewed simply, is now recognized as a complex, multifaceted concept. Part H of IDEA has clearly established, as the federal policy of the United States, the right of families of infants and toddlers with disabilities to be the planners and recipients of individualized services, if they so choose. As in other areas and at other times in history, federal policy has been developed prior to the widespread establishment of the concepts and practices which have been mandated by the legislation. Hence, interventionists and state policymakers across the United States are currently struggling to operationalize and implement these important, yet challenging concepts. Early interventionists from all disciplines are much like choreographers who have been commissioned to cooperatively develop a new dance. Each has knowledge of many different steps, positions, and movements; however, they need to combine these steps in a new and innovative way, while often inventing new steps as well. The intended outcome is a dance that is beautiful, unique, and flows easily.

The threshold is exciting. As a result of the advancements beginning in the 1970s, no longer do interventionists simply ask "Is early intervention effective?" or "Which intervention is the most effective?" Instead they are interested in determining which interventions are effective, with which children, with which type of families, and under which circumstances. Intervention with children and families has come a long way in a relatively short time, but many challenges remain, as interventionists attempt to address the complexities of each family.

REFERENCES

Bailey, D., & Simeonsson, R. (1988). Home-based early intervention. In S. Odom & M. Karnes (Eds.), *Early intervention for infants and children with handicaps; An empirical base* (pp. 199–216). Baltimore: Paul H. Brookes Publishing Co.

Beckman-Bell, P. (1981). Child-related stress in families of handicapped children. *Topics in Early Childhood Special Education, 7*(2), 59–71.

Best, J., & Roberts, G. (1976). Early cognitive development in hearing impaired children. *American Annals of the Deaf, 121,* 560–564.

Bettelheim, B. (1967). *The empty fortress: Infantile autism and the birth of the self.* New York: The Free Press.

Bidder, B., Bryant, G., & Gray, O.P. (1975). Benefits to Down's Syndrome children through training their mothers. *Archives of Disease in Childhood, 50,* 383–386.

Blacher, J., & Meyers, C.T. (1983). A review of attachment formation and disorder of handicapped children. *American Journal of Mental Deficiency, 87,* 359–371.

Bloom, B. (1964). *Stability and change in human characteristics.* New York: John Wiley.

Braswell, W.R. (1977). Intervention with handicapped infants: Correlates of progress. *Mental Retardation, 15*(4), 18–22.

Bristol, M., & Shopler, E. (1989). The family in the treatment of autism. In *American Psychiatric Association, treatments of psychiatric disorders: A task force report of the American Psychiatric Association* (pp. 249–266). Washington, DC: American Psychiatric Association.

Bronfenbrenner, U. (1974). Is early intervention effective? In M. Guttenbag & E. Struening (Eds.), *Handbook of evaluation and research* (pp. 519–603). Beverly Hills: Sage Publications.

Bronfenbrenner, U. (1976). The experimental ecology of education. *Educational Researcher, 5,* 5–15.

Bronfenbrenner, U. (1977). Toward an experimental ecology of human development. *American Psychologist, 32,* 513–531.

Bronfenbrenner, U. (1979). *The ecology of human develop-*

ment: Experiments by nature and design. Cambridge: Harvard University Press.

Colletta, N. (1981). Social support and the risk of maternal rejection by adolescent. *Journal of Psychology, 109,* 191–197.

Dokecki, R.R., & Heflinger, C.A. (1989). Strengthening families of young children with handicapping conditions: Mapping backward from "street level." In J.J. Gallagher, P.L. Trohanis, & R.M. Clifford (Eds.), *Policy implementation and PL 99-457: Planning for young children with special needs* (pp 59–84). Baltimore: Paul H. Brookes Publishing Co.

Dumas, J.E., & Wahler, R.G. (1983). Predictions of treatment outcome in parent training: Mother insularity and socioeconomic disadvantage. *Behavioral Assessment, 5,* 501–513.

Dunst, C.J., & Trivette, C.M. (1990). Assessment of social support in early intervention programs. In S.J. Meisels & J. P. Shonkoff (Eds.), *Handbook of early childhood intervention* (pp. 326–349). Cambridge: Cambridge University Press.

Dunst, C.J., Trivette, C.M., Alexander, J.A., Gatens, M.C., Parkey, C., & Mankinen, M.N. (in preparation). *A social systems approach to documenting the benefits of child-centered interventions.* Morganton, NC: Center for Family Studies, Western Carolina Center.

Education for All Handicapped Children Act of 1975, PL 94-142. (August 23, 1977). Title 20, U.S.C. 1401 et seq: *U.S. Statutes at Large, 89,* 773–796.

Education of the Handicapped Act Amendments of 1986, PL 99-457. (October 8, 1986). Title 20, U.S.C. 1400 et seq: *U.S. Statutes at Large, 100,* 1145–1177.

Frodi, A. (1981). Contribution of infant characteristics to child abuse. *American Journal of Mental Deficiency, 85,* 341–349.

Gallagher, J.J. (1990). The family as a focus for intervention. In S.J. Meisels & J.P. Shonkoff (Eds.), *Handbook of early childhood intervention* (pp. 540–559). Cambridge: Cambridge University Press

Gallagher, J.J., & Bristol, M. (1987). Families of young handicapped children. In M. Wang, M. Reynolds, & H. Walberg (Eds.), *The handbook of special education research and practices* (Vol. III). Oxford, England: Pergamon Press.

Griest, D.L., & Forehand, R. (1982). How can I get any parent training done with all these other problems going on? The role of family variables in child behavior therapy. *Child and Family Behavior Therapy, 4*(1), 73–80.

Gross, A.M., Eudy, C., & Drabman, R.S. (1982). Training parents to be physical therapists with their physically handicapped child. *Journal of Behavioral Medicine, 5,* 321–327.

Hunt, J. McV. (1961). *Environment and experience.* New York: Roland Press.

Individuals with Disabilities Education Act of 1990, PL 101-476. (October 30, 1990). Title 20, U.S.C. 1400 et seq: *U.S. Statutes at Large, 104,* 1103–1151.

Kaiser, C., & Hayden, A. (1984). Clinical research and policy issues in parenting severely handicapped infants. In J. Blacher (Ed.), *Severly handicapped young children and their families: Research in review* (pp. 275–317). New York: Academic Press.

Kelly, J.F. (1982). Effects of intervention on caregiver infant interaction when the infant is handicapped. *Journal of the Division for Early Childhood, 5,* 53–63.

Kirk, S.A. (1958). *Early education of the mentally re-tarded.* Urbana: University of Illinois Press.

Kraus, M.W., & Jacobs, F. (1990). Family assessment: purposes and techniques. In S.J. Meisels & J.P. Shonkoff (Eds.), *Handbook of early childhood intervention* (pp. 303–325). Cambridge: Cambridge University Press.

Lombardino, L., & Mangan, N. (1983). Parents as language trainers: Language programming with developmentally delayed children. *Exceptional Children, 49,* 358–361.

Maistro, A.A., & German, M.L. (1981). Maternal locus of control and developmental gain demonstrated by high risk infants: A longitudinal analysis. *Journal of Psychology, 109,* 213–221.

Mash, E. (1984). Families with problem children. In A. Doyle, D. Gold, Y.D. Moskowitz (Eds.), *Children in families with stress* (pp. 65–84). San Francisco: Jossey-Bass.

McCubbin, H.I., Joy, C.B., Cauble, A.E., Comeau, J.K., Patterson, J.M., & Needle, R.H. (1980). Family stress and coping: A decade review. *Journal of Marriage and the Family, 42,* 855–871.

McCubbin, H.I., McCubbin, M.A., Patterson, J.M., Cauble, A.E., Wilson, L.R., & Warwick, W. (1983). CHIP: Coping health inventory for parents: An assessment of parental coping patterns in the care of the chronically ill child. *Journal of Marriage and the Family, 45,* 359–370.

McCubbin, H.I., & Patterson, J.M. (1981). *Systematic assessment of family stress, resources and coping: Tools for research, education and clinical intervention.* St. Paul: Family Social Science.

McCubbin, H.I., & Patterson, J.M. (1982). The Family stress process: The Double ABCX Model of adjustment and adaptation. In H.I. McCubbin, M.B. Sussman, & J.M. Patterson (Eds.), *Social stress and the family: Advances and developments in family stress theory and research* (pp. 7–38). New York: Haworth Press.

McMahon, R.J., Forehand, R., Griest, D.L., & Wells, K.C. (1981). Who drops out of treatment during parent behavior training? *Behavioral Counseling Quarterly, 1,* 79–85.

Meisels, S.J., & Shonkoff, J.P. (Eds.). (1990). *Handbook of early childhood intervention.* Cambridge: Cambridge University Press.

Mercer, J.R., & Richardson, J.G. (1975). "Mental Retardation" as a social problem. In N. Hobbs (Ed.), *Issues in the classification of children: Vol. 11, A sourcebook on categories, labels, and their consequences* (pp. 463–496). San Francisco: Jossey-Bass.

Minuchin, S. (1974). *Families and family therapy.* Cambridge: Harvard University Press.

Moos, R.H., & Moos, B.S. (1976). A typology of family social environments. *Family Process, 15,* 357–370.

Olson, D.H., Russell, C.S., & Sprenkle, D.H. (1983). Circumplex model of marital and family systems: VI. Theoretical update. *Family Process, 22,* 69–83.

Olson, D.H., Sprenkle, D.H., & Russell, C.S. (1979). Circumplex model of marital and family systems: I. Cohesion and adaptability dimensions, family types and clinical applications. *Family Process, 18,* 3–28.

Piper, M.C., & Ramsay, M.K. (1980). Effects of early home environment on the medical development of Down Syndrome infants. *American Journal of Mental Deficiency, 5,* 39–44.

Rhodes, W. (1977). The transformation of caregiving: A

proposal. In J. Paul, D. Stedman, & G. Neufield (Eds.), *Deinstitutionalization* (pp. 80–93). Syracuse, NY: Syracuse University Press.

Sameroff, A.J. (1983). Developmental systems: Contexts and evolution. In W. Kessen (Ed.), *Handbook of child psychology: Vol. I, History, theories, and methods* (pp. 238–294). New York: Wiley.

Sameroff, A.J. (1987). The social context of development. In N. Eisenberg (Ed.), *Contemporary topics in developmental psychology* (pp. 273–291). New York: Wiley.

Sameroff, A.J., & Chandler, M.J. (1975). Reproductive risk and the continuum of caretaking casualty. In F.D. Horowitz, M. Hetherington, S. Scarr-Salapatek, & G. Siegel (Eds.), *Review of child development research* (Vol. 4, pp. 187–244). Chicago: University of Chicago Press.

Sameroff, A.J., & Friese, B.H. (1990). Transactional regulation and early intervention. In S.J. Meisels & J.P. Shonkoff (Eds.), *Handbook of early childhood intervention* (pp. 119–149). Cambridge: Cambridge University Press.

Sharav, T., Collins, R., & Shlomo, L. (1985). Effects of maternal education in prognosis of development in children with Down Syndrome. *Pediatrics, 76,* 387–391.

Simeonsson, R.J., & Bailey, J.B. (1990). Family dimensions in early intervention. In S.J. Meisels & J.P. Shonkoff (Eds.), *Handbook of early childhood intervention* (pp. 428–444). Cambridge: Cambridge University Press.

Simeonsson, R.J., Cooper, D.H., & Scheiner, A.P. (1982). A review and analysis of the effectiveness of early intervention programs. *Pediatrics, 69,* 635–641.

Skeels, H.M., & Dye, H.B. (1939). A study of the effects of differential stimulation of children. *Proceedings of the American Association on Mental Deficiency, 44,* 114–136.

Skinner, B.F. (1938). *The behavior of organisms: An experimental analysis.* New York: Appleton.

Stedman, D.J., & Eichorn, D.H. (1964). A comparison of the growth and development of institutionalized and home-reared mongoloids during infancy and early childhood. *Journal of Mental Deficiency, 69,* 391–401.

Stile, S., Cole, J., & Garner, A. (1979). Maximizing parental involvement in programs for exceptional children: Strategies for education and related service personnel. *Journal of the Division for Early Childhood, I,* 68–82.

Stoneman, Z., Brody, G.H., & Abbott, D. (1983). In-home observations of young Down Syndrome children with their mothers and fathers. *American Journal of Mental Deficiency, 87,* 591–600.

Trivette, C.M., & Dunst, C.J. (in preparation). *Caregiver styles of interaction: Child, parent, family, and extra-family influences.*

Turnbull, A.P., Brotherson, M.J., & Summers, J.A. (1985). The impact of deinstitutionalization on families: A family systems approach. In R.H. Bruininks & K.C. Lakin (Eds.), *Living and learning in the least restrictive environment* (pp. 26–52). Baltimore: Paul H. Brookes Publishing Co.

Walsh, F. (Ed.). (1980). *Normal family processes.* New York: Guildford Press.

Werner, E.E. (1990). Protective factors and individual resilience. In S.J. Meisels & J.P. Shonkoff (Eds.), *Handbook of early childhood intervention* (pp. 97–116). Cambridge: Cambridge University Press.

Wiegerink, R., & Posante, R. (1977). Consumerism. In J. Paul, D. Stedman, & G. Neufield (Eds.), *Deinstitutionalization* (pp. 63–79). Syracuse, NY: Syracuse University Press.

Winton, P. (1986). The developmentally delayed child within the family context. In B. Keogh (Ed.), *Advances in special education* (Vol. 5, pp. 219–255). Greenwich, CT: JAI Press.

Winton, P., & Turnbull, A.P. (1981). Parent involvement as viewed by parents of preschool handicapped children. *Topics in Early Childhood Special Education, I,* 11–19.

Section III

RESEARCH

Chapter 11

Knowns and Unknowns
in the Outcomes of Drug-Dependent Women

Robin L. Hansen, M.D.
Gordon L. Ulrey, Ph.D.
University of California, Davis

RECOGNITION OF PERINATAL DRUG USE IN-creased significantly during the 1980s and 1990s. With this recognition has come concern about the effects of passive exposure to the developing fetus. Multiple complications have been described and related to drug use, including: low birth weight, prematurity, placental abruption, cerebral infarctions, congenital malformations, stillbirth, neonatal withdrawal syndromes, sudden infant death syndrome, and neurobehavioral abnormalities. However, the existing literature on the effects of perinatal drug exposure in humans has been based on very selective screening criteria, relatively small sample sizes, and inadequate controls (Gomby & Shiono, 1991; Neuspiel & Hamel, 1991; Strauss & Allred, 1986). Therefore, our current understanding of the risk profile for increased morbidity and mortality related to drug use, as well as the contribution of other confounding factors known to affect fetal development, must be viewed with caution.

There are many forms of perinatal drug use, some of which are legally tolerated, such as cigarette and alcohol use. Although there is clear evidence that both of these drugs have adverse effects on fetal development and are the most commonly used drugs during pregnancy (Gomby & Shiono, 1991; Zuckerman 1991), it is the use of illegal drugs such as crack co-caine, crystal amphetamine, PCP, and LSD during pregnancy that has been the focus for most of the reported scientific literature and media concern during the 1980s and 1990s.

Recognition of the strengths and weaknesses in the studies currently available is critical since research outcome significantly influences public policy. Despite the many unanswered questions about the impact of prenatal substance exposure, the press has provided substantial "media hype" in portraying drug-exposed infants as brain-damaged, unlovable, and unteachable addicts—"neurochemical time-bombs" waiting to explode (Greer, 1990). Labels such as "crack babies" and "addicted infants" have become commonplace. This chapter will review the literature on the perinatal impact of drug use and discuss the implications for future research needs and public policy issues.

PREVALENCE

Estimates of the actual prevalence rates of prenatal substance abuse are central to the concerns raised about the impact of prenatal drug use on infant outcome. These estimates are also critical for determining public policy guidelines and adequate planning for allocation and development of needed resources. Gomby and Shiono (1991) reviewed 27 recent studies of exposure rates from across the United States. They assessed that as many as 73% of pregnant 12- to 34-year-olds have used alcohol sometime during their pregnancies, and 37.6% have smoked cigarettes. Estimates of the number of cocaine-exposed infants from the 1990 NIDA Survey are approximately 4.5%, with different studies ranging from 1% to 58%. Reviewing the available studies, it is ascertained that across the country, the closest estimates of prenatal cocaine exposure are between 2% and 3% and for marijuana between 3% and 12%; approximately 739,200 women each year use one or more illegal substances during their pregnancies.

It is clear that estimates vary widely due to regional differences in drug use and in the sensitivity of methods used to identify drug use or exposure. In addition, estimates of exposure rates do not inform us as to the number of infants harmfully affected by their exposure.

Many of the methodologic problems in determining prevalence rates, as well as actual risks from exposure, relate directly to issues of identification of drug use, which are enmeshed in ethical and legal dilemmas. Social stigmatization, the threat of criminal prosecution, and issues of personal freedom and privacy significantly influence identification of substance-using women. Complications related to illegal drug use are neither specific for or limited to those drugs. There are numerous confounding factors which are known to impact on developmental outcomes such as smoking, alcohol use, poor prenatal care, low socioeconomic status, or poor reproductive history, present in many of the pregnancies identified with illicit drug use. The prevalent use of inconsistent or biased screening methods to identify women or infants exposed to drugs has limited the ability to evaluate the contribution of these confounding factors to adverse perinatal and developmental outcome. Existing studies have employed a variety of different techniques which create significant concern about variances in the samples studied.

The use of maternal admission of drug use to identify exposed infants has the advantages of being inexpensive, less fraught with controversy, and able to identify previous drug use. However, maternal admission of drug use has repeatedly been shown to be inaccurate in identifying exposed infants (Frank et al., 1988; Gillogley, Evans, Hansen, Samuels, & Batra, 1990; Hansen, Evans, Gillogley, Hughes, & Krener, in press). Urine toxicology screening has been used in many situations to identify illicit drug use in pregnant women and exposed infants, despite the major limitations of representing only a brief time in perinatal history and not reflecting frequency or amount of use. The sensitivity of screening methods and individual rates of drug metabolism vary, but detection of cocaine and amphetamine metabolites in the urine is generally possible up to 3 days after use, while marijuana use may be detected up to 10 days after ingestion (Zuckerman, Frank, Hingson, et al., 1989). Additionally, the use of selective criteria to determine who is screened, further limits the accuracy of urine toxicology testing by missing significant numbers of women and infants who are not tested (Hansen et al., in press).

Zuckerman et al. (1989) compared the results of history taking for perinatal drug use with urine toxicology testing in a group of women who knew they were being screened for marijuana and cocaine. Twenty-four percent of the women who used cocaine during pregnancy denied illicit drug use. Significant differences in fetal growth of toxicology-positive women disappeared when self-reported drug use alone was used to define exposure. In a 1-year study of universal toxicology screening at the time of delivery in a single hospital-based obstetrical service, approximately one-third of the women testing positive for cocaine denied any history of drug use, and just over one-half of the women testing positive for amphetamines denied use (Gillogley et al., 1990). In a countywide study that included all obstetrical services in Sacramento County, California, for a 1-month period, 9.2% of the urine screens were positive. Urines were screened for amphetamines, cocaine, opiates, marijuana, alcohol, benzodiazepines, and PCP. Of those women with positive screens, only 33%

would have been screened by existing hospital protocols. In addition, only 18% of those testing positive reported any drug use during pregnancy.

It is evident from these results that the limitations inherent in identifying exposed women and infants have significant implications for the interpretation of existing data on the effects of illicit drug use. In particular, the use of selective screening criteria has the inherent risk of underdetection, and therefore misrepresentation, of the complications of perinatal drug use. Population-based data are required for accurate determination of actual risk for perinatal and long-term complications related to drug use.

Several population-based studies have been done that help examine some of the confounds of different identification procedures. For example, Chasnoff, Landress, and Barrett (1990) investigated the prevalence of drug use during pregnancy by screening all women presenting for prenatal care in Pinellas County, Florida, for a 1-month period. Urine toxicological screening for alcohol, opiates, cocaine, and cannabinoids was done blindly. No significant differences were found in the prevalence of positive toxicology screens between private and public clinics (13.1% vs. 16.3%), nor between white and black women (15.4% vs. 14.1%). Despite similar rates of substance abuse, black women were reported to health authorities at approximately 10 times the rate for white women ($p < .0001$). Such biases in reporting will clearly influence perceived outcomes.

Universal urine toxicology testing over a 1-year period was done for cocaine, amphetamines, and opiates at the University of California, Davis Medical Center (UCDMC) Obstetrical Service (Gillogley et al., 1990). The obstetrical population at UCDMC is primarily urban and insured by Medi-Cal (Medicaid) or not at all. Ethnicity is diverse: 46% caucasian, 21.8% Hispanic, 21.7% black, 5% Asian, and 5.5% various other groups. Of the 1643 women admitted, 20.5% had positive results. Cocaine alone was detected in 139 screens (46%) and amphetamine/methamphetamine in 106 (35%). More than one of these chemicals were detected in 35 screens (12%), while only 19 screens were positive for opiates alone. Two hundred ninety-nine patients with positive toxicology results were matched for race and discharge date with patients having negative toxicology and drug history.

Various screening criteria were examined in the group of universally screened women to determine if accurate selective screening criteria could be documented (Hansen et al., in press). Using the criteria of known history of drug use or no prenatal care, 74.6% (223) of the universally screened positive women would have been identified, while 33% of the negative women would have been screened as well. The 223 positive women who would have been screened using these criteria represent 13.6% of the total group screened (223/1643).

In this universal screening sample, the two criteria of known history of drug use or no prenatal care had a sensitivity of 74.6% and specificity of 67%. The positive predictive value was 63.4%, with a negative predictive value of 77.5%. Adding smoking to these two criteria improves the sensitivity to 93.6% and the negative predictive value to 90.7%, although it decreases the specificity to 47.3% and the positive predictive value to 57.6%. The addition of current preterm labor or prior preterm birth to the criteria does not significantly change any of these values. Smoking proved to be the single finding most strongly correlated with a positive urine toxicology result.

Toxicology positive women in the Davis study were significantly older, of higher gravidity, and had much less prenatal care than control patients ($p < .001$). They were also significantly more likely to report smoking and alcohol use ($p < .001$). In addition, the positive mothers were less likely to be married ($p < .02$). All of these factors represent significant confounds that must be considered in determining the contribution of illicit drug exposure to outcome.

In summary, from this study, as well as a review of others, it can be concluded that the method of identification is a critical variable. The use of universal screening appears to have the important advantage of higher reliability in detecting which children have been exposed.

However, resistance to universal screening remains because of concerns about privacy, the potential for prosecution and/or removal of the infant, cost, and issues about appropriate follow-up procedures and guidelines. New methods for identification of illicit drug use, such as hair analysis and meconium testing, can detect use for longer periods during gestation; yet investigators and practitioners must continue to struggle with decisions about who to screen and the bias introduced by those decisions.

PERINATAL AND NEONATAL OUTCOME

Perinatal complications that have been associated with substance use during pregnancy include prematurity, stillbirth, abruptio placentae, fetal distress, and intrauterine growth retardation (Burkett, Yasin, & Palow, 1990; Chasnoff, Burns, Schnoll, & Burns, 1985; Chasnoff, Hunt, Kletter, & Kaplan, 1989; Dombrowski, Wolfe, Welch, & Evans, 1991; Neerhof, MacGregor, Retzky, & Sullivan, 1989; Oro & Dixon, 1987; Zuckerman et al., 1989). However, the methods used to identify substance use in women were quite variable, with inadequate controls and sample sizes in most studies to control for other biological and environmental confounding variables. Additionally, because it is unusual for women to use only one drug during pregnancy, isolating the effects of a single drug is extremely difficult. There are conflicting or ambiguous findings reported in existing outcome studies.

Gillogley et al. (1990) found significant differences in the incidence of premature labor between ($p < 0.006$) users and nonusers. No significant differences were found between the two groups in the incidence of premature rupture of membranes, abruptio placentae, intrauterine fetal death, and fetal distress. Neerhof et al. (1989) also failed to detect an increase in abruptio placentae in their prevalence study on cocaine abuse during pregnancy, while Dombrowski et al. (1991) found that the incidence was nearly doubled.

Conflicting results exist similarly in the literature regarding the effects of prenatal substance exposure on infant outcome. Studies are confounded by the same methodologic shortcomings and variables discussed in the prevalence and obstetrical outcome studies. Small sample sizes, differing identification procedures, and inadequate control for possible confounds are common.

Zuckerman (1991) emphasizes the contribution of biologic variables that further confound our understanding of the effects of prenatal substance exposure. Genetic or other biologic factors in either the mother or the fetus may render some fetuses more susceptible or vulnerable to any given insult, including prenatal substance exposure. The frequency, amount, and gestational timing of exposure are other important variables in determining the potential effects on the fetus, although accurately quantifying them is extremely difficult.

Cocaine has consistently been found across studies to be associated with impaired fetal growth— most commonly in birth weight and head circumference. The presumed mechanism for this impairment is the physiological effect of cocaine in restricting placental blood flow. Zuckerman et al. (1989) used multivariate analysis to investigate the contribution of other variables associated with cocaine use in their population to low birth weight, such as cigarette or marijuana use and poor nutrition. They concluded that it is the cumulative effect of multiple substances and other risk factors that has the most significant adverse effect on the newborn.

Gillogley et al. (1990) found that birthweight, length, head circumference, Apgars, and gestational age were significantly lower in the infants born to toxicology positive mothers screened for cocaine, amphetamines, and opiates. These differences persisted in all but Apgar scores when differences in prenatal care, smoking, and prior preterm births were controlled. In controlling for gestational age, significant differences remained between groups for birthweight and head circumference. This is consistent with previous reports (Chasnoff, Lewis, Griffith, & Willey, 1989; Cherukuri, Minkoff, Feldman, Parekh, & Glass, 1988;

Fulroth, Phillips, & Durand, 1989; Hadeed & Siegel, 1989; Neerhof et al., 1989; Petitti & Coleman, 1990; Ryan, Ehrlich, & Finnegan, 1987).

The incidence of congenital anomalies in substance exposed infants has varied across studies. While Zuckerman et al. (1989) and Bingol, Fuchs, Diaz, Stone, & Gromisch (1987) found an increase in major or multiple anomalies in cocaine users, Neerhof et al. (1989) found an increase in anomalies only in infants with exposure to multiple substances. Anomalies reported in cocaine–exposed infants have been postulated to be related to vascular constriction and disruption of previously normal development (Hoyme et al., 1990). Limb reduction anomalies, hypospadias, and other genitourinary anomalies have been ascribed to cocaine use in the first trimester (Chasnoff, Chisum, & Kaplan, 1988; Hoyme et al., 1990). No differences were found by Gillogley et al. (1990) in the incidence of congenital anomalies between exposed infants or controls.

Neuspiel and Hamel (1991) recently reviewed the literature on the effects of cocaine on infant behavior. Most of the behavioral studies were found to be flawed by inadequate comparison groups, insufficient measurement of exposure, lack of consideration of confounding effects, nonblind examinations, and/or behavioral outcome measures without clinical relevance. Koren, Graham, Shear, and Einarson (1989) also found a bias in the reporting of results. A review of 58 abstracts related to the gestational effects of cocaine submitted to the Society for Pediatric Research from 1980 to 1989 revealed that only one of nine studies (11%) showing no effect was accepted for presentation, compared to 28 of 49 (57%) showing positive effects ($p = 0.013$). Because authors may be less likely to submit negative results for review, this study may actually underestimate the degree of bias against reporting negative results.

The existence of a true abstinence or withdrawal syndrome from cocaine or amphetamines has been questioned. Most studies are limited by the lack of drug-free controls and nonblinded examiners. Hadeed and Siegel (1989) found no differences in withdrawal symptoms in cocaine-exposed infants compared to nonexposed, using blinded examiners. Jitteriness was found to be significantly associated with marijuana, but not cocaine exposure, in infants evaluated by examiners unaware of exposure status (Parker et al., 1990). Chasnoff and his colleagues (Chasnoff, 1989; Chasnoff et al., 1985; Chasnoff, Griffith, MacGregor, Dirkes, & Burns, 1989) reported differences in performance on the Neonatal Behavioral Assessment Scale (Brazelton, 1984), comparing cocaine-exposed infants to infants exposed to opiates or nonexposed controls. Cocaine-exposed infants showed increased irritability, tremulousness, state lability, and poor state organization. However, these studies are limited by selection problems and inadequate consideration of confounding variables. Eisen et al. (1991) found that cocaine-exposed infants had impaired performance on the habituation cluster of the NBAS and higher scores on their Neonatal Stress Scale. Multivariate analysis revealed that maternal alcohol use and obstetric complications were the only significant variables that contributed to stress behaviors. Cocaine exposure continued to be the significant variable accounting for differences in habituation.

The majority of infants exposed to opiates prenatally do exhibit a characteristic withdrawal syndrome at birth (Finnegan, 1985). Withdrawal symptoms usually manifest within 72 hours after birth, although they may begin as long as 10 days after birth. Most commonly, these infants show hyperirritability, jitteriness, increased muscle tone, gastrointestinal dysfunction, tachypnea, increased temperature, poor feeding, and seizures. Acute symptoms generally last 2–8 weeks. Subacute symptoms may last as long as 6 months, with persistent irritability, altered sleep patterns, and feeding difficulties. Low birth weights and small head circumferences have also been associated with opiate exposure. No increase in the incidence of congenital anomalies has been reported (Zuckerman, 1991).

Few studies are available on the effects of

prenatal marijuana exposure, despite its common use in pregnancy. The few studies done have failed to identify major birth defects or consistent effects on fetal growth or behavior (Zuckerman, 1991). Zuckerman et al. (1989) have shown a lowering of birth weight due to marijuana use during pregnancy, consistent with the indirect effect of decreasing placental oxygen delivery through marijuana's direct effects on increasing maternal carbon monoxide levels and reducing oxygen exchange in the lungs. As previously noted, this association would have been missed if it relied solely on self-reported use rather than combining reported use with urine toxicology.

Dixon and Bejar (1989) found abnormalities on cranial sonography in 35% of infants exposed prenatally to cocaine and/or amphetamines, compared to 28% of an ill comparison group and 5% of normal infants. Brain lesions found in the exposed infants included white matter cavities and densities, acute infarcts, intraventricular, subarachnoid and subependymal hemorrhages, and enlargement of the ventricles. No clinical neurological abnormalities were associated with these findings and the long term significance of these lesions is unknown. Single cases of intracranial hemorrhage associated with cocaine exposure have been reported (Chasnoff, Bussey, Savich, & Stack, 1986; Spires, Gordon, Chondhuri, Maldonado, & Chan, 1989; Tenorio, Nazvi, Bickers, & Hubbird, 1988).

Transient changes in electroencephalograms (EEGs) were reported by Doberczak, Shanzer, Senie, and Kandall (1988) in cocaine-exposed infants, with bursts of sharp waves and spikes found at 1 week of age that resolved by 3–12 months. There were no seizures or other clinical symptoms associated with the EEG abnormalities. Prolonged interpeak and absolute latencies in auditory brainstem responses were found in 18 cocaine-exposed infants compared to 18 nonexposed infants in the first week of life by Shih, Core-Wesson, and Reddix (1988). However, the studies were not blinded for review, other confounding variables were not controlled, and follow-up studies were not done, so the significance of these differences remains

unknown. Salamy, Eldredge, Anderson, and Bull (1990) found similar increases in ABR transmission times which had reverted to normal by 3–6 months.

Earlier concerns that cocaine exposure significantly increased the risk of sudden infant death syndrome (SIDS) in exposed infants (Chasnoff, Burns, & Burns, 1987; Durand, Espinoza, & Nickerson, 1990) have not been substantiated in other studies (Bauchner & Zuckerman, 1990). Chasnoff, Hunt, Kletter, and Kaslan (1989), and Davidson et al. (1986) have shown abnormal pneumograms in substance-exposed infants, although the value of pneumograms in predicting SIDS is questioned (Waggener, Southall, & Scott, 1987). Control for confounding factors such as cigarette smoking, ethnicity, and birthweight was not done. The effect of opiate exposure on the risk of SIDS is also unclear, although it has been estimated at 2%–3% in heroin and methadone exposed infants (Chavez, Ostrea, Stryker, & Smialek, 1979; Finnegan, 1979; Hunt & Brouilette, 1987; Rajegowda, Kandall, & Falcigeria, 1978; Rosen & Johnson, 1988).

In summary, the authors' review of perinatal and neonatal outcome studies of drug-exposed infants suggests that identification of a linear relationship between a specific drug and adverse impact on outcome has not been established. Both biological and environmental variables interact to determine risk. However, the high incidence of complications and compromise in neonatal outcome indicate that drug exposure has contributed to increased risks for both mother and infant. The studies to date strongly support the need for further well-controlled studies because of the extremely high incidence of morbidity and mortality in the drug-exposed groups.

LONGITUDINAL OUTCOME

Longitudinal follow-up of drug-exposed infants has been limited by the same confounds noted in the studies of perinatal outcome, in addition to the tremendous difficulty in maintaining contact with families characterized by high mobility, financial instability, inconsistent use of social support and medical services, high rates of familial violence, and continued drug use. Follow-up studies have found behavioral, attentional, and organizational problems after infancy. However, existing studies have not adequately addressed factors related to the postnatal environment, which may in fact be more significant in developmental outcome than prenatal factors such as drug exposure. Most studies have gathered data from poor, nonwhite women and their children who have multiple factors present in their lives, other than prenatal drug exposure, that place the children at significant risk for poor developmental outcome.

Research on the development of opiate-exposed infants is more common than those of other drugs, primarily because heroin addiction in pregnant women was recognized for many years before drugs such as cocaine and amphetamines. Most studies within the first 2 years of life have shown no consistent significant differences between exposed and nonexposed children on traditional developmental assessments such as the Bayley Scales of Infant Development (Kaltenbach & Finnegan, 1984, 1986, 1987; Strauss & Reynolds, 1983). Inconsistent differences in performance on particular subscales of the Bayley have been reported both within and across studies. Wilson and her colleagues have compared the development of heroin- and methadone-exposed infants to nonexposed controls up to 6 years of age, with differing results. At 1 year of age, infants in all three groups scored within normal ranges on the Bayley, with methadone infants scoring the lowest (Wilson, Desmond, & Waite, 1981). At 3–6 years of age, one study found heroin-exposed children had more developmental and behavioral problems than nonexposed comparison children (Wilson, McCreary, Kean, & Baxter, 1979), while another study found no differences between heroin, methadone, and non-exposed children (Wilson, 1989) when examined between 3–5 years of age. Lifschitz, Wilson, O'Brian-Smith, and Desmond (1985) found an increased incidence of low-average and mildly retarded intellectual performance in heroin- and methadone-exposed infants compared to a nonexposed group between 3 and 6 years of age. Regression analysis demonstrated that the amount of prenatal care, prenatal risk score, and home environment were most predictive of intellectual performance and that the degree of maternal narcotic use was not a significant factor. Follow-up into school age with a subgroup of heroin-exposed children indicated that 65% had repeated one or more grades or were receiving special education services (Wilson, 1989).

Follow-up studies of cocaine- and polydrug-exposed infants have increased since the late 1980s although they are limited in the number of infants studied, adequate control groups, and considerations of confounding variables. Developmental scores have been reported to be within the normal to low-average range by Rodning, Beckwith, and Howard (1990) at UCLA and Chasnoff and his associates at the Center for Perinatal Addiction at Northwestern Hospital in Chicago (Chasnoff, Griffith, Freier, & Murray, 1992).

Normal developmental scores were also found on the Bayley Scales of Infant Development in a large group of infants exposed to cocaine and/or amphetamines followed at the University of California, Davis through 24 months (Hansen et al., in press). However, qualitative differences were recognized by clinic staff in attention and organizational strategies seen in these infants. The normal scores on the Bayley may partly be due to the structure imposed on the infant's behavior by the examiner in performing the test. In addition, Bayley scores have shown little predictive value for subsequent developmental outcome in other groups of high-risk infants (Fagan & Singer, 1983).

A subgroup of 36 infants with positive toxicology screens at birth for either cocaine or amphetamines were compared to a group of 26 nonexposed infants on a standardized test of visual recognition memory, the Fagan Test of Infant Intelligence (FTII). Visual recognition memory has been shown to be more predictive of later cognitive outcome in other groups of high-risk infants than the Bayley (Fagan & Montie, 1988; Fagan, Singer, Montie, & Shepherd, 1986; Gotlieb, Biasini, & Bray, 1988). Significant differences were found between the exposed and nonexposed infants in both the mean scores and in the percentage of infants testing at risk ($p < 0.01$), with exposed infants showing less preference for novelty (Struthers & Hansen, 1992). The long-term significance of these differences remains to be studied, but the findings suggest that investigators must explore new ways to tease out subtle differences in these children.

A comparison of polydrug-exposed infants with nonexposed high-risk premature infants at 18 months showed that the drug-exposed infants had very disorganized play and significantly less representational play. They were also felt to be less securely attached to their caregivers than were the comparison group (Rodning, Beckwith, & Howard, 1989, 1990). Preliminary results from the Center for Perinatal Addiction at 3 years of age indicate that 60% of the substance-exposed children studied were felt to be normal with respect to language and behavioral organization (Griffith, 1990). Problems with expressive language, attention, and behavioral organization of varying severity were found in the remaining children.

Children enrolled in an intervention program within the Los Angeles Unified School District for 3- to 5-year olds with prenatal drug exposure have been reported by staff to show poor emotional modulation, attentional problems, speech and language delays, disorganization, and poor social skills (D. Kronstadt, personal communication, 1991). These difficulties are felt by program staff to be the result of multiple risk factors, of which prenatal substance exposure is but one.

Fried and Watkinson (1990) have followed 130 children for whom prenatal exposure to marijuana, cigarettes, and alcohol had been ascertained. At 48 months, significantly lower scores in verbal and memory domains of the McCarthy Scales of Children's Abilities (1972) were associated with maternal marijuana use after adjusting for confounding variables. This data suggests a long-term effect of marijuana upon complex behavior that was not appreci-

ated in earlier assessments, and which needs to be studied further.

Some exposed children at school age are demonstrating poor attention, difficulty processing information, and behavioral problems that interfere with their learning (Howard, Beckwith, Rodning, & Kropenske, 1989). However, more than half of the children participating in the LA preschool program are now in regular classrooms, assisted as needed with tutoring or special education resources.

The research to date indicates that most investigators now agree that there is no "typical profile" that holds true for prenatally exposed children. Which effects are primarily related to prenatal drug exposure and which are secondarily related to environmental variables has not been adequately examined. The severity of problems within individual children, and the percentage of exposed children with problems remain unanswered questions. Clearly, the difficulties described in prenatally exposed children are not specific for drug exposure. These children have unique strengths and weaknesses, which may or may not impact on their educational abilities.

IMPLICATIONS FOR RESEARCH AND POLICY

Substance abuse during pregnancy clearly places the fetus at risk for multiple complications of growth and development. The actual risk for abnormal fetal development and neonatal outcome related to maternal drug use during pregnancy has been obscured by methods of screening, issues of sample selection and size, and inadequate control for confounding variables. Most studies of perinatal drug use have reported data from risk- or complication-determined toxicology testing. Inherent in these methods is the potential for misrepresentation of results, primarily by under-detection of actual drug exposure as well as relative "overdetection" of complication rates.

Prematurity and intrauterine growth retardation have been the most consistent findings across studies. However, no specific effects on neurobehavioral or developmental outcome have been consistently related to individual illicit drug use. Associated confounding variables have, to date, been inadequately studied —both prenatal variables, as well as variables in the postnatal environment such as continued drug exposure, poor nutrition, and inadequate medical care; parental dysfunction; and family violence. Large population–based studies with suitable control groups are required to adequately answer questions about the prevalence, impact, and long-term consequences of prenatal substance use.

Appropriate outcome measures must be further investigated. The effects of prenatal drug exposure are likely to vary with the timing, frequency, and duration of exposure as well as with the contribution of individual and environmental differences. Global measures such as the Bayley Scales of Infant Development may not identify specific areas of dysfunction; measures focused on isolated tasks are frequently less robust in terms of standardization, validity, and predictability for long-term significance. Comprehensive evaluations that include assessment of social-emotional status and environmental variables, in addition to cognitive skills, are crucial in determining both outcome and appropriate intervention strategies. These children must be evaluated using a biopsychosocial risk model rather than a deficit model. Intervention strategies must be based on the recognition that fetal exposure compromises or jeopardizes developmental pro-cesses, but that organismic and environmental forces can contribute to positive developmental outcomes.

As further research continues, intervention resources must be provided to those women and children already identified with multiple needs related to substance use and exposure. Treatment facilities must be available to pregnant and parenting women, with access to prenatal care and health and developmental services provided to their infants. Even without clear answers to the questions about developmental and behavioral outcome in exposed infants, intervention services can be developed based upon existing knowledge of effective developmental and educational strategies used in other high-risk groups of children and their families.

Issues of confidentiality, labelling, and resource allocation loom large for the medical, educational, and social services systems. These issues have significant implications for researchers as well as public policy. If comprehensive identification of prenatal drug use is to be used primarily for criminalization and prosecution, little will be gained in our understanding or our treatment of drug abusing women and their children. Fewer women will seek prenatal or obstetrical care and their infants will be further at risk. Children labelled as "crack babies" or "drug addicts" will further suffer from social and educational stigmatization based on inappropriate generalizations and stereotypes that have the potential for self-fulfilling prophecy.

REFERENCES

Bauchner, H., & Zuckerman, B. (1990), Cocaine, SIDS and home monitoring. *Journal of Pediatrics, 117,* 904–906.

Bingol, N., Fuchs, M., Diaz, V., Stone, R.K., & Gromisch, D.S. (1987). Teratogenicity of cocaine in humans. *Journal of Pediatrics, 110,* 93–96.

Brazelton, T.B. (1984). *Neonatal Behavioral Assessment Scale* (2nd ed). Clinics in Developmental Medicine No. 88. Philadelphia: J.B. Lippincott.

Burkett, G., Yasin, S., & Palow, D. (1990). Perinatal implications of cocaine exposure. *Journal of Reproductive Medicine, 35(1),* 35–42.

Chasnoff, I.J. (1989, December). *Cocaine: Two-year follow-up of infants.* Paper presented at the National Asso-ciation for Perinatal Addiction Research and Education Conference, Miami, FL.

Chasnoff, I.J., Burns, K.A., & Burns, W.J. (1987). Cocaine use in pregnancy: Perinatal morbidity and mortality. *Neurotoxicology and Teratology, 9,* 291–293.

Chasnoff, I.J., Burns, W.J., Schnoll, S.H., & Burns, K.A. (1985). Cocaine use in pregnancy. *New England Journal of Medicine, 313,* 666–669.

Chasnoff, I.J., Bussey, M.E., Savich, R., & Stack, C.M. (1986). Perinatal cerebral infarction and maternal cocaine use. *Journal of Pediatrics, 108,* 456–459.

Chasnoff, I.J., Chisum, G.M., & Kaplan, W.E. (1988). Maternal cocaine use and genitourinary tract malformations. *Teratology, 37,* 210–204.

Chasnoff, I.J., Griffith, D.R., Freier, C., & Murray, J. (1992). Cocaine/polydrug use in pregnancy: Two-year follow-up. *Pediatrics, 89,* 284–289.

Chasnoff, I.J., Griffith, D.R., MacGregor, S., Dirkes, K., & Burns, K.A. (1989). Temporal patterns of cocaine use in pregnancy: Perinatal outcome. *Journal of the American Medical Association, 261,* 1741–1744.

Chasnoff, I.J., Hunt, C.E., Kletter, R., & Kaplan, D. (1989). Prenatal cocaine exposure is associated with respiratory pattern abnormalities. *American Journal of Diseases of Children, 143,* 583–587.

Chasnoff, I.J., Landress, H.J., & Barrett, M.E. (1990). The prevalence of illicit drug or alcohol use during pregnancy and discrepancies in mandatory reporting in Pinnellas County, Florida. *New England Journal of Medicine, 332,* 1202–1206.

Chasnoff, I.J., Lewis, D.E., Griffith, D.R., & Willey, S. (1989). Cocaine and pregnancy: Clinical and toxicological implications for the neonate. *Clinical Chemistry, 35,* 1276–1278.

Chavez, C., Ostrea Jr., E., Stryker, J., & Smialek, C. (1979). SIDS among infants of drug dependent mothers. *Journal of Pediatrics, 95,* 407–409.

Cherukuri, R., Minkoff, H., Feldman, J., Parekh, A., & Glass, L. (1988). A cohort study of alkaloidal cocaine ("Crack") in pregnancy. *Obstetrics and Gynecology, 72,* 147–151.

Davidson, S.L., Schuetz, S., Krishna, V., Bean, X., Wingert, W., Washsman, L., & Keens, T.G. (1986). Abnormal sleeping ventilatory pattern in infants of substance abusing mothers. *American Journal of Diseases of Children, 140,* 1015–1020.

Dixon, S., & Bejar, R. (1989). Echoencephalographic findings in neonates associated with maternal cocaine and methamphetamine use: Incidence and clinical correlates. *Journal of Pediatrics, 115,* 770–778.

Doberczak, T.M., Shanzer, S., Senie, R.T., & Kandall, S.R. (1988). Neonatal neurologic and electroencephalographic effects of intrauterine cocaine exposure. *Journal of Pediatrics, 113,* 254–358.

Dombrowski, M.P., Wolfe, H.M., Welch, R.A., & Evans, M.I. (1991). Cocaine abuse is associated with abruptio placentae and decreased birth weight, but not shorter labor. *Obstetrics and Gynecology, 77,* 139–141.

Durand, D.J., Espinoza, A.M., & Nickerson, B.G. (1990). Association between prenatal cocaine exposure and sudden infant death syndrome. *Journal of Pediatrics, 117,* 909–911.

Eisen, L.N., Field, T.M., Bandstra, E.S., Roberts, J.P., Morrow, C., Larson, S.K., & Steele, B.M. (1991). Perinatal cocaine effects on neonatal stress behavior and performance on the Brazelton Scale. *Pediatrics, 88,* 477–480.

Fagan, J.F., & Montie, J.E. (1988). Behavioral assessment of cognitive well-being in the infant. In J.F. Kavanagh, (Ed.). *Understanding mental retardation: Research accomplishments and new frontiers* (pp. 207–221). Baltimore: Paul H. Brookes Publishing Co.

Fagan, J.F., & Singer, L.T. (1983). Infant recognition memory as a measure of intelligence. In L.P. Lipsett (Ed.). *Advances in infancy research* (Vol. 2, pp. 31–78). Norwood, NJ: Ablex.

Fagan, J.F., Singer, L.T., Montie, J.E., & Shepherd, P.A. (1986). Selective screening device for the early detection of normal or delayed cognitive development in infants

at risk for later mental retardation. *Pediatrics, 78,* 1021–1026.

Finnegan, L.P. (1979). In utero opiate dependence and SIDS. *Clinical Perinatology, 6,* 163.

Finnegan, L.P. (1985). Effects of maternal opiate abuse on the newborn. *Federation Proceedings, 44,* 2317.

Frank, D.A., Zuckerman, D.S., Amaro, H., Aboagye, K., Bauchner, H., Cabral, H., Fried, L., Hingson, R., Kayne, H., Leverson, S.M., Parker, S., Reece, H., & Vinci, R. (1988). Cocaine use during pregnancy: Prevalence and correlates. *Pediatrics, 82,* 888–895.

Fried, P.A., & Watkinson, B. (1990). 36 and 48-month neurobehavioral follow-up of children prenatally exposed to marijuana, cigarettes, and alcohol. *Journal of Developmental and Behavioral Pediatrics, 11,* 49–58.

Fulroth, R., Phillips, B., & Durand, D.J. (1989). Perinatal outcome of infants exposed to cocaine and/or heroin in utero. *American Journal of Diseases of Children, 143,* 905–910.

Gillogley, K.M., Evans, A.T., Hansen, R.L., Samuels, S.J., & Batra, K.K. (1990). The perinatal impact of cocaine, amphetamine, and opiate use detected by universal intrapartum screening. *American Journal of Obstetrics and Gynecology, 163,* 1535–1542.

Gomby, D.S., & Shiono, P.H. (1991). Estimating the number of substance-exposed infants. *The Future of Children, 1,* 17–25.

Gotlieb, S.J., Biasini, P.J., & Bray, N.W. (1988). Visual recognition memory in IUGR and normal birth-weight infants. *Infant Behavior and Development, 11,* 223–228.

Greer, J.V. (1990). The drug babies. *Exceptional Children,* 382–384.

Griffith, D.R. (1990). *Developmental follow-up of cocaine-exposed infants to three years.* Paper Presented at the International Society for Infant Studies. Montreal.

Hadeed, A.J., & Siegel, S.R. (1989). Maternal cocaine use during pregnancy: Effect on the newborn infant. *Pediatrics, 84,* 205–210.

Hansen, R.L., Evans, A.T., Gillogley, K.M., Hughes, C.S., & Krener, P.G. (in press). Perinatal toxicology screening. *Journal of Perinatology.*

Howard, J., Beckwith, L., Rodning, C., & Kropenske, V. (1989). Development of young children of substance-abusing parents. *Zero to Three, 9,* 8–12.

Hoyme, H.E., Jones, K.L., Dixon, S.D., Jewett, T., Hanson, J.W., Robinson, L.K., Msall, M.E., & Allanson, J.E. (1990). Prenatal cocaine exposure and fetal vascular disruption. *Pediatrics, 85,* 743–747.

Hunt, C.E., & Brouilette, R.T. (1987). Sudden infant death syndrome. *Journal of Pediatrics, 110,* 669.

Kaltenbach, K., & Finnegan, L.P. (1984). Developmental outcome of children born to methadone-maintained women: A review of longitudinal studies. *Neurotoxicology and Teratology, 6,* 271–275.

Kaltenbach, K., & Finnegan, L.P. (1986). Neonatal Abstinence Syndrome, pharmacotherapy and developmental outcome. *Neurotoxicology and Teratology, 8,* 353–355.

Kaltenbach, K., & Finnegan, L.P. (1987). Perinatal and developmental outcome of infants exposed to methadone in-utero. *Neurotoxicology and Teratology, 9,* 311–313.

Koren, G., Graham, K., Shear, H., & Einarson, T. (1989). Bias against the null hypothesis: The reproductive hazards of cocaine. *Lancet, 2,* 1440–1442.

Kronstadt, D. (1991). Complex developmental issues of prenatal drug exposure. *The Future of Children, 1,* 36–49.

Lifschitz, M.H., Wilson, G.S., O'Brian-Smith, E., & Desmond, M.M. (1985). Factors affecting head growth and intellectual function in children of drug addicts. *Pediatrics, 75,* 268–274.

McCarthy Scales of Children's Abilities. (1972). New York: The Psychological Corporation.

Neerhof, M.G., MacGregor, S.N., Retzky, S.S., & Sullivan, T.P. (1989). Cocaine abuse during pregnancy: Peripartum prevalence and perinatal outcome. *American Journal of Obstetrics and Gynecology, 161,* 633–638.

Neuspiel, D.R., & Hamel, S.C. (1991). Cocaine and infant behavior. *Journal of Developmental and Behavioral Pediatrics, 12,* 55–64.

Oro, A.S., & Dixon, S.D. (1987). Perinatal cocaine and methamphetamine exposure: Maternal and neonatal correlates. *Journal of Pediatrics, 111,* 571–578.

Parker, S., Zuckerman, B., Bauchner, H., Frank, D., Vinci, R., & Cabral, H. (1990). Jitteriness in full-term neonates: Prevalence and correlates. *Pediatrics, 85,* 17–23.

Petitti, D.B., & Coleman, C. (1990). Cocaine and the risk of low birth weight. *American Journal of Public Health, 80,* 25–28.

Rajegowda, B.K., Kandall, S.R., & Falcigeria, L. (1978). Sudden unexpected death in infants of drug dependent mothers. *Early Human Development, 2,* 219.

Rodning, C., Beckwith, L., & Howard J. (1989). Prenatal exposure to drugs: Behavioral distortions reflecting CNS impairment? *Neurotoxicology, 10,* 629–634.

Rodning, C., Beckwith, L., & Howard, J. (1990). Characteristics of attachment organization and play organization in prenatally drug exposed toddlers. *Development and Psychopathology, 1,* 277–289.

Rosen, T.S., & Johnson, H.L. (1988). Drug addicted mothers, their infants and SIDS. *Annals of New York Academy of Science,* 89–95.

Ryan, L., Ehrlich, S., & Finnegan, L. (1987). Cocaine abuse in pregnancy: Effects on the fetus and newborn. *Neurotoxicology and Teratology, 9,* 295–299.

Salamy, A., Eldredge, L., Anderson, J., & Bull, D. (1990). Brain-stem transmission time in infants exposed to cocaine in utero. *Journal of Pediatrics, 17,* 627–629.

Shih, L., Core-Wesson, B., & Reddix, B. (1988). Effects of maternal cocaine abuse on the neonatal auditory system. *International Journal of Pediatric Otorhinolaryngology, 15,* 245–251.

Spires, M.C., Gordon, E.F., Chondhuri, M., Maldonado, E., & Chan, R. (1989). Intercranial hemorrhage in a neonate following prenatal cocaine exposure. *Pediatric Neurology, 5,* 324–326.

Strauss, M.G., & Allred, L.J. (1986). Methodological issues in detecting specific long-term consequences of perinatal drug exposure. *Neurobehavioral Toxicology and Teratology, 8,* 368–373.

Strauss, M.E., & Reynolds, K.S. (1983). Psychological characteristics and development of narcotic-addicted infants. *Drug and Alcohol Dependence, 12,* 381–393.

Struthers, J.M., & Hansen, R.L. (1992). Visual recognition memory in drug-exposed infants. *Journal of Developmental and Behavioral Pediatrics, 13,* 108–111.

Tenorio, G.M., Nazvi, M., Bickers, G.H., & Hubbird, R.H. (1988). Intrauterine stroke and maternal polydrug abuse. *Clinical Pediatrics, 27,* 565–567.

Waggener, T.B., Southall, D.P., & Scott, L.A. (1987). Analyses of breathing patterns in prospective populations does not predict susceptibility to SIDS. *Pediatric Research, 22,* 506A.

Wilson, G.S. (1989). Clinical studies of infants and children exposed prenatally to heroin. *Annals of New York Academy of Sciences, 562,* 183–194.

Wilson, G.S., Desmond, M.M., & Wait, R.B. (1981). Follow-up of methadone-treated women and their infants: Health, development and social implications. *Journal of Pediatrics, 98,* 716–722.

Wilson, G.S., McCreary, R., Kean, J., & Baxter, J.C. (1979). The development of preschool children of heroin-addicted mothers: A controlled study. *Pediatrics, 63,* 135–141.

Zuckerman, B. (1991). Drug-exposed infants: Understanding the medical risk. *The Future of Children, 1,* 26–35.

Zuckerman, B., Frank, D.A., Hingson, R., Amaro, H., Levenson, S.M., Kayne, H., Parker, S., Vinci, R., Aboagye, K., Fried, L.E., Cabral, H., Timperi, R., & Bauchuer, H. (1989). Effects of maternal marijuana and cocaine use on fetal growth. *New England Journal of Medicine, 320,* 762–768.

Chapter 12

Influence of Perinatal Risk Factors (Preterm Birth, Low Birth Weight, and Oxygen Deficiency) on Movement Patterns
An Animal Model and Premature Human Infants

C. ROBERT ALMLI, PH.D.
Washington University School of Medicine, St. Louis, Missouri

---

BRAIN INJURY IN THE PREMATURE/LOW birth weight neonate is an enormous clinical problem because these premature infants are at high risk for a variety of neurodevelopmental problems including developmental delays, motor dysfunction, learning disabilities, and behavior disorders. The two major variants of brain injury sustained by premature infants are intraventricular hemorrhage (IVH, including germinal matrix-subependymal hemorrhage) and hypoxic-ischemic encephalopathy (HIE) to brain parenchyma (e.g., periventricular leukomalacia) (Hill & Volpe, 1989; Volpe, 1987). Although both of these forms of brain injury can be imaged by cranial ultrasonography (Guzzetta, Shackelford, Volpe, Perlman, & Volpe, 1986), they are often found to be "clinically silent" during the early neonatal period. Conventional neurological assessments during the early neonatal period have not proven particularly reliable or consistent in identifying specific neurobehavioral dysfunctions (and the severity thereof) associated with

variants of the above brain injury patterns (Hill, 1989; Volpe, 1987, 1989a, 1989b).

The reasons for this problem in early clinical recognition are likely to be related to a variety of issues including: limitations on invasive neurological testing of sick infants during the neonatal period (Volpe, 1987), the differential effects of injury to immature and rapidly growing nervous systems (Almli, 1984, 1990; Almli & Finger, 1988; Almli & Fisher, 1977), and developmental changes in cerebral representations of movements in the newborn versus the child (Almli, 1990; Almli & Dyer, 1990; Almli & Fisher, 1977; Almli & Mohr, 1990; Sarnat, 1989).

With regard to the issue of changing cerebral representations of movement, Sarnat (1989) has recently presented a strong argument in favor of cortical and subcortical motor areas as being functionally important in the neonate. Although these brain motor areas are clearly immature during the perinatal period, they may subserve different needs or functions in the

The author gratefully acknowledges Nancy M. Mohr and Martina Dyer for their participation in the human and animal research, and expresses appreciation to the staff of St. Louis Children's Hospital (St. Louis, MO) for their encouragement and support of the research with the premature infants.

newborn than in the older infant or child. These developmental changes in neuromotor organization and function may underlie some of the difficulties of conventional neurological assessment of premature infants with brain damage during the neonatal period.

These issues and problems underscore the continuing need for the development of evaluation and assessment procedures that would allow for early identification of those neonates eminently at-risk for motoric dysfunction. The problem is especially critical for fragile premature neonates for whom invasive neurological assessment may be contraindicated (Hill, 1989; Hill & Volpe, 1989; Volpe, 1987). Because motoric development follows a biologically determined course, analysis of certain early motor patterns may be useful in identifying neuromotor dysfunction during the neonatal period, as well as serving as early predictors of developmental outcome (Anders, Keener, & Kraemer, 1985; Fukumoto, Mochizuki, Takeishi, Nomura, & Segawa, 1981; Hill, 1989; Korner et al., 1985; Prechtl, 1984, 1988). This chapter describes research on an early type of motor pattern, the *cyclic spontaneous movement pattern*, and the potential use of this measure for identification of neurobehavioral dysfunction in premature infants suffering brain injury. Identification of motor deficits during the neonatal period is important because it provides the opportunity for institution of appropriate early interventions during a time of great neuroplasticity and nervous system growth (Almli, 1984, 1990; Almli & Finger, 1988). Early identification and intervention would potentially facilitate the infant's attainment of maximal motor function, and also provide the parents/caregivers the opportunity to make optimal adaptations to any of the infant's acute or enduring deficits.

CYCLIC SPONTANEOUS MOVEMENT PATTERNS

The cyclic spontaneous movement (CSM) pattern has been described for embryos, fetuses, and neonates of a variety of vertebrate species, including humans (Almli & Dyer, 1989; Almli

& Mohr, 1990; Corner, 1977; de Vries, Visser, & Prechtl, 1982; Hamburger, 1971; Robertson, 1987, 1989; Smotherman, Robinson, & Robertson, 1988), and appears to be representative of rhythmic or cyclic phenomena (e.g., circadian, sleep-wake, kicking-stepping) common to many biological systems (Rapp, 1987; Rusak & Zucker, 1975; Thelen, Bradshaw, & Ward, 1981). Because of the ubiquitous nature of this movement pattern during immaturity, it has been suggested as a potential neurobehavioral index of nervous system function and integrity during early periods of nervous system development (Almli & Dyer, 1990; Almli & Mohr, 1990; Cioni, Ferrari, & Prechtl, 1988; Prechtl, 1988; Prechtl & Nolte, 1984).

The CSM pattern is distinguished by the *cyclic* and *spontaneous* nature of movements of all body segments including head, arms, legs, and trunk. The pattern is cyclic in that periods of relatively high levels of motoric activity are separated by periods of relatively low levels of motoric activity, with alternating periods of activity occurring on a non-random basis. Cyclic spontaneous movement patterns at 0.5–3.0 cycles/minute have been described for most every species studied (Corner, 1977). This movement pattern is also thought to occur *spontaneously*, without the application of any known external sensory stimulation, and does not appear to be "reflexive" or "intentional" in the traditional sense. The concept of spontaneous movement was advanced by neuroembryologists (Hamburger, 1971; Holt, 1931; Preyer, 1895) to distinguish this type of early movement pattern from stimulation-induced reflexive movements, and to highlight the importance of this movement pattern in subsequent neurobehavioral development.

Neural Control of Spontaneous Movements

Research on the development of neural mediation of CSM patterns indicates that local spinal/cranial neurons generate spontaneous movement patterns, and that brainstem and forebrain mechanisms come to regulate these patterns during subsequent development (Almli & Dyer, 1990; Almli & Mohr, 1990; Dyer,

Strauss, & Almli, 1990; Corner, 1977; deVries et al., 1982; Hamburger, 1971; Oppenheim, 1975; Robertson & Smotherman, 1990). Almli and colleagues (Almli & Dyer, 1990; Almli & Mohr, 1990; Dyer et al., 1990) have suggested that "forebrain" influences on CSM patterns develop relatively early in gestation, and as cortical and subcortical motor systems become increasingly mature during the postnatal period, the CSM pattern becomes integrated, regulated, and/or inhibited in some unknown fashion. The hypothesis of early supraspinal influence on spontaneous movement patterns is supported by in utero studies of anencephalic fetuses displaying abnormal spontaneous movement patterns as early as 16–35 weeks gestational age (Visser, Laurini, deVries, Bekedam, & Prechtl, 1985).

Functional Significance of Spontaneous Movement Patterns

The functional significance of the CSM pattern in neurobehavioral development can only be speculated upon at this time; however, this early movement pattern does appear to have important consequences during development. The CSM pattern may play a role in developmental neuronal modeling by influencing neuronal death and synaptic elimination processes (Thompson, 1983), which are important for the establishment of functional neural circuitry and reflex arcs (e.g., probabilistic epigenesis; Gottlieb, 1970; Holt, 1931). The CSM pattern may also be beneficial in preventing congenital limb abnormalities and deformities that would be associated with fetal immobility or akinesia (Moessinger, 1989). Furthermore, CSM patterns during the early postnatal period may regulate the infant's interactions with an invariant stimulus environment by periodically shifting periods of "inactive focused attention" and "active scanning" during waking periods. This periodic and predictable movement pattern may also communicate infant "well-being," as well as elicit caregiver–infant interaction. Thus, the CSM pattern may play a significant role in a variety of neurobehavioral developmental processes by influencing development of neuronal circuitry patterns, bone-joint-

muscle characteristics, behavioral states, and attentional processes, as well as social interactions. Disruption of CSM patterns could potentially have negative consequences for the fetus or neonate that would be far-reaching and diverse.

BRAIN INJURY AND SPONTANEOUS MOVEMENT PATTERNS

The author's research has concentrated on study of the development of spontaneous movement patterns and the effects of early nervous system injury on spontaneous movement patterns in both a *rat model of premature birth* and *human infants born prematurely*. Few quantitative studies of CSM patterns of premature human infants are available in the research literature; none of the human studies have quantitatively studied CSM patterns of individual body segments, and none have assessed relations between perinatal neuropathology, CSM patterns, and developmental outcome.

Preterm and Full-Term Neonatal Rat Studies

Preterm rats were delivered prematurely by C-section at 20 (pre-20) or 21 (pre-21) days of gestation and full-term rats were allowed normal vaginal delivery at 21–22 (full-21) days of gestation. The neonatal rats of the three gestational age groups were housed in incubators and studied during the first 24 hours of postnatal life. At 1–2 hours postnatal, spontaneous movements of individual neonatal rats were videotaped while in incubators, followed by an oxygen deprivation (asphyxia) or control treatment. At 1 hour (6 hours postnatal) and 19 hours (24 hours postnatal) following asphyxia or control treatment, the neonates were videotaped a second and third time, followed by sacrifice and brain analyses (histological and neurochemical).

For the videotaping and analysis of spontaneous movements, a high-resolution video recording/playback system with single-frame and slow-motion (0.1 sec real time) capability was used. The timing of the video playback system was synchronized with the time-base of a computer (for preservation of "real time"), and spontaneous movements (types, counts, and durations) of individual body segments were scored directly to the computer. Mouth movements scored were openings/closings. Head movements scored were medial/lateral, rotational, and extensions/flexions of the head/neck. Forelimb movements, scored separately, included flexion, extension, or rotation at the shoulder, elbow, or wrist. Hindlimb movements, scored separately, included flexor, extensor, or rotational movements originating at, or distal to, the pelvis. Trunk movements of three types were scored separately and included trunk-twitch (quick, spasm-like movements of the trunk), trunk-extension (arching or elongation of the trunk), and trunk-flexion (lateral/ventral flexions of the trunk). Intra- and inter-scorer reliabilities for movements of individual body segments were above $r = 0.900$.

Specially developed computer software programs provided both quantification and graphic reconstruction of numbers (counts) and durations (0.25 sec resolution) of spontaneous

movements, as well as time series and spectral analysis (FFT) of spontaneous movement periodicity. Figure 1 shows representative time-series and spectral plots of CSM patterns for a neonatal rat (pre-21) and a premature human infant (born at 29 weeks gestational age). The time-series plot was quantified for periodicity of movement bursts (peaks) by calculating the average period between bursts/peaks that exceeded a critical value (critical value = the mean + 2 standard deviations of the mean for numbers of movements/5-sec bin). The spectral plot was quantified by identifying a significant/dominant peak (deviation from randomness or background noise) and calculating the center frequency of the peak (cycles/minute), the periodicity (seconds), the percentage power within the peak (% power), and the value (cycles/minute) that represents half of the total power in the spectral plot (50% power measure; total spectrum = 100% power).

Results of studies of CSM patterns with preterm and full-term rat neonates have been presented at scientific meetings (Almli & Dyer,

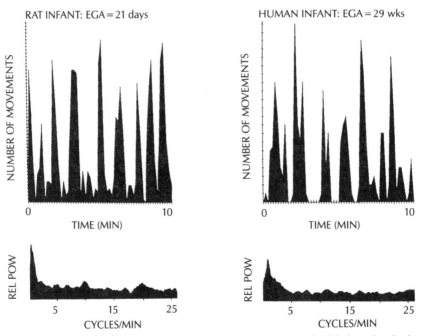

Figure 1. Time-series and spectral plots of spontaneous movements of total body segments (head, limbs, and trunk) of a prematurely delivered rat infant (left) and a prematurely delivered human infant (right). The time-series plots (top) show numbers of movements/10-second bin as a function of time (total time = 10 minutes). The spectral plots (bottom) show relative power (total black area under the curve = 100% power) as a function of frequencies of movement in cycles/minute. See text for explanation of infant characteristics, testing conditions, and quantification of the time-series and spectral plots.

1989, 1990; Dyer et al., 1990). The left side of Figure 1 shows time-series (top) and spectral (bottom) plots of CSM patterns of total body movements for a pre-21 neonatal rat on the day of C-section delivery. The time-series plot shows the cyclic nature of spontaneous movements, with a burst of movement occurring at an average periodicity of 67 seconds. Spectral analysis computed on this same data yielded a dominant peak, containing 44% of the power, centered at 0.75 cycles/min (periodicity = 80 sec). The 50% power value equaled 1.9 cycles/minute, showing that half of the neonates motor activity was contained within a frequency band of 0–1.9 cycles/minute. Similar quantitative values were obtained for the analysis of spontaneous movement patterns of individual body segments, indicating that movements of all body segments were in-phase and synchronized with one another (i.e., movements of all body segments were synchronized for active and inactive phases).

Comparisons of these quantitative measures of CSM patterns revealed no differences between the three gestational age groups for percent power, center frequency, or periodicity of the dominant peak in the spectra, or for the 50% power measure. These results indicate that CSM patterns are stable during these developmental time periods, and that CSM measures accurately characterize movement patterns of neonatal rats delivered prematurely or at full-term.

For the preterm (pre-20 and pre-21) and full-term (full-21) neonates, the time required to achieve the asphyxia criterion (three successive gasps separated by at least 15 sec) decreased as a function of gestational age (i.e., pre-20 = 92 minutes, pre-21 = 82 minutes, and full-21 = 42 minutes), and there were no differences between males and females within any of the age groups. Asphyxia criterion time was negatively correlated with birth body weight ($r = 0.814$, $p < .05$), which differed between gestational age groups. These results indicate that resistance, or tolerance, to asphyxia increases as a function of earlier gestational ages and lower birth weights.

Brain analyses of the asphyxiated neonates

revealed that the treatment was associated with brain hemorrhages (e.g., subependymal, intraventricular, intraparenchymal, subarachnoid hemorrhages) and elevated brain neurotransmitters (i.e., dopamine and serotonin in the hippocampus, caudate-putamen, and nucleus accumbens). The brain hemorrhages in the asphyxiated neonatal rats were similar to those of human infants born prematurely (Pape & Wigglesworth, 1979; Volpe, 1987).

Analysis of spontaneous movements of the premature and full-term neonatal rats showed that certain characteristics of spontaneous movement patterns were altered by the asphyxia treatment. For total numbers of movements (sum of mouth, head, forelimbs, hindlimbs, and trunk movements), the asphyxiated pre-20 neonates did not differ from control neonates, while the asphyxiated pre-21 and full-21 neonates displayed a reduction in total body movements in comparison to controls. This reduction in total movement activity was due to decreased movements of only the head, forelimbs, and hindlimbs, not the mouth or trunk.

In contrast to the age-related effects on numbers of movements, asphyxia treatment disrupted CSM patterns for all age groups. Figure 2 shows spectral plots for pre-21 neonates (left-control, right-asphyxia) for total body CSM patterns at 2, 6, and 24 hours postnatal. For these three measurement periods, the pre-21-Control neonate (Figure 2, left) displayed clear dominant peaks in the spectral plots centered at 0.75–1.50 cycles/minute (periodicity = 40–80 seconds, percent power = 39%–49%, 50% power = 2.1–3.0 cycles/minute). The pre-21-Asphyxia neonate (Figure 2, right) displayed similar CSM pattern quantifications at 2 hours postnatal (pre-treatment); however, at 1 hour and 19 hours post-asphyxia, there were no clear dominant peaks in the spectral plots (i.e., no dominant periodicity of movement was displayed). The spontaneous movement activity of the asphyxiated neonate was distributed across the entire 0–30 cycles/minute frequency domain and appeared to be randomly generated. Separate spectral analyses computed for movements of individual body seg-

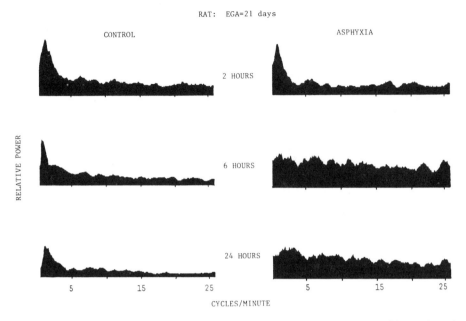

Figure 2. Spectral plots of spontaneous movement of total body segments at 2, 6, and 24 hours postnatal for rat infants who were delivered prematurely at 21 days gestational age (left = control, right = asphyxia). The 6-hour and 24-hour plots of the asphyxia rat were 1 hour and 19 hours post-treatment, respectively. Plot descriptions are as in Figure 1. See text for explanation of infant characteristics, asphyxia treatment, and quantification of spectral plots.

ments also showed a lack of consistent periodicity in movement patterns, as well as a lack of phase synchronization of movements between different body segments. This asphyxia-induced disruption of CSM patterns was also found for both the pre-20 and full-21 groups, indicating that the measure of CSM patterns is sensitive to perinatal brain injury (asphyxia and brain hemorrhage) in both premature and fullterm rats during the early neonatal period.

The effects of asphyxia on spontaneous movement patterns of neonatal rats indicate that the display of normal CSM patterns is dependent upon an intact and normally functioning nervous system. It is also important to note that neonatal reflexes (e.g., withdrawal, placing) remained relatively intact for the asphyxiated neonates, indicating that CSM patterns may be more sensitive to neonatal neural injury than are reflexes. These findings for premature and full-term neonatal rats provided the impetus and foundation for the study of CSM patterns in premature human infants suffering brain injury.

Premature Human Neonate Studies

Videotapings of spontaneous movements of premature infants (birth weights ≤1,500 grams) were made while the neonates occupied their own incubators/beds in the Neonatal Intensive Care Unit (NICU) at the St. Louis Children's Hospital in St. Louis, Missouri. The infants were *undisturbed* during the taping; no placement, manipulation, or stimulation of the infant was involved or required prior to, during, or following the videotaping. The videotapings of the infants were quantitatively analyzed for spontaneous movement patterns (types, numbers, durations, and cyclicity of movements) of individual body segments (head, arms, legs, and trunk) with the aid of a computer-assisted movement analysis system as described above. Infants' movement patterns were studied weekly (first test at 5–7 days postnatal) from birth until discharge from the NICU. Infants were subsequently evaluated (e.g., medical, sensory, motor, psychometric developmental assessments) at the Newborn Medicine Follow-up Clinic at Children's Hospital.

The neonates studied had an average birth weight of 1,047 grams and an average gestational age at birth of 28.9 weeks. At initial testing (5–7 days postnatal) they weighed 987 grams. The neonates received their initial cranial ultrasound scan within the first 3 days postnatal, and this was repeated at approximately 5–7 day intervals as indicated. Brain injury was identified, described, and graded by location and size, as well as ventricular size, according to established criteria (Guzetta et al., 1986).

Preliminary research on CSM patterns of human infants born prematurely indicates that the measurement of neonatal CSM patterns may represent a valid and reliable neurobehavioral index of nervous system integrity and function (Almli & Mohr, 1990; Cioni et al., 1988; Prechtl, 1988). Figure 1 (right) presents time-series and spectral plots of CSM patterns for total body (sum of head, limbs, and trunk) movement of an infant born at 29 weeks gestational age (birth weight = 1,095 grams) and tested at 7 days postnatal. This male infant was negatively diagnosed for brain hemorrhage or bronchopulmonary dysplasia, but had positive diagnoses for prematurity, hyperbilirubinemia, and respiratory distress syndrome. The time-series plot shows a clear cyclicity of movement with a calculated average periodicity of 75 sec. The spectral plot of the same movement data shows a dominant peak containing 34% power and centered at 1.03 cycles/minute (period = 58 seconds, 50% power = 2.35 cycles/minute). Similar quantifications of CSM patterns were found for the individual body segments of this neonate, indicating phase synchronization between movements of different body segments.

Studies of premature neonates (*without* diagnosed brain injury) reveals that CSM patterns for the total body, and for individual body segments, are relatively stable at 0.75–1.5 cycles/minute for neonates born at 24–32 weeks gestational age and tested during the first week of postnatal life. Furthermore, these quantitative CSM patterns appear to be stable for selected individual infants who were studied through approximately term-age, and between different

behavioral states such as sleep (quiet and active) and waking (crying/distressed infants have not been tested) (Prechtl, 1974). Comparison of CSM patterns between supine or prone positioning reveals an effect on the number of movements (i.e., higher numbers of movements in supine than prone); however, the CSM pattern persists at a normal periodicity.

Research with premature infants with ultrasound-diagnosed brain injury (hemorrhagic and/or ischemic) indicates that some types of brain injury are associated with altered or disrupted CSM patterns. Figure 3 shows time-

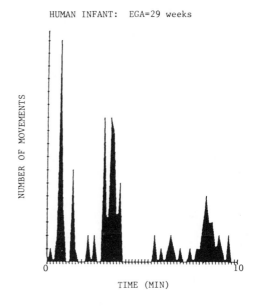

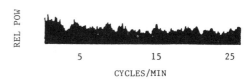

Figure 3. Time-series and spectral plots of total body segment movements of a brain-injured, premature human infant born at 29 weeks gestational age and tested at 7 days postnatal. Plot descriptions are as in Figure 1. Compare to "control" infant in Figure 1 (right). See text for explanation of infant characteristics and quantification of time-series and spectral plots.

series and spectral plots of a premature neonate (female, born at 1,030 grams at 29 weeks, tested at 7 days postnatal), who sustained bilateral intraventricular hemorrhage with intraparenchymal involvement (consistent with periventricular leucomalacia). Compared to the control infant (Figure 1), the brain-injured neonate (Figure 3) displayed an irregular pattern of total body movement activity in the time-series plot (top), and no clear dominant peak in the spectral plot (bottom). This loss of consistent cyclicity of spontaneous movement for the total body was also found for each of the individual body segments. The spontaneous motor ouput of this neonate was devoid of the normal cyclic pattern, and appeared to be generated randomly, without phase synchronization between body segments. The only quantification applicable to this "flat" spectral plot was the measure of 50% power (10.36 cycles/minute compared to the range of 1.5–4.0 cycles/minute for neonates without brain injury), which indicated that the neonate with brain injury demonstrated movements that were distributed broadly across a wide frequency domain of 0–30 cycles/minute. Subsequent movement studies revealed similar disruptions of CSM patterns in this infant who was eventually diagnosed as developmentally delayed with spasticity and hypertonicity at a 3-month corrected age follow-up.

It is important to note that current research indicates that relatively extensive brain hemorrhage and/or intraparenchymal involvement are associated with disruption of CSM patterns, whereas small hemorrhages, or those confined to the germinal matrix, may spare CSM patterns. Additional research is necessary to determine any potential relations between severity and locus of neuropathology and CSM pattern disruption. Also noteworthy are the findings that different aspects of spontaneous movements may be influenced by brain injury. Comparison of neonates sustaining at least bilateral IVH with control neonates revealed that the neonates with brain injury displayed reduced numbers of movements of the head, legs, and trunk. Most of the neonates with more moderate brain injury displayed relatively normal follow-up evaluations. Overall, these results indicate that premature infants with more extensive brain injuries display altered CSM patterns during the early neonatal period and subsequent motor problems identified during follow-up visits. The infants with more moderate brain injury may display a transient reduction in motor output (numbers of movements of certain body segments) during the neonatal period and an essentially normal follow-up evaluation.

Premature infants with selected medical diagnoses, *excluding* brain injury, have also been included in preliminary studies of CSM patterns to determine any potential effects of these diagnoses on early spontaneous movement patterns. For example, infants with diagnoses including prematurity, hyperbilirubinemia, and respiratory distress syndrome do not consistently display disruption of spontaneous movement patterns. However, infants who will ultimately be diagnosed with bronchopulmonary dysplasia already display relatively high levels of motor activity of the limbs as early as 5–7 days postnatal. Despite the high levels of extremity motor output, these infants continued to display essentially normal CSM patterns. These preliminary results indicate that certain medical diagnoses may influence some movement characteristics (e.g., numbers of limb movements), yet have little or no influence on other characteristics of movement (e.g., CSM patterns). Additional research is necessary to determine how the various medical diagnoses associated with prematurity may influence early spontaneous movement patterns.

DISCUSSION AND SUMMARY

Overall, research with newborn rats (premature and full-term) and premature human infants indicates that CSM patterns are a relatively stable and consistent characteristic of motor output during the neonatal period. This holds for infants at different gestational ages at birth, different levels of motor output, between males and females, for supine and prone body positions, and for selected medical diagnoses such as respiratory distress syndrome.

In contrast, the results for both rat and human neonates indicate that CSM patterns may be altered or disrupted by some types of perinatal nervous system injury (e.g., asphyxia, hemorrhagic, and/or ischemic injury). Certain types of perinatal brain injuries are associated with alterations in numbers and timing of movement of specific body segments, while more extensive brain injuries appear to be additionally associated with disruption of the CSM pattern. The disruption of the CSM pattern is in the form of movements of body segments losing their consistent periodicity, and a loss of phase synchronization between segments. Thus, neonates sustaining extensive brain injury display spontaneous movements of body segments that are relatively unpredictable for numbers, timing, and pattern, and therefore appear to be of poor quality. Those neonates displaying disrupted CSM patterns also appear to be the infants most likely identified as motorically delayed and/or dysfunctional during later postnatal follow-up. While certain types of brain injury disrupt spontaneous movement patterns, it is also possible that CSM patterns may be influenced by other biological and environmental conditions (e.g.,

meningitis or intrauterine drug/smoking exposure), which are currently under study. Nevertheless, the current results support the hypothesis that CSM patterns may serve as an index of nervous system integrity and function, as these movement patterns are sensitive to certain types of nervous system injury. Therefore, the measure of CSM patterns may prove useful in the early identification of neuromotor dysfunction in brain-injured premature neonates, and potentially in the early prediction of later developmental outcome.

An important advantage of CSM measurement, as a neurodevelopmental assessment of very young, small, and/or sick neonates, is that the measurement and analysis of CSM is relatively *non-invasive* to the infant (i.e., measurement of CSM requires no manipulation, stimulation, or disturbance of the infant, as is typically required by neurological testing of reflexes or muscle tone). Thus, the CSM measure has the potential to be used, with few or no contraindications, as early as the day of birth, and as frequently as desired under a variety of changing biological and environmental conditions.

REFERENCES

Almli, C.R. (1984). Early brain damage and time-course of behavioral dysfunction: Parallels with neural maturation. In S. Finger & C.R. Almli (Eds.), *Early brain damage: Vol. 2, Neurobiology and behavior* (pp. 99–116). New York: Academic.

Almli, C.R. (1990). Normal sequential behavioral and physiological changes throughout the developmental arc. In D.A. Umphred (Ed.), *Neurological rehabilitation* (pp. 79–109). St. Louis, MO: Mosby.

Almli, C.R., & Dyer, M. (1989). Extrauterine motor development of "fetal rat" delivered by C-section. *Neuroscience Abstracts, 15*, 70.

Almli, C.R., & Dyer, M. (1990). Diffuse nervous system injury alters cyclic, spontaneous movements of newborn, fullterm and preterm rats. *Neuroscience Abstracts, 16*, 333.

Almli, C.R., & Finger, S. (1988). Toward a definition of recovery of function. In S. Finger, T.E. LeVere, C.R. Almli, & D.G. Stein (Eds.), *Brain injury and recovery: Theoretical and controversial issues* (pp. 1–14). New York: Plenum.

Almli, C.R., & Fisher, R.S. (1977). Infant rats: Sensorimotor ontogeny and effects of substantia nigra destruction. *Brain Research Bulletin, 2*, 425–459.

Almli, C.R., & Mohr, N.M. (1990, July). *Cyclic, spontaneous movement patterns of human infants born prematurely.* Paper presented at the meeting of the Inter-

national Society for Developmental Psychobiology, Cambridge, England.

Anders, T.F., Keener, M.A., & Kraemer, H. (1985). Sleep-wake state organization, neonatal assessment and development in premature infants during the first year of life. II. *Sleep, 8*, 193–206.

Cioni, G., Ferrari, F., & Prechtl, H.F.R. (1988). Posture and spontaneous motility in fullterm infants. *Early Human Development, 18*, 247–262.

Corner, M.A. (1977). Sleep and the beginnings of behavior in the animal kingdom—studies of ultradian motility cycles in early life. *Progress in Neurobiology, 8*, 279–295.

de Vries, J.I.P., Visser, G.H.A., & Prechtl, H.F.R. (1982). The emergence of fetal behaviour. I. Qualitative aspects. *Early Human Development, 7*, 301–322.

Dyer, M., Strauss, E.A., & Almli, C.R. (1990). The effects of spinal transection on motor cyclicity in neonatal rats. *Neuroscience Abstracts, 16*, 331.

Fukumoto, M., Mochizuki, N., Takeishi, M., Nomura, Y., & Segawa, M. (1981). Studies of body movements during night sleep in infancy. *Brain Development, 3*, 37–43.

Gottlieb, G. (1970). Conceptions of prenatal behavior. In L.R. Aronson, E. Tobach, D.S. Lehrman, & J.S. Rosenblatt (Eds.), *Developmental evolution of behavior* (pp. 111–137). San Francisco: W.H. Freeman & Co.

Guzzetta, F., Shackelford, G.D., Volpe, S., Perlman, J.M., & Volpe, J.J. (1986). Periventricular intraparenchymal echodensities in the premature newborn: Critical determinant of neurological outcome. *Pediatrics, 78*, 995–1006.

Hamburger, V. (1971). Development of embryonic motility. In E. Tobach, L.R. Aronson, & E. Shaw (Eds.), *The biopsychology of development* (pp. 45–66). New York: Academic Press.

Hill, A. (1989). Assessment of the fetus: Relevance to brain injury. *Clinics in Perinatology, 16*, 413–434.

Hill, A., & Volpe, J.J. (1989). Perinatal asphyxia: Clinical aspects. *Clinics in Perinatology, 16*, 435–457.

Holt, E.B. (1931). *Animal drive and the learning process.* New York: Holt.

Korner, A.F., Zeanah, C.H., Linden, J., Berkowitz, R.I., Kraemer, H.C., & Agras, W.S. (1985). The relation between neonatal and later activity and temperament. *Child Development, 56*, 38–42.

Moessinger, A.C. (1989). Morphological consequences of depressed or impaired fetal activity. In W.P. Smotherman & S.R. Robinson (Eds.), *Behavior of the fetus* (pp. 163–173). Caldwell: Telford Press.

Oppenheim, R.W. (1975). The role of supraspinal input in embryonic motility: A reexamination in the chick. *Journal of Comparative Neurology, 160*, 37–50.

Pape, K.E., & Wigglesworth, J.S. (1979). *Haemorrhage, ischemia and the perinatal brain.* Philadelphia: J.B. Lippincott.

Prechtl, H.F.R. (1974). The behavioral states of the newborn infant (a review). *Brain Research, 76*, 185–212.

Prechtl, H.F.R. (1984). Continuity and change in early neural development. In H.F.R. Prechtl (Ed.), *Continuity of neural functions from prenatal to postnatal life* (Clinics in Developmental Medicine No. 94) (pp. 1–15). Philadelphia: J.B. Lippincott.

Prechtl, H.F.R. (1988). Developmental neurology of the fetus and the newborn. In F. Kubli, N. Patel, W. Schmidt, & O. Linderkamp (Eds.), *Perinatal event and brain damage in surviving children* (pp. 50–57). Berlin: Springer-Verlag.

Prechtl, H.F.R., & Nolte, R. (1984). Motor behaviour of preterm infants. In H.F.R. Prechtl (Ed.), *Continuity of neural functions from preterm to postnatal life* (pp. 79–91). Oxford: Blackwells.

Preyer, W. (1895). *Specielle physiologie des embryo* (Special physiology of the embryo). Leipzig: Grieben.

Rapp, P.E. (1987). Why are so many biological systems periodic? *Progress in Neurobiology, 29*, 261–273.

Robertson, S.S. (1987). Human cyclic motility: Fetal-newborn continuities and newborn state differences. *Developmental Psychobiology, 20*, 425–442.

Robertson, S.S. (1989). Mechanism and function of cyclicity in spontaneous movement. In W.P. Smotherman & S.R. Robinson (Eds.), *Behavior of the fetus* (pp. 77–94). Caldwell: Telford Press.

Robertson, S.S., & Smotherman, W.P. (1990). The neural control of cyclic motor activity in the fetal rat (Rattus Norvegicus). *Physiology and Behavior, 47*, 121–126.

Rusak, B., & Zucker, I. (1975). Biological Rhythms and animal behavior. *Annual Review of Psychology, 26*, 137–171.

Sarnat, H.B. (1989). Do the corticospinal and corticobulbar tracts mediate functions in the human newborn? *The Canadian Journal of Neurological Sciences, 16*, 157–160.

Smotherman, W.P., Robinson, S.R., & Robertson, S.S. (1988). Cyclic motor activity in the fetal rat (Rattus Norvegicus). *Journal of Comparative Psychology, 102*, 78–82.

Thelen, E., Bradshaw, G., & Ward, J.A. (1981). Spontaneous kicking in month-old infants: Manifestation of a human central locomotor program. *Behavioral and Neural Biology, 32*, 45–53.

Thompson, W. (1983). Synapse elimination in neonatal rat muscle is sensitive to pattern of muscle use. *Nature, 302*, 614–616.

Visser, G.H.A., Laurini, R.N., de Vries, J.I.P., Bekedam, D.J., & Prechtl, H.F.R. (1985). Abnormal motor behaviour in anencephalic fetuses. *Early Human Development, 12*, 173–182.

Volpe, J.J. (1987). *Neurology of the newborn* (2nd ed.). Philadelphia: W.B. Saunders.

Volpe, J.J. (1989a). Intraventricular hemorrhage and brain injury in the premature infant: Neuropathology and pathogenesis. *Clinics in Perinatology, 16*, 361–386.

Volpe, J.J. (1989b). Intraventricular hemorrhage and brain injury in the premature infant: Diagnosis, prognosis, and prevention. *Clinics in Perinatology, 16*, 387–411.

Chapter 13

Neonatal Behavior

Physiological, Temperamental,
and Developmental Correlates in Infancy

EMANUEL TIROSH, M.D.
Bnai Zion Medical Center and Technion-Israel Institute of Technology, Haifa, Israel
ANAT SCHER, PH.D.
Haifa University, Haifa, Israel

THE NEONATAL BEHAVIORAL ASSESSMENT Scale (NBAS) (Brazelton, 1984) evaluates the infant's potential for self-organization and state control as a response to his or her environment. The NBAS has been employed in numerous studies for the purpose of characterizing infants' innate endowment. A large number of studies addressed more specifically the validity of the NBAS. Such studies beyond their validation purpose may delineate the intercorrelation existing between and within different physiological and behavioral systems and then enhance the understanding of a variety of observed processes in infancy and childhood.

In this chapter, two types of correlative research are presented: *concurrent*—employing two measures simultaneously and evaluating the degree of their correlation; and *predictive*—employing two measures separated in time. (It should be emphasized that most neonatal studies to date have investigated "at-risk" infants, whereas the following report involves normal full-term infants only.) In the first of the following three studies, concurrent paradigm was employed, whereas the predictive approach is represented in the two other prospective studies.

Unlike most neonatal autonomic research to date, which investigated heart rate variability and respiratory sinus arrhythmia (Harper, Huppenbrouwers, & Sterman, 1976; Porges, McCabe, & Young, 1982; Richards, 1987; Richards & Cameron, 1989), the scope of the first study was to evaluate the correlation between respiratory habituation and behavioral excitability. The neonatal behaviors reflecting arousal, as assessed by the NBAS, consist of peak of excitement, rapidity of buildup, and irritability. Subsequent cluster analysis added lability of state to the preceding three items.

It has been argued that although the respiratory rate can be the same during a quiet behavioral state and distress, the changing amplitude of the respiratory excursion might give additional information (Miller, Hollingsworth, & Sanders, 1985). The main hypothesis of the first study was that infants characterized as highly aroused or alternatively, with less state control, would manifest delayed respiratory habituation to repeated stimuli. The second study examines the correlation between neonatal behaviors and later temperament. Infant temperament is often defined as a biologically

This study was supported by grants from the fund for Basic Research Administration, the Israeli Academy of Sciences, the Israel Foundation Trustees, and the Technion and Haifa University Collaborative Research Fund.

based disposition, which is stable over a long period of time (Goldsmith, Bradshaw, & Reiser-Danner, 1986). The NBAS appears to tap early temperamental aspects of behavior (Green, Bax, & Tsitsikan, 1989; Isabelle, Ward, & Belsky, 1985; Peters-Martin & Wachs, 1984). Some studies have addressed the relationship between the NBAS and later temperamental attributes (Crockenberg & Smith, 1982; Hubert, Wachs, Peters-Martin, & Cansdour, 1982; Isabelle et al., 1985; Matheny, Riese, & Wilson, 1985; Sostek & Anders, 1977). Neonatal state control has been found to be significantly correlated with high rhythmicity, good adaptability, and positive approach at 6 months (Green et al., 1989). The purpose of this study was to assess the relationship between the different NBAS items and the infants' temperament at 4 months of age as perceived by his or her mother.

The third study examined the same relationship, as well as three other dimensions: 1) developmental outcome at 3 and 9 months of age, 2) growth patterns, and 3) health aspects. The two latter dimensions were followed for the first 12 months of life. Unlike the previous two studies, the neonatal behavior in this study was assessed with the Einstein Neonatal Neurobehavioral Assessment Scale (ENNBAS) (Kurtzberg, Vaughan, & Daun, 1974). Despite the difference between the two scales, they overlap in both content and administration technique. The following not-mutually-exclusive hypotheses underlying the third study were:

1. Neonatal neurobehavioral attributes may be related to a more general innate imprint from which not only later development and temperament, but also growth and immunity, are influenced.
2. Neurobehavioral attributes may affect growth patterns and disease rate.

STUDY I

Methods

Subjects   Thirty-two full-term infants, products of normal deliveries and with Apgar scores of 8 or above at 1 minute and 10 at 5 minutes,

were consecutively recruited for the study. Seven infants were excluded from the study due to suspected illness or inappropriate state during the procedure.

Procedure   The full NBAS was administered between 36 and 48 hours of age. Within 3–4 hours following the NBAS, the infants underwent the polygraphic study consisting of respiratory chest movement (belt), electrocardiogram, electro-oculogram, and arm and leg movement. When the infants were in state I–II (Brazelton, 1984), up to 10 2-seconds-long stimuli of sound (60 decibel) and light (64 J/flash) were delivered. A closed circuit video system enabled continuous observation of the behavioral state. Stimuli were operated by remote control and were automatically registered (Figure 1).

Each subsequent stimulus was delivered following 6 seconds of recorded baseline respiratory pattern with an average of 20 seconds interstimulus interval. Periods of 6 seconds pre-stimulus and 6 seconds post-stimulus were analyzed. This interval was selected because it represented periods of reactive attention (Fox & Porges, 1985; Porges et al., 1982). The amplitude of each inspiration was measured, and mean and SD were derived. No significant difference in respiratory rate, associated with a definite difference in pattern, was observed and this rate was not included in the analysis. Stimuli with movement artifacts, as well as excursions of 20% or less (possible artifacts), were excluded from the analysis. Computer ranking of decreasing pre- and post-stimulus magnitude of difference in mean and SD was used to define habituation (i.e., the stimulus with the greatest similarity between the pre- and post-stimulus patterns indicated habituation). The NBAS arousal variables and respiratory habituation were subjected to Spearman rank correlation analysis whereas the Pearson product moment correlation was used to analyze the neurobehavioral items.

Results

The correlations between the arousal items and respiratory habituation ranged from .16 to .44. The correlations between the different NBAS

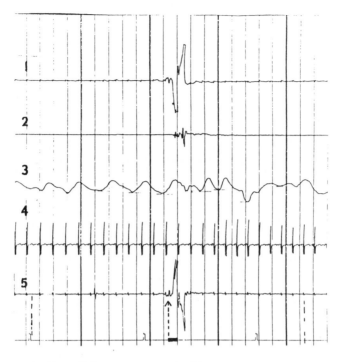

1. Upper limb movement   4. Heart rate
2. Lower limb movement   5. Ocular movement
3. Respiration   6. Arrow and blackened are -
                               Stimulus onset and duration

Figure 1. Polygraphic record of pre- and post-stimulus periods. (1 = upper limb movement, 2 = lower limb movement, 3 = respiratory, 4 = heart rate, 5 = ocular movement, arrow and blackened area = stimulus onset and duration.) (From E. Tirosh, M. Davidovich, M. Jaffe, A. Berger, & A. Cohen [1991]. Relationship between neonatal excitability and respiratory habituation. *Journal of Perinatology, 11* [4] , 344. Copyright © 1991. Reprinted by permission of Appleton & Lange, Inc.)

arousal items were higher (Table 1), as were the correlations between the pre- and post-stimulus mean respiratory amplitudes ($r = .82, p < .0001$).

STUDY II

Methods

Subjects Forty-seven consecutive, healthy, full-term babies, products of uneventful pregnancies, participated in the study. Their Apgar scores ranged between 8 and 9 after 1 minute and 10 after 5 minutes. Eighty percent of the mothers were of the middle socioeconomic class, 15% were upper-middle class, and 5% were of the lower class. Seven infants were excluded from the study because of missing data or hospitalization.

Procedure Out of the six NBAS clusters (Lester, Als, & Brazelton, 1982), the cluster of reflexes was omitted. Since an earlier study in Israel (Tirosh, Abadi, & Berger, 1988) revealed a different cluster structure from the one previously reported, analysis of the items was preferred rather than their summary scores. When the infants were 4 months (± 7 days) old their mothers were requested to complete the Infant Characteristic Questionnaire (ICQ) (Bates, Bennett-Freeland, & Lounsbury, 1979). The Stepwise Regression Analysis procedure was used for statisical analysis.

Results

The NBAS items of cuddliness, consolability, and defense were significantly predictive of the temperamental factor of unpredictability. The

Table 1. Mean (SD) and correlations of the four arousal items and respiratory habituations

Item	Mean (SD)	Peak of excitement	Rapidity of buildup	Lability of state	Stimulus light	Sound
Irritability	5.3 (1.4)	.31 (.11)	.42 (.03)	.60 (.001)	.17 (NS)	.21 (NS)
Peak of excitement	6.6 (0.9)		.34 (.08)	.33 (.1)	.44 (.03)	.16 (NS)
Rapidity of buildup	5.6 (0.8)			.36 (.7)	.13 (NS)	.38 (.07)
Lability of state	4.8 (1.2)				.32 (NS)	.17 (NS)

more optimal the infants behavioral responses, the more predictable were they perceived by their mothers (Table 2). Items representing autonomic stability, regulation of state, and orientation predicted the infants' nonadaptability 4 months later. The total temperamental score was best predicted by items representing the behavioral cluster of state regulation (i.e., cuddliness, consolability) and defense out of the motor cluster ($r = .56$, $p < .05$).

STUDY III

Methods

Subjects   A total of 118 full-term, healthy infants were sequentially recruited for this study. Their Apgar scores ranged between 8 and 10 at 1 minute and 9 and 10 at 5 minutes. Fifteen percent were upper-middle class, 71% middle class, and 14% lower-middle class and lower class. The ENNABS (Kurtzberg et al., 1974) was administered between 36 and 48 hours of age. This assessment consists of 22 items representing the following four factors: 1) orientation, 2) active mobility, 3) reflexive response, and 4) passive tone. Additionally, the observer scores general behavioral impressions based on the whole assessment. Following interobserver reliability ascertainment between the two researchers administering the assessment, only three clusters remained for later analysis: 1) activity, 2) reflexes, and 3) orientation. The Bayley Scale of Infant Development (Bayley, 1969) and the ICQ (Bates et al., 1979) were administered at 3 and 9 months of age. Periodic body length, weight, and head circumference were documented, as well as the infant's health history during the first 12 months of life. The anthropometric data were plotted on a standard percentile curve (Hamill, 1977).

The data were subject to Pearson product moment correlation, followed by regression analysis which included the following independent variables: maternal age, education, ethnic origin, infants' sex, birth order, and ENNBAS scores. Percentile change was defined as a dif-

Table 2. Regression analysis of NBAS and later temperament (N = 40)

Step/predictor	R	F	#	P
Fussy/difficult				
1—Cuddliness	−.23	10.23	2.76	.002
Unadaptable				
1—Tremor	−.39	22.07	4.22	.0001
2—Startles	−.47	4.85	1.00	.034
3—Consolability	−.55	6.05	.91	.019
4—Inanimate visual-auditory	−.72	18.20	1.4	.0002
Unpredictable				
1—Cuddliness	−.24	10.90	3.90	.0002
2—Consolability	−.37	7.00	2.70	.01
3—Defense	−.47	6.20	3.80	.01

ference between age-specific head circumference and weight percentiles and those obtained at birth, and the difference between the length percentile and that obtained at 1 month of age.

Results

The ENNBAS activity cluster was modestly correlated with the Mental Developmental Index (MDI) at 3 months of age ($r = .38, p < .001$). The orientation cluster was correlated, although in a negative direction with the 9 month Psychomotor Developmental Index (PDI) ($r = .28, p < .01$). The remaining correlations were accounted for by other intervening variables such as maternal origin and birth order. The 3 month temperamental factors of fussy/difficult and nonadaptability were correlated with the cluster of orientation ($r = .22, p < .03$) and irritability ($r = .19, p < .02$) respectively. The correlation between age-specific changes in growth percentiles and ENNBAS clusters are presented in Table 3. By and large, it appears that the better the infant scored in the activity and the reflex clusters, the lower growth rate during the first 12 months of life. Analysis of covariance with infants' sex and birth weight as covariates indicated that the significant relationship between attributes of neonatal behavior and head circumference remains valid at the ages of 1 and 3 months only (activity: $F = 3.6, p < .003$, orientation $F = 3.2, p < .007$, and reflexes F 2.2, $p < .05$). Gastrointestinal disease rate was significantly

and negatively correlated with the cluster of reflexes ($r = .45, p < .003$). The orientation cluster was positively correlated with respiratory disease rate ($r = .34, p < .02$) as well as gastrointestinal disease rate ($r = .36, p < .01$).

DISCUSSION

The data generated by all three studies suggest that neonatal behaviors are correlated, and thus predictive of other physiological developmental and behavioral processes.

The results of the first study indicate that respiratory regulation is related to the basic arousal pattern. It is possible, as argued by Woodson (1983) that behavioral responses are adaptive reactions to changes in physiological activity and are not a reflection of an underlying state. Yet, an equally plausible explanation is that the behavioral pattern serves as a signal to the environment to reduce the stimulus because of a slow habituation process.

Not surprisingly, the correlations within the neurobehavioral and autonomic domains are stronger than those revealed between them. This pattern of correlations probably reflects the true balance of relationships within and between the different systems under study.

The second study corroborates previous observations of the predictive value of mother-infant interaction (Waters, Vaughn, & Egeland, 1980) and of infants' temperamental attributes by the neonatal behaviors (Crockenberg & Smith,

Table 3. Correlations between changes in growth curves and ENNBAS clusters (p)

Age (in months)	Activity			Reflexes			Orientation		
	Wt	L	Hc	Wt	L	Hc	Wt	L	Hc
1	−.24 (.01)	NA —	— —	−.18 (.04)	NA —	— —	— —	NA —	— —
3	−.20 (.03)	— —	−.33 (.01)	−.28 (.005)	— —	— —	−.20 (.04)	— —	−.19 (.05)
6	−.18 (.04)	−.23 (.02)	−.22 (.03)	−.21 (.04)	.23 (.02)	−.20 (.03)	— —	— —	— —
9a	— —	−.26 (.02)	— —	−.31 (.004)	−.26 (.02)	−.21 (.05)	— —	— —	— —
12	— —	— —	— —	−.37 (.001)	−16 (.01)	— —	— —	— —	— —

Wt = weight, L = length, Hc = head circumference, NA = not applicable.

1982; Green et al., 1989). Of particular interest was the finding that cuddliness, consolability, and defense response were the most sensitive overall predictors of the infants' temperament 4 months later. This observation supports previous findings (Capute, Derivan, Shauvel, & Rodriguez, 1975; Isabelle et al., 1985). The overall conclusion from this study is that a transaction between the neurobehavioral disposition of the infant and the parental perception of his or her temperament does exist.

The third study focused on developmental, growth, and health aspects during the first 12 months of life. No previously published investigations which address the relationship of the latter two characteristics with neonatal behaviors exist. Despite the rather modest correlations between the growth patterns and the three neonatal neurobehavioral clusters, their consistency across ages contributes to their validity. An optimal neonatal neurobehavioral status can be attributed to an increased body size resulting from a more nurturing intrauterine environment. The infant's birth size is not necessarily his or her constitutional/genetic size, and an overall gradual regression trend is observed. Alternatively, it is possible that a more optimal neurobehavioral status at birth is followed by increased activity and energy expenditure during the initial course of development and associated with a decelerative, however physiological, growth rate.

The cluster of reflexes and orientation were found to correlate with disease rate in an opposite direction. The authors cannot account for this trend or rule out a possible spurious result. Of interest, however, is that more optimal orientation was inversely correlated with both 9 month Psychomotor Development Index and disease rate. The possible differential significance of orientation vis-a-vis later Mental Development Index and Psychomotor Develop-ment Index and health should be considered in future research. The results of the above studies invoke several methodological questions, not the least of which is that of reliability. High interobserver agreement was ascertained prior to the administration of the ENNABS and during the research process. Yet *a posteriori* analysis of the data controlling for the observer revealed a significant difference on some of the items. The possible observer bias should be considered not only at the start but also at the conclusion of the study. It appears that measures which seemingly tap similar attributes in fact might produce different results. Until a criterion validity is established, different behavioral measures should not be used interchangeably. The homogeneous "healthy" nature of the samples probably accounts for the rather modest correlations obtained in the three studies. It is suspected that the inclusion of a more heterogeneous group of infants, particularly those at risk, would have resulted in statistical evidence for stronger relationships. Finally, in both the first and the third study the "law of initial values" (Wilder, 1958) is of great relevance. The post-stimulus mean amplitude was bound to be determined to a large extent by the pre-stimulus amplitude and, likewise, the future growth patterns of the infants was largely dependent on their size at birth.

It is therefore proposed that the same law might apply to a wider set of physical, developmental, and temperamental variables which depend to different degrees on the initial neonatal endowments.

In summary, the results of this investigation not only point to the interrelations between different neonatal characteristics but also illuminate their potential contribution to development, temperament, and health in the course of the first year of life.

REFERENCES

Bates, T.E., Bennett-Freeland, C.A., & Lounsbury, M.C. (1979). Measurement of infant difficultness. *Child Development, 50,* 794–803.

Bayley, N. (1969). *Manual for the Bayley Scale of Infant Development.* New York: The Psychological Corporation.

Brazelton, T.B. (1984). *Neonatal Behavioral Assessment Scale* (Spastic International Medical Publication). London: Blackwell Scientific.

Capute, A.J., Derivan, A.P., Shauvel, P.J., & Rodriguez, A. (1975). Infantile autism I. A prospective study of the diagnosis. *Developmental Medicine and Child Neurol-*

ogy, *17*, 58–62.

Crockenberg, S.B., & Smith, B. (1982). Antecedents of mother-infant interaction and infant irritability in the first three months of life. *Infant Behavior and Development, 5*, 105–119.

Fox, N.A., & Porges, S.W. (1985). The relation between neonatal heart period patterns and developmental outcome. *Child Development, 56*, 28–37.

Goldsmith, H.H., Bradshaw, D.L., & Reiser-Danner, L.A. (1986). Temperamental dimensions as potential development influence on attachment. In J.V. Lerner & R.M. Lerner (Eds.), *Temperament and psychosocial interaction during infancy and childhood: New directions in child development* (pp. 5–34). San Francisco: Jossey Bass.

Green, J., Bax, M., & Tsitsikan, H. (1989). Neonatal behavior and early temperament: A longitudinal study of the first six months of life. *American Journal of Orthopsychiatry, 59*, 82–93.

Hamill, P.W. (1977). *NCHS growth curves for children from birth to 18 years.* United States Department of Health, Education and Welfare Publication (PHS), 78-1650.

Harper, R.M., Hoppenbrouwers, T., & Sterman, M.B. (1976). Polygraphic studies of normal infants during the first six months of life. I. Heart rate and variability as a function of state. *Pediatric Research, 10*, a45–a51.

Hubert, N., Wachs, T.D., Peters-Martin, P., & Cansdour, M.J. (1982). The study of early temperament: Measurement and conceptual issues. *Child Development, 53*, 571–600.

Isabelle, R.A., Ward, M.J., & Belsky, J. (1985). Convergence of multiple sources of information on infant individuality: Neonatal behavior, infant behavior and temperament reports. *Infant Behavior and Development, 8*, 283–291.

Kurtzberg, G., Vaughan, J.R., & Daun, C. (1974). Neurobehavioral performance of low-birth weight infants at 40 weeks conceptional age: Comparison with normal full-term infants. *Developmental Medicine and Child Neurology, 41*, 590–607.

Lester, B.M., Als, H., & Brazelton, T.B. (1982). Regional obstetric anasthesia and newborn behavior: A reanalysis toward synergistic effects. *Child Development, 53*, 688–692.

Matheny, A.P., Riese, M.L., & Wilson, R.S. (1985). Rudiments of infant temperament: Newborn to nine months. *Developmental Psychology, 21*, 486–494.

Miller, B.D., Hollingsworth, B.A., & Sanders, L.W. (1985). Assessment of infant-caregiver interaction using cardiac respiratory and behavioral monitoring: Conceptual and technical issues in a new methodology. *Journal of the American Academy of Child Psychiatry, 24*, 286–297.

Peters-Martin, P., & Wachs, T.D. (1984). A longitudinal study of temperament and its correlates in the first 12 months. *Infant Behavior and Development, 7*, 285–298.

Porges, S.W., Arnold, W.R., & Forbes, E.J. (1973). Heart variability: An index of attentional responsivity in human newborns. *Developmental Psychology, 8*, 85–92.

Porges, S.W., McCabe, P.M., & Young, B.G. (1982). Respiratory heart interactions: Psychophysiological implications for pathophysiology and behavior. In J. Caccioppo & R. Petty (Eds.), *Perspective in cardiovascular psychology* (pp. 223–264). New York: Guilford.

Richards, J.E. (1987). Infant visual sustained attention and respiratory sinus arrhythmia. *Child Psychiatry, 58*, 488–496.

Richards, J.E., & Cameron, D. (1989). Infant heart rate variability and behavioral states. *Infant Behavior and Development, 12*, 45–56.

Sostek, A.M., & Anders, T.F. (1977). Relationships among the Brazelton neonatal scale, Bayley infant scales, and early temperament. *Child Development, 48*, 320–328.

Tirosh, E., Abadi, J., & Berger, A. (1988). Comparison of early neonatal behaviour in two Israeli ethnic groups. *Israel Journal of the Medical Sciences, 24*, 676–680.

Tirosh, E, Davidovich, M., Jaffe, M., Berger, A., & Cohen, A. (1991). Relationship between neonatal excitability and respiratory habituation. *Journal of Perinatology, 11*(4), 343–346.

Waters, E., Vaughn, B.F., & Egeland, B.R. (1980). Individual differences in infant-mother attachment relationships at age one: Antecedents in neonatal behaviour in an urban, economically disadvantaged sample. *Child Development, 51*, 201–214.

Wilder, J. (1958). Modern psychopathology and the law of initial values. *American Journal of Psychotherapy, 12*, 199–221.

Woodson, R.H. (1983). Newborn behavior and the transition to extrauterine life. *Infant Behavior and Development, 6*, 139–144.

Chapter 14

Intrauterine Growth Retardation: Diagnosis and Neurodevelopmental Outcome

Shaul Harel, M.D.
Miriam Kutai, M.D.
Tel Aviv Medical Center, Tel Aviv, Israel
Abraham Tomer, M.D.
Edith Tal-Posener, M.D.
Yael Leitner, M.D.
Aviva Fatal, M.D.
University of Tel Aviv, Tel Aviv, Israel
Ariel Jaffa, M.D.
Serlin Maternity Hospital, Tel Aviv Medical Center, Tel Aviv, Israel
Ephraim Yavin, Ph.D.
The Weizmann Institute of Science, Rehovot, Israel

INTRAUTERINE GROWTH RETARDATION (IUGR) is a condition that occurs in 3%–10% of all pregnancies (Lockwood & Weiner, 1986). The significance thereof is well recognized due to its variability in etiology, natural history, and influence on short- and long-term outcome. These are reflected in high rates of neonatal mortality and neurodevelopmental disabilities (Allen, 1986). The most commonly used definition of IUGR is one that includes infants who weigh less than 2,500g and are below the tenth percentile for gestational age (Brar & Rutherford, 1988). Intrauterine growth–retarded neonates constitute 33% of all low birth weight infants (Band, 1978). Intrauterine growth retardation is more prevalent among children with mental retardation or cerebral palsy, as well as in those having minimal brain dysfunction or speech or learning disabilities (Allen, 1986; Low et al., 1982). It is more common in a low socioeconomic population, among certain ethnic groups, inhabitants of high altitude, smokers, and as a family trait (Lockwood & Weiner, 1986).

Brain damage due to intrauterine insults may not be clinically evident until late in development. It is therefore crucial to follow small for gestational age (SGA) newborns who are at risk for neurodevelopmental handicaps, and who may need special intervention. In order to fulfill this goal, several steps must be taken: 1) IUGR must be diagnosed by a reliable index as soon as possible in utero; 2) etiological assessment of environment, family, and mother

This chapter was condensed (with some modifications and additional data) from two papers published in *International Pediatrics*, 1991,6, 109–120.

This research was made possible through a grant from The Gulton Foundation, New York, U.S.A.

must be made; 3) as the baby is born, his or her neurobehavioral state must be studied with a valid, sensitive, and predictive examination; and 4) finally, the baby must be followed longitudinally in order to detect, as early as possible, any neurodevelopmental abnormalities.

It is the purpose of this chapter to discuss the diagnosis of IUGR and to review some methodological dilemmas that relate to neurodevelopmental outcome. This chapter also presents some preliminary results of a wider research project which prospectively follows IUGR infants from pregnancy through school age, with biometric-ultrasonic, physiologic (placental and fetal blood flow), biochemical (vasoactive prostanoid substances), and pathological (placental) indices. These infants will have repeated follow-up neurobehavioral and neurodevelopmental examinations.

DIAGNOSIS

Pathogenesis and Classification

Traditionally, IUGR is classified into "symmetrical or early," "asymmetrical or late," and "intermediate" types. The major differences between the first two types are summarized in Table 1.

The different classifications of IUGR types are mainly based on the major phases of normal fetal growth as described by Rosso and Winick (1974) and Winick (1971). During early fetal life (first 16 weeks), virtually all growth is due to increases in cell number (hyperplasia). Increases in cell size (hypertrophy) become dominant during the latter part (from 32 weeks) of gestation. An intrauterine insult throughout the periods of both hyperplastic and hypertrophic growth will result in fewer and smaller cells.

Intrauterine growth retardation induced by intrauterine infection, genetic causes, congenital malformation, environmental insults, and severe malnutrition usually results in early "symmetric" restriction of fetal growth, uniformly affecting all body organs including the brain. Vascular-induced IUGR results in a later restriction leading to an "asymmetrical" newborn, with greater affection of body than brain growth. The latter particularly affects organs such as the skeleton, liver, thymus, spleen, and adrenals, while vital organs such as the brain and the heart are selectively protected and relatively spared (Holt, Cheek, Mellitis, & Hill, 1975; Minkowsky, 1973).

In the last trimester of human pregnancy, the body of the fetus may gain 2,500 g in weight, while the brain gains approximately 250 g (about 7 cm in head circumference by Lubchenco Intrauterine Growth Curves, 1970). When growth is retarded at that time by vascular-induced IUGR, assuming that the brain is far less affected than the body, this continuing sparing effect of brain weight must be expected to result in a substantial increase in the brain:body ratio. Usually, the higher the brain:body ratio, the more severe the IUGR process is, and the greater the risk for the brain to be affected. Therefore, vascular IUGR may cause a severe decrease in body weight gain, mild decrease in brain weight gain, but only minor changes in head circumference. It could be speculated that the mild decrease in brain mass growth during the critical period of the "brain growth spurt," in the last trimester of pregnancy, is partially explained by the sparing effect on cell proliferation, protein synthesis, and myelination. In spite of this sparing effect on quantitative brain development, qualitative changes in synaptic formation, receptor and neurotransmitter development could still be affected and influence neurodevelopment and function.

Since the consequences of experimental vascular placental insufficiency on the fetal human brain is not feasible, an experimental animal model is in order. A number of experimental models of laboratory animals are currently available for studying placental insufficiency (Chanez, Privat, Flexor, & Drian, 1985; Creasy, Barrett, Deswilt, Kahanpaa, & Rudolph, 1972; Emmanovilides, Townsend, & Bauer, 1968; Harel et al., 1978; Hill, Myers, Scott, & Cheek, 1971; Ho & Guy, 1971; Roux, 1971; Van Marthens, Harel, & Zamenhof, 1975; Wigglesworth, 1964).

Table 1. Classification of IUGR

	Type I: Symmetrical	Type II: Asymmetrical
Incidence	25%	75%
Social background	Low socio-economic status	More affluent society
Etiology	Congenital infections (T.O.R.C.H.) Genetic and malformations Environmental insults (x rays, drugs, alcohol, smoking) Severe malnutrition	Uteroplacental pathology and insufficiency Maternal disorders
Timing of insult	< 28 weeks gestation	> 28 weeks gestation
Growth process		
Cell number	Decreased (hypoplastic)	Normal
Cell size	Normal	Decreased (hypotrophic)
Brain size	Decreased	Relatively normal ("brain sparing")
Liver, thymus size	Decreased	Decreased
Placental growth	Frequently normal	Decreased
Ultrasonography		
PI	Normal	Decreased
BPD/HC	Small	Early—normal, late—reduced
AC	Small	Small
FL	Decreased	Relatively normal
EFW	Decreased	Decreased
HC:AC	Normal	Early—increased, late—reduced
IUCI	Normal	Increased
Fetal behavior	Abnormal—early	Abnormal—late
Doppler ultrasonography		
Umbilical-utero placental resistance index	Increased	Increased
Carotid resistance index	Increased, no "brain sparing"	Decreased—early, "brain sparing" increased(?)—late, failure of "brain sparing"
Postnatal catch-up growth	Poor	Relatively good

From Harel, S., Tal-Posener, E., Kutai, M., Tomer, A., Jaffa, A., Zuk, L., and Yavin, E. (1991). Intrauterine growth retardation and brain development: Part I: Pre- and perinatal diagnosis. *International Pediatrics, 6,* 110; reprinted by permission. Adapted and modified from Brar and Rutherford (1988).

PI = ponderal index; BPD/HC = biparietal diameter/head circumference; AC = abdominal circumference; FL = femur length; EFW = estimated fetal weight; HC:AC = head circumference:abdominal circumference; IUCI = intrauterine cephalization index.

Generally, fetuses subjected to vascular-induced placental insufficiency exhibit reduced body weight gain and have significantly smaller brains compared to control animals of the same age, although a sparing mechanism for the brain was indicated (Battaglia, 1970). Intrauterine growth–retarded animals are more prone to neurological dysfunction in early postnatal life. Light microscopy and ultrastructural studies indicate that IUGR animals have a reduced number of cells and exhibit lesser synaptic connections. The rabbit, which is a perinatal developer (Harel, Watanabe, Linke, & Schain,

1972), has previously been studied in our laboratory with regard to several morphological (Harel, Yavin, Barak, Tomer, & Binderman, 1981), biochemical (Harel, Shapira, Tomer, Donahue, & Quilligan, 1985), and neurological parameters (Harel et al., 1978; Teng et al., 1976).

Accumulation of clinical data has strongly implied an association between prolonged maternal vascular disease from various causes and IUGR resulting in an "asymmetrical" SGA newborn (Minkowsky, 1973). One-third of SGA infants result from maternal problems of circulation, of which hypertension and toxemia are the most common. Preeclampsia, a hypertensive disorder specific to pregnancy, is associated with proteinuria, edema, and at times, coagulation abnormalities. In toxemic conditions, numerous placental infarcts, atheromatous changes in the decidual spiral arteries, or failure of the normal physiological dilatation of the placental spiral arteries, may be sufficient to decrease perfusion of the placenta below that which is adequate to meet the needs of the fetus. This process of increased vasoconstriction, platelet aggregation, and reduced uteroplacental blood flow is particularly likely to increase toward the latter part of the third trimester. Research findings produced in the 1980s showed that umbilical arteries of infants born to preeclamptic women produce prostacyclin in a much lower quantity than do those of infants whose mothers are normal (Dadak, Kefalides, Sinzeringer, & Giorgow, 1982). In preeclamptic pregnancy, however, the placenta produces seven times more thromboxane than prostacyclin (Walsh, 1985). An increasing volume of related research suggests that on the one hand, a decrease in production of prostacyclin, a potent vasodilator, and inhibitor of platelet aggregation during pregnancy, and on the other hand, an increase in thromboxane, a potent vasoconstrictor, and stimulator of platelet aggregation, may play a significant role in causing inadequate placental perfusion and could contribute to the clinical manifestations of preeclampsia, as well as adversely affect the growth of the fetus (Walsh, 1985). The thromboxane/prostacyclin imbalance also appears in the maternal and fetal circulation (Walsh, 1985). Therefore, the distribution of blood flow within the fetus might be altered, inducing possible secondary systemic effects. It has been found that the earlier the onset of preeclampsia, the worse the prognosis of intrauterine growth (Long, Abell, & Beischer, 1980).

Clinical Manifestations

Dysmature SGA infants are more often asymmetrically growth-retarded, being primarily underweight, and therefore appear thin and wasted. The skin is loose, often dry, and frequently scaling. There is little subcutaneous tissue (decrease in skin fold thickness). While weight is low, quite often length is not affected, and head size is usually relatively normal. Hair on the head tends to be sparse. These babies are usually alert and active and seem hungry (Sweet, 1986). As many as 65% of SGA infants in the delivery room are likely to present with one or more severe and often life-threatening problems (Ounsted, Moar, & Scott, 1981). These include: asphyxia, hypoglycemia, polycythemia, and hypothermia (Table 2). The postnatal growth is characterized by the observation that if catching up has not occurred by 3 years of age, the child will remain small (Drillien, 1970; Fitzhardinge & Steven, 1972). The long-term morbidity includes problems in the area of cognition, language, hearing, motor function, attention, and behavior.

Fetal Assessment for IUGR

The various biometric, behavioral, and blood flow parameters are summarized in Table 3. The diagnosis of IUGR is dependent on accurate evaluation of the gestational age. In the prenatal period, this can be attained by obtaining the exact date of the last menstrual period and ultrasonographic biometric parameters. In the postnatal period gestational age can be assessed by using a combination of physical and neurological signs (Dubowitz, Dubowitz, & Goldberg, 1970).

It is now, in 1993, believed that although IUGR is difficult to diagnose, an early accurate diagnosis and fetal growth assessment could be

Table 2.   Risk factors associated with IUGR

Congenital anomalies
Birth asphyxia
Hypoglycemia
Hypocalcemia
Hypothermia
Polycythemia
Coagulation disturbances
Meconium aspiration
Persistent fetal circulation

From Harel, S., Tal-Posener, E., Kutai, M., Tomer, A., Jaffa, A., Zuk, L., and Yavin, E. (1991). Intrauterine growth retardation and brain development: Part I: Pre- and perinatal diagnosis. *International Pediatrics*, 6, 111; reprinted by permission.

Table 3. Fetal assessment for IUGR

Ultrasonography
1. Biometric parameters
    Biparietal diameter
    Head circumference (HC)
    Abdominal circumference (AC)
    Crown-heel length (CHL)
    Femur length (FL)
    HC:AC ratio
    Estimated fetal weight (EFW)
    Ponderal index = $EFW:FL^3$
    Intrauterine cephalization index = HC:EFW
    Fetal biophysical score (movement, breathing, heart rate, tone, amniotic fluid volume)
2. Fetal behavior
    Motor activity
    Behavioral states

Doppler
1. Uteroplacental blood flow (umbilical and uterine resistance index)
2. Cerebral blood flow (carotid resistance index)

From Harel, S., Tal-Posener, E., Kutai, M., Tomer, A., Jaffa, A., Zuk, L., and Yavin, E. (1991). Intrauterine growth retardation and brain development: Part I: Pre- and perinatal diagnosis. *International Pediatrics, 6,* 111; reprinted by permission.

crucial for the reduction of mortality and morbidity. Several biometric parameters or indices (Table 3) have been devised and used, mainly by obstetricians, for early detection, diagnosis, or follow-up of IUGR pregnancies: thoracic and abdominal circumference (AC), weight, head circumference (HC), and length (Quaschino et al., 1986), in utero ponderal index (PI) (Yagel et al., 1986), mid-arm circumference to head circumference ratio (Patterson & Pouliot, 1987), mean hemoglobin concentration (Huisman & Aarnoudse, 1986), height of the frontal lobes (Battisti, Bach, & Gerard, 1986), and the transverse cerebellar diameter (Reece, Goldstein, Pilu, & Hobbins, 1987).

Since the current classical definition of IUGR based only on birth weight below 2,500 g has certain limitations, Sabbagha et al. (1976) and Sabbagha (1978) have expanded the IUGR definition to include certain other criteria which are relevant to the outcome of the IUGR process.

The following criteria by Sabbagha included three groups of fetuses. Group 1 includes fetuses with a biparietal diameter (BPD) falling in the range percentile 90–75 who have a 3.5% birth predictability of IUGR. Group 2 includes fetuses with a BPD falling in the range percen-

tile 75–25 who have a 10% birth predictability of IUGR. Group 3 includes fetuses with BPD falling in the range percentile 25 or less who have a 52.1% birth predictability of IUGR. Therefore, an early diagnosis of IUGR can be made when the growth rate of the above biometric parameter declines from one percentile group range to another, after at least two consecutive ultrasound measurements (Sabbagha, 1978; Sabbagha et al., 1976).

In trying to assess the influence of adverse conditions in utero that may affect body growth, brain growth, or both, the brain weight:body weight ratio can be used as an index for the severity of the IUGR process. Based on this ratio, a *cephalization index* (CI) has been proposed to express the degree of brain maturity and possible vulnerability in relation to gestational age and IUGR (Harel, Tomer, Barak, Binderman, & Yavin, 1985; Harel, Yavin, Tomer, Barak, & Binderman, 1985). The *intrauterine cephalization index* (IUCI), the ratio between head circumference and estimated fetal weight, can be calculated and determined in each Sabbagha percentile group range. Therefore, a "symmetrical" IUCI defines the head circumference and the estimated fetal weight within the same group range. "Asymmetrical" IUCI defines the head circumference and the estimated fetal weight in two different group ranges.

The *fetal biophysical score* (FBS), which involves measurement of several fetal biophysical parameters in concert, has been found useful to predict fetal compromise (Hill & Volpe, 1989a). Reduction in quantity and quality of *fetal motor activity* (Bekedam, Visser, de Vries, & Prechtl, 1985), and delay in the appearance of *behavioral states* (van Vliet, Martin, Nijhuis, & Prechtl, 1985) have also been described in the growth-retarded fetuses.

Doppler ultrasound has been applied to assess blood flow in both the umbilical and uteroplacental circulation. This technique can contribute much to the understanding of pathophysiology of pregnancy-induced hypertension and fetal growth retardation (Gabbe, 1988; Maulik & McMellis, 1987). In the mid-1980s, measurement of the fetal carotid artery reflecting cerebral blood flow has been facilitated by color doppler ultrasonography. In the growth-retarded fetus, resistance was found to be decreased in the cerebral circulation and increased in the umbilical-uteroplacental vasculature, suggesting an increase in peripheral vascular resistance and a compensatory reduction in vascular resistance in the fetal brain (i.e., a "brain sparing" effect in the presence of a chronic fetal insult) (Hill & Volpe, 1989b; Vladimiroff, Tonge, & Stewart, 1986).

NEURODEVELOPMENTAL OUTCOME

Methodology and Considerations

Choosing a Reliable Index To Identify IUGR Pre- and Perinatally Indices of IUGR and their predictive values are summarized in Table 4.

Ponderal Index (PI) The in utero PI (the ratio of the estimated fetal weight to the third power of the femur length), was found to be sensitive to neonatal distress (Yagel et al., 1987). Nevertheless, the in utero PI was not highly specific or sensitive for detecting IUGR, as measured after birth (Brown, Miller, Gabert, & Kissling, 1987).

Some investigators related their follow-up on IUGR babies to the postnatal PI. Children who were born with a low postnatal PI suffered more from neurodevelopmental abnormalities at school age, such as motor and perceptual difficulties, compared with those born with a normal PI (Calame et al. 1986). In another study, low PI newborns scored less in the Brazelton neonatal behavior assessment scales (Als, Tronick, Adamson, & Brazelton, 1976). Although they did well in Denver screening tests at a later stage, they indeed had behavioral and sleep problems. Another follow-up study also failed to show a difference in the performance in the Denver test among IUGR children between those born with a low and normal PI (Tenovou et al., 1988).

Biparietal Diameter (BPD) and Head Circumference The growth rate of the BPD in utero was a better predictor of developmen-

tal outcome (Fancourt, Campbell, & Harvey, 1976; Harvey, Prince, Bunton, Parkinson, & Campbell, 1982). Children whose BPD growth decelerated before the 26th week of pregnancy achieved less in cognitive, perceptual, and motor skills, compared with control, although not in subnormal levels (mean development quotient [DQ] of 93 compared to 102 in the control).

Head to Abdominal Circumference The head to abdominal circumference ratio, especially when combined with the ponderal index, was sensitive as well (Patterson & Pouliot, 1987).

Birth Weight Most of the follow-up studies on IUGR babies related their findings to the birth weight, though this parameter is accepted as nonspecific and nonsensitive. Among 20,000 children, severe mental retardation could be significantly related to birth weight under the 10th percentile (Rantakallio, 1985), yet less severe disabilities could not. This collosal study included a nonhomogeneous population so that any conclusions must be drawn very cautiously. Nevertheless, review of collaborative studies of the National Institute of Health did confirm that birth weight, as a single biologic parameter, could later predict the neurodevelopmental outcome of children, aside from the socio-economical and cultural background (Harel, Tomer, & Rabinovitz, 1989). In contrast, a follow-up study of children born with appropriate and inappropriate low-birth weight to gestational age, could not find differences in learning ability, motor and language skills, and attention span, between the two groups (Low et al., 1982).

Adolescents who were born as full-term babies with low birth weight (SGA) achieved less than the control group in cognitive, verbal, reading, and arithmetic skills. Yet, their scores were not in the subnormal range (Westwood, Kramer, Munz, Lovett, & Watters, 1983). In another study, similar differences between children born SGA and appropriate for gestational age (AGA) were not found (Als et al., 1976). In a study of twins, the smaller of the twins scored consistently less than their heavier

Table 4. Indices of IUGR and their predictive value

Index	Prediction	Outcome	Author
In utero ponderal index (PI)	Sensitive, nonspecific	Perinatal morbidity	Yagel, Zacut, Igelstein, Palti, Hurwitz, and Rosen (1987)
Postnatal PI	Significant	Learning, perception, motor skills	Calame, Fawer, Claeys, Arrazola, Ducret, and Jaunin (1986)
Postnatal PI	Significant	Brazelton assessment scale, behavioral trends in babies	Als, Tronick, Adamson, and Brazelton (1976)
Postnatal PI	Insignificant	Performance on Denver test	Tenouvo, Kero, Korventranta, Piekkala, Sillanpaa, and Erkkola (1988)
Postnatal PI	Nonspecific, VLBW	Physical growth	Brandt (1985)
Head circumference (HC)	Significant	When affected before 26 weeks, lower cognitive skills	Fancourt, Campbell, and Harvey (1976)
Biparietal diameter (BPD)	Significant	When affected before 26 weeks, lower mental function and motor skills	Harvey, Prince, Bunton, Parkinson, and Campbell (1982)
Head circumference: abdominal circumference (HC:AC)	Significant	Perinatal mortality	Patterson and Pouliost (1987)
birth weight (BW)	Significant in preterm and term	Rate of mortality, severe mental retardation	Rantakallio (1985)
	Insignificant in preterm and term	School achievement and IQ	
BW	Insignificant	Learning, motor skills, language, hyperactivity, attention span	Low, Galbraith, Muir, Killen, Pater, and Karchmar (1982)
BW	Significant	Growth and learning skills	Westwood, Kramer, Munz, Lovett, and Watters (1983)
BW	Insignificant in term	Learning skills	Als, Tronick, Adamson, and Brazelton (1976)
BW	Significant in term, insignificant premature	Performance on Denver test	Tenouvo, Kero, Korvenranta, Piekkala, Sillanpaa, and Erkkola (1985)
BW	Significant in smaller of monozygous co-twins	Delayed growth and reduced intelligence	Henrichsen, Skinhoj, and Andersen (1986)
Very low birth weight (VLBW)	Insignificant in premature	Neurodevelopmental disability	Haas, Asprion, Buchwald-Saal, and Mentzel (1986)
VLBW	Insignificant in premature	DQ	Arad and Nezer (1990)
VLBW	Significant in premature	Motor, visual, and perceptual skills	Matilainen, Heinonen, Siren-Tiusanen, Jokela, and Launiala (1987)
	Insignificant	School achievement	
VLBW	Significant in premature	Neurodevelopmental problems	Calame, Fawer, Claeys, Arrazola, Ducret, and Jaunin (1986)

(continued)

Table 4.   (continued)

Index	Prediction	Outcome	Author
BW	Insignificant	Perinatal, morbidity	Patterson, Prihodar, Gibbs, and Wood (1986)
BW	Significant	Motor, language, and cognitive skills, not after 4 years of age	Gerhard, Vollmar, Runnenbaum, and Kubli (1987)
Skin fold thickness	Significant	Development and performance at school age	Hill, Verniaud, Deter, Pennyson, and Reppig (1984)
Cephalization index	Significant for term only	Severe neurodevelopmental disability	Harel, Tomer, Barak, Binderman, and Yavin (1985)

From Harel, S., Tal-Posener, E., Kutai, M., Tomer, A., Jaffa, A., Zuk, L., and Yavin, E. (1991). Intrauterine growth retardation and brain development: Part II: Neurodevelopmental outcome. *International Pediatrics*, 6, 115; reprinted by permission.

brothers, although again not in the subnormal levels (Henrichsen, Skinhoj, & Andersen, 1986).

It appears that the prognostic validity of certain IUGR indices differs between full term and premature babies (Patterson, Prihoda, Gibbs, & Wood, 1986). The birth weight alone was not a significant prognostic factor among very low birth weight (VLBW) babies (Arad & Nezer, 1990; Haas, Asprion, Buchwald-Saal, & Mentzel, 1986). Other studies reported low achievements in several tests of children born as premature SGA as compared with premature AGA, especially concerning motor visual and perceptual skills (Matilainen, Heinonen, Siren-Tiusanen, Jokela, & Launiala, 1987), and neurodevelopmental problems (Calame et al., 1986). In the latter study, school failure could not be related to SGA versus AGA among children born prematurely. Tenovou et al. (1988) also found that while preschool children born as full-term SGA babies performed less well than their AGA peers in the Denver screening tests, such differences were not demonstrated among prematurely born children.

Skin Fold Thickness   The postnatal diagnosis of IUGR is not less perplexing. Hill et al. (1984), found that the clinical assessment of poor subcutaneous fat and general "thin" appearance were better predictors of later outcome than birth weight percentiles. Weight percentiles are not consistent predictors. Forty-

five percent of Hill's IUGR newborns weighed above 10th percentile.

The Cephalization Index (CI)   The cephalization index or the head circumference to body weight ratio is a rational index for asymmetric IUGR, reflecting brain vulnerability. The higher the brain:body ratio, or the CI, the more severe the IUGR process and the greater the risk for the brain to be affected (Harel, Tomer, et al., 1985; Harel, Yavin, et al., 1985). In other processes leading to symmetric IUGR, the CI does not increase as all organs are uniformly affected. The CI can be measured in utero as the ratio of head circumference to estimated fetal weight. In two previous studies the CI in IUGR animal and human newborns was assessed. In the first study on an experimental ischemic rabbit model (Harel, Yavin, et al., 1985), the results showed that the CI can be used as an indicator for the degree to which brain maturity and possible vulnerability are affected by vascular-induced IUGR. These restricted IUGR newborn rabbits disclosed neurodevelopmental problems such as learning disabilities (Teng et al., 1976), and delay in neuromotor skills acquisition (Harel et al., 1978). In a retrospective human clinical study (Harel, Tomer, et al., 1985), the newborn CI was correlated with long-term neurodevelopment. A trend could be delineated: the higher the CI, reflecting a greater degree of brain vulnerability, the later the gestational age, the more severe the clinical pathology—especially the likelihood of cerebral palsy and severe psychomotor retardation (Figure 1).

Assessment of the Socio-familial, Environmental, Pregnancy, Labor, and Neonatal Risk

A fruitful "optimality concept" as a method of risk scoring, which has proven its practicability and efficiency, was introduced by Prechtl (1982). He pointed out the following facts: pre- and perinatal complications are poorly defined; a clear distinction from the normal is often difficult; complications may vary from mild to se-

vere; and they rarely occur alone, sometimes being conditional on other risk factors. For instance, toxemia of pregnancy is not only high blood pressure, but also weight gain, edema, protein in urine, SGA newborn, hypoglycemia, and seizures. Another example is a single young unmarried mother who could also be conditional for other risk factors such as: low socio-economic status, previous abortions, poor sanitary care during pregnancy, cigarette smoking, alcohol or drug intake, prematurity and low birth weight, high rate of perinatal complications, incompetent mother. It is difficult, therefore, to define a certain condition as

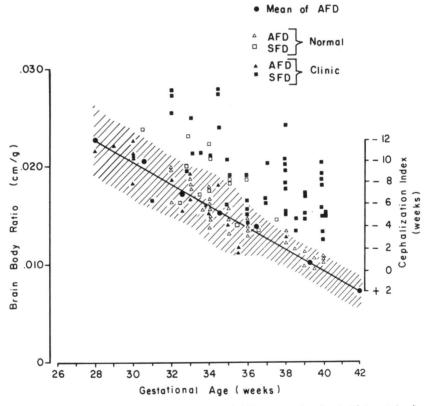

Figure 1. Brain(cm):body(g) ratios at birth, from three categories of children, were plotted against their gestational age. The first category, mean of AFD (●), consists of 70 normal newborns at different gestational ages (weeks) whose H.C.:BoW ratios were obtained at 3 days. The mean values were used to draw the "normal" line. The shaded area represents ± 2 SE. From this "normal" curve it is possible to extrapolate on the y-axis a cephalization index (CI = weeks) that expresses brain maturity and possible vulnerability (see text). The second category, "normal," consists of 44 (Δ) AFD and (□) SFD children (below 2,500 g) from a "well baby care" station, showing normal development after 1 year of age. The third category, "clinic," consists of 14 (▲) AFD and 47 (■) SFD children referred to a neuropediatric service for a variety of reasons, selected only because their birth weight was below 2,500 g. Most children (36/44) in the "normal" category follow the curve in the normal range (± 2SE—shaded area). All the AFD "clinic" children displayed "mild" symptomatology not clearly related to brain damage and their CI fell within the normal range. In the SFD "clinic" children, a trend could be delineated: in the later gestational age (38–40 weeks), the higher the CI (reflecting a greater degree of brain vulnerability), the more severe was the clinical pathology, especially the likelihood of brain damage such as cerebral palsy and severe psychomotor retardation ($P < 0.01$).

positively pathological or abnormal. It is sim-
pler to define an optimal range for a specific
condition. This concept is also useful since it
takes into account the cumulative effect of several coincidental, unfavorable factors. Therefore, the more meaningful the clinical event is,
the more nonoptimal conditions are present,
and the more at risk the infant is. One can thus
compose a risk questionnaire consisting of
items well defined, with regard to the condition
in question. Each item can be in an optimal or
suboptimal state. The definition of when an
item is "optimal" and when it is "suboptimal"
must be completely clear. In the normal population, most of the items will be "optimal,"
with the exception of a small random number
of items. In a true pathological condition, this
number will increase significantly, due to accumulation of damaging interrelated factors.
Thus, each item simply gets one point when it
is suboptimal, and at the end of the questionnaire, one simply counts these points. The total
number of the suboptimal items is defined as
the risk score. Prechtl's method is advantageous in several ways: 1) phenonema are di-
chotomically scored, without having to deal
with the problems of rating; therefore, more validity and reproducibility of the results are expected; 2) the final score is numerical; therefore, accessible to simple statistical analysis;
and 3) it is sensitive, but not specific, because
no special attention is given to the different
suboptimal items, only to the final score.

Assessment of the
Neonatal Neurobehavioral State

The classical neurobehavioral assessments of
the newborn (NBAN) are based on items collected by well-known investigators. The motor–
tone items are derived from the studies of
Thomas, Chesni, and Saint-Anne Dargassies
(1960) and Amiel-Tison and Grenier (1980),
and were later adopted by Dubowitz and Dubowitz (1981). The five arousal states and their
influence on the newborn's performance were
defined by Prechtl and Beintema (1964). They
added items concerning spontaneous activity,

reflexes, postures, and responses. With these
examinations Prechtl and Beintema could define hyperexcitable, apathic, and hemisyn-
dromes. Brazelton (1973) shed light on higher
functions and emphasized the response and habituation to animate and inanimate stimuli, as
well as the concept of organization and modulation of the newborn's responses to the changing environment (Als & Brazelton, 1981).

Combinations based on these tests are reported. Allen and Caputo (1989) reported on
ability to detect risk for cerebral palsy with
specificity of 69% and sensitivity of 80%. Dubowitz et al. (1984) emphasized the prognostic
importance of the NBAN as compared with ultrasonographic studies of intraventricular hemorrhage. The abovementioned studies demonstrated several weaknesses: they require
scoring for each item on different scales (Brazelton, 1973; Dubowitz et al., 1984; Prechtl &
Beintema, 1964), or nonnumerical scoring
(Dubowitz et al., 1984), which makes it difficult to achieve consistency between examiners;
some works have items for subjective impression (Allen & Caputo, 1989); and their predictive value is not clear.

Preliminary Research Results

The authors' research project was based on the
following methods, taking into consideration
the methodological approaches as previously
discussed.

A population of IUGR newborns is being
followed-up from the prenatal stage to postnatally. The study group comprised 52 newborns, born between September 1989 and June
1991, at the Serlin Maternity Hospital of the Tel
Aviv Medical Center. Since asymmetric IUGR
is the most common in our population, the criteria for choosing them were any newborn who
weighed less than the 10th percentile for his
gestational age, and any whose CI was above
the normal range previously published (Harel,
Tomer, et al., 1985). The control group consisted of 94 AGA term newborns who were randomly selected at the nursery during the period
mentioned above. The social, familial, preg-

nancy, and labor history, as well as the neonatal course, is under consideration, all by optimality questionnaires.

The study group was assessed in utero, pre- and postnatally, in three ways: 1) biometric ultrasonographic measurements, 2) optimality high risk questionnaires, and 3) the NBAN. The control group was followed in the same way. However, since they were followed from birth only, no ultrasonographic information is available.

The questionnaires and NBAN were composed according to Prechtl's "optimality concept." The four high-risk questionnaires included socio-familial, obstetric, ultrasonographic, and neonatal.

In order to examine the newborns in an objective and reproducible way, the best neurobehavioral representative items from each of the well-established newborn examinations (Amiel-Tison & Grenier, 1980; Brazelton, 1973; Dubowitz & Dubowitz, 1981; Prechtl & Beintema, 1964), were collected and adopted, organizing them in an order that follows the expected changes in the baby's arousal state (as was found after a short run in normal newborns), and scoring them according to Prechtl's optimality concept. Nonreproducible items were avoided and an attempt was made to avoid repeating similar ones; items representing most aspects of the neurodevelopmental spectrum were included. The benefits of this approach are comprehensiveness, easy scoring, and quantitative analysis. Such an examination can be easily utilized in a busy newborn clinic for daily use, and demands only 15 minutes of the physician's time.

The NBAN included 48 items, adopted from the classical NBAN, as mentioned above, and covered the spectrum of tone, spontaneous movements and postures, responses and habituation to animate and inanimate stimuli, primary reflexes, and items related to neurological pathology. The newborns were examined at 24–48 hours after birth, and for prematures, at least at 37 weeks postconception. The environmental conditions (light, noise, temperature) were kept at optimal range. The babies were examined 1.5–2 hours after meals in order to have them in an optimal and controlled arousal state.

Intraexaminer variability of the NBAN was checked by repeating the NBAN of 20 of the control newborns on two separate occasions by the same physician. Interexaminer variability was checked by having each of the 20 newborns examined by three physicians on three different occasions.

The biometric parameters characterizing each group are presented in Table 5, showing significant differences in all of them. The deviation of the CI of the IUGR group in relation to standard values corrected for gestational age, as published previously (Harel, Tomer, et al., 1985), was also significant.

The risk scores of the questionnaires and NBAN of the control and study groups are presented in Table 6, showing significant differences in all but the socio-familial questionnaire. Although a higher prevalence of IUGR in the low socio-economic population was expected, the similarity of the socio-familial questionnaire was anticipated, as the population comes from social environments which receive similar pre- and perinatal medical care.

As shown in Table 7, a differentiation was

Table 5. Biometric parameters of the two groups

Group	n	Control	n	IUGR	P
Gestational age (w)	95	39.15 ± 4.42	52	36.13 ± 5.83	<0.01
Birth weight (g)	95	3352 ± 395	51	1796 ± 431	<0.01
Height (cm)	95	44.31 ± 16.55	52	38.06 ± 13.43	<0.05
Head circumference (cm)	95	33.21 ± 7.28	52	29.58 ± 4.78	<0.01
CI (cm/g × 10²)	95	1.00 ± 0.24	51	1.76 ± 0.39	<0.01

From Harel, S., Tal-Posener, E., Kutai, M., Tomer, A., Jaffa, A., Zuk, L., and Yavin, E. (1991). Intrauterine growth retardation and brain development: Part II: Neurodevelopmental outcome. *International Pediatrics, 6*, 118; reprinted by permission.

Table 6. Mean risk scores of the two groups[a]

Group	n	Control	n	IUGR	P
Sociofamilial risk score	95	10.52 ± 7.54	52	11.46 ± 7.39	N.S.
Obstetrical risk score	95	13.88 ± 7.38	52	20.64 ± 8.28	<0.01
Ultrasonographic risk score	—		33	42.09 ± 23.28	—
Neonatal risk score	95	0.78 ± 2.55	51	23.38 ± 10.87	<0.01
Total mean risk score[b]	95	9.42 ± 4.38	51	18.30 ± 6.07	<0.01
Neurobehavioral score	95	5.30 ± 3.40	51	10.37 ± 7.38	<0.01

From Harel, S., Tal-Posener, E., Kutai, M., Tomer, A., Jaffa, A., Zuk, L., and Yavin, E. (1991). Intrauterine growth retardation and brain development: Part II: Neurodevelopmental outcome. *International Pediatrics, 6,* 119; reprinted by permission.

[a]Presented are the mean percentage ± standard deviations of suboptimal items out of the total number of items in each questionnaire.

[b]Total mean risk score is the mean percentage ± standard deviation of suboptimal items in sociofamilial, obstetrical, and neonatal risk questionnaires.

attempted between the premature and the term newborns in the IUGR group. There was a significant difference in all parameters and risk scores besides the sociofamilial risk score and the neurobehavioral score.

CONCLUSIONS

The following conclusions have been drawn from this preliminary study:

1. An asymmetric IUGR population can be successfully identified by measuring their CI, pre- and postnatally. This parameter may reflect a degree of brain maturity and vulnerability probably due to damage caused to the fetus in utero and perinatally, as reflected by high-risk questionnaires,

composed according to Prechtl's "optimality concept."

2. A neurobehavioral examination of the newborn, also based on Prechtl's "optimality concept," with items representing the best classical known examinations, can identify increased risk and differentiate IUGR from normal newborns. This neurobehavioral examination has proved to be valid in inter- and intra-examiner comparisons.

Finally, in order to estimate the predictive value of the risk questionnaires, the CI and the NBAN, an increasing number of patients are required, additional physio-biochemical parameters will be used and further longitudinal studies will be performed. However, in spite of this comprehensive approach, the warning

Table 7. The difference between IUGR-PREM and IUGR-TERM groups

	n	IUGR-PREM	n	IUGR-TERM	P
Mean birth weight (g)	19	1364 ± 269	29	2081 ± 271	<0.01
Mean head circumference (cm)	19	28.24 ± 1.51	29	31.39 ± 1.43	<0.01
Mean CI (cm/gr × 10[2])	19	2.13 ± 0.35	25	1.53 ± 0.19	<0.01
Socio-familial risk score	19	12.00 ± 7.18	29	10.75 ± 7.56	N.S.
Obstetric risk score	19	25.86 ± 6.40	29	17.36 ± 8.12	<0.01
Ultrasound risk score	11	61.64 ± 18.23	20	33.04 ± 18.28	<0.01
Neonatal risk score	19	31.64 ± 8.45	29	18.32 ± 9.45	<0.01
Total mean risk score	19	22.87 ± 4.08	29	15.48 ± 5.48	<0.01
Neurobehavioral score	19	9.64 ± 7.02	29	10.12 ± 6.85	N.S.

From Harel, S., Tal-Posener, E., Kutai, M., Tomer, A., Jaffa, A., Zuk, L., and Yavin, E. (1991). Intrauterine growth retardation and brain development: Part II: Neurodevelopmental outcome. *International Pediatrics, 6,* 119; reprinted by permission.

The risk scores are presented as the percentage ± standard deviations of suboptimal items out of total number of items in each Risk Questionnaire and in the neurobehavioral score.

of Prechtl (1982) should be remembered,: " . . . to judge the validity of the neonatal examination only on the criterion of long term prediction of neurological impairment is misleading and was certainly overemphasized in the past. There are too many factors which influence the prognosis of early signs in an unpredictable way" (p. 47).

REFERENCES

Als, H., & Brazelton, T.B. (1981). A new model of assessing the behavioural organization in preterm and fullterm infants. *Journal of the American Academy of Child Psychiatry*, 20, 239–262.

Als, H., Tronick, E., Adamson, L., & Brazelton, B.T. (1976). The behaviour of the full term yet underweight newborn infant. *Developmental Medicine and Child Neurology*, 18, 590–602.

Allen, M.C. (1986). Developmental outcome and follow-up of the small-for-gestational-age children. *Seminars in Perinatology*, 8(2), 123–156.

Allen, M.C., & Capute, A.J. (1989). Neonatal neurodevelopmental examination as a predictor of neuromotor outcome in premature infants. *Pediatrics*, 83(4), 498–506.

Amiel-Tison, C., & Grenier, A. (Eds.). (1980). *Neurologic evaluation of the newborn and the infant*. Paris: Masson Publishing USA.

Arad, I., & Nezer, D. (1990). Growth and development of very-low-birth-weight infants. *Harefuah*, 118(1), 1–5.

Band, H. (1978). Neonatal problems of infants with intrauterine growth retardation. *Journal of Reproductive Medicine*, 21, 359–364.

Battaglia, F.C. (1970). Intrauterine growth retardation. *American Journal of Obstetrics and Gynecology*, 106, 1103–1114.

Battisti, O., Bach, A., & Gerard, P. (1986). Brain growth in sick newborn infants: a clinical and real-time ultrasound analysis. *Early Human Development*, 13(1), 13–20.

Bekedam, D.J., Visser, G.H.A., de Vries, J.J., & Prechtl, H.F.R. (1985). Motor behaviour in the growth retarded fetus. *Early Human Development*, 12, 155–165.

Brar, H.S., & Rutherford, S.E. (1988). Classification of intrauterine growth retardation. *Seminars in Perinatology*, 12 (1), 2–10.

Brazelton, T.B. (1973). Neonatal behavioural assessment scale. In *Clinical Developmental Medicine 50*, London: Heinemann.

Brown, H.L., Miller, J.M., Gabert, H.A., & Kissling, G. (1987). Ultrasonic recognition of the small for gestational age fetus. *Obstetrics and Gynecology*, 69(4), 631–635.

Calame, A., Fawer, C.L., Claeys, V., Arrazola, I., Ducret, S., & Jaunin, L. (1986). Neurodevelopmental outcome and school performance of very-low-birth weight infants at 8 years of age. *European Journal of Paediatrics*, 145(6), 461–466.

Chanez, C., Privat, A., Flexor, M.A., & Drian, M.J. (1985). Release of polyunsaturated fatty acids from phospholipids and alteration of brain membrane integrity by oxygen-derived free radicals. *Journal of Neuroscience Research*, 12, 595–605.

Creasy, R.K., Barrett, C.T., Deswilt, M., Kahanpaa, K.V., & Rudolph, A.M. (1972). Experimental intrauterine growth retardation in the sheep. *American Journal of Obstetrics & Gynecology*, 112, 566–573.

Dadak, C., Kefalides, A., Sinzeringer, H., & Giorgow, W. (1982). Reduced umbilical artery prostacyclin formation in complicated pregnancies. *American Journal of Obstetrics & Gynecology*, 144, 792–795.

Drillien, C.M. (1970). The small for date. Etiology and prognosis. *Pediatric Clinics of North America*, 17, 19–24.

Dubowitz, L.M.S., & Dubowitz, V. (1981). The neurological assessment of the preterm and fullterm newborn infants. *Clinics in Developmental Medicine, No. 79*, London: Spastics International Medical Publication, Blackwell (UK); Philadelphia: J.B. Lippincott (USA).

Dubowitz, L.M.S., Dubowitz, V., & Goldberg, C.G. (1970). Clinical assessment of gestational age of the newborn infant. *Journal of Pediatrics*, 77, 1–10.

Dubowitz, L.M.S., Dubowitz, V., Palmer, P.G., Miller, G., Fawer, C.I., & Levene, M.I. (1984). Correlation of neurologic assessment in the preterm newborn infant with outcome at 1 year. *Journal of Pediatrics*, 155, 452–456.

Emmanovilides, G.C., Townsend, D.E., & Bauer, R.A. (1968). Effects of single umbilical artery ligation in the lamb fetus. *Pediatrics*, 42, 919–927.

Fancourt, R., Campbell, S., & Harvey, D. (1976). Follow-up study of small-for date babies. *British Medical Journal 1*, 1435–1437.

Fitzhardinge, P., & Steven E. (1972). The small-for-date infant. I. Later growth patterns. *Pediatrics*, 49, 671–681.

Gabbe, S.G. (Guest ed.). (1988). Obstetric ultrasound update. In *Clinical Obstetrics and Gynecology*, 31(1), 1–2.

Haas, G., Asprion, B., Buchwald-Saal, M., & Mentzel, H. (1986). Obstetrical and neonatal risk factors in very low birth weight infants related to their neurological development. *European Journal of Pediatrics*, 145, 341–346.

Harel, S., Shapira, Y., Hartzler, J., Teng, E.L., Quilligan, E., & Van der Meulen, J.P. (1978). Neuromotor development in relation to birth weight in rabbit. *Biology of the Neonate*, 33, 1–7.

Harel, S., Shapira, Y., Tomer, A., Donahue, M.J., & Quilligan, E. (1985). Vascular induced intrauterine growth retardation: Relations between birth weight and the development of biochemical parameters in young rabbits. *Israel Journal of Medical Sciences*, 21, 829–832.

Harel, S., Tal-Posener, E., Kutai, M., Tomer, A., Jaffa, A., Zuk, L., & Yavin, E. (1991). Intrauterine growth retardation and brain development; Part I: Pre and perinatal diagnosis. *International Pediatrics*, 6, 109–120.

Harel, S., Tomer, A., Barak, Y., Binderman, J., & Yavin, E. (1985). The Cephalization Index: A screening device for brain maturity and vulnerability in normal and intra-uterine growth-retarded newborns. *Brain and Development, 7(6)*, 580–584.

Harel, S., Tomer, A., & Rabinovitz, G. (1989). The high-risk infant: A classical model for prevention, identification, assessment and treatment of children with risk for developmental disabilities: A plan for interaction of community and medical center resources. In J.H. French, S. Harel, & P. Casaer (Eds.), *Child neurology and developmental disabilities: Selected proceedings of the Fourth International Child Neurology Congress* (pp. 199–207). Baltimore: Paul H. Brookes Publishing Co.

Harel, S., Watanabe, K., Linke, I., & Schain, R.J. (1972). Growth and development of the rabbit brain. *Biology of the Neonate, 21*, 381–399.

Harel, S., Yavin, E., Barak, Y., Tomer, A., & Binderman, I. (1981). The cephalization index: A new developmental indicator for brain maturity. In M. Monset-Couchard & A. Minkowski (Eds.), *Physiological and biochemical basis for perinatal medicine* (pp. 314–322). Basel: S. Karger.

Harel, S., Yavin, E., Tomer, A., Barak, Y., & Binderman, I. (1985). Brain:body ratio and conceptional age in vascular-induced intrauterine growth retarded rabbits. *Brain and Development, 7*, 575–579.

Harvey, D., Prince, J., Bunton, J., Parkinson, C., & Campbell, S. (1982). Abilities of children who were small for gestational age babies. *Pediatrics, 69(3)*, 296–300.

Henrichsen, L., Skinhoj, S., & Andersen, G.E. (1986). Delayed growth and reduced intelligence in 7–19 year old intrauterine growth retarded children, compared with their monozygous co-twins. *Acta Paediatrica Scandinavica, 75*, 31–35.

Hill, A., & Volpe, J.J. (1989a). Commentary on chapter 6. In A. Hill & J.J. Volpe (Eds.), *Fetal neurology: International review of child neurology series* (pp. 117–119). New York: Raven Press.

Hill, A., & Volpe, J.J. (1989b). Commentary on chapter 7. In A. Hill & J.J. Volpe (Eds.), *Fetal neurology: International review of child neurology series* (pp. 139–141). New York: Raven Press.

Hill, D.E., Myers, A.B., Scott, R.E., & Cheek, D.B. (1971). Fetal growth retardation produced by experimental placental insufficiency in the rhesus monkey. *Biology of the Neonate, 19*, 68–82.

Hill, R.M., Verniaud, W.M., Deter, R.L., Pennyson, L.M., & Reppig, G.M. (1984). The effect of intrauterine malnutrition on the term infant—a 14 year progressive study, McCulley, L.B., Hill, L.L. *Acta Paediatrica Scandinavica, 73*, 482–487.

Ho, W., & Guy, J.A. (1971). Cellular growth in experimental intrauterine growth retardation in rats. *Journal of Nutrition, 101*, 1631–1633.

Holt, A.B., Cheek, D.B., Mellitis, D., & Hill, D.E. (1975). In D.B. Cheek (Ed.), *Fetal and postnatal cellular growth: Hormones and nutrition* (pp. 23–24). New York: John Wiley & Sons.

Huisman, A., & Aarnoudse, J.G. (1986). Increased 2nd trimester hemoglobin concentration in pregnancies later complicated by hypertension and growth retardation. Early evidence of a reduced plasma volume. *Acta Obstetrics and Gynecology Scandinavica, 65* (6), 605–608.

Lockwood, C.J., & Weiner, S. (1986). Assessment of fetal growth. *Clinical Perinatology, 13* (1), 3–35.

Long, P.A., Abell, D.A., & Beischer, N.A. (1980). Fetal growth retardation and preeclampsia. *British Journal of Obstetrics and Gynecology, 87*, 13–18.

Low, J.A., Galbraith, R.S., Muir, D., Killen, H., Pater, B., & Karchmar, J. (1982). Intrauterine growth retardation: a study of long term morbidity. *American Journal of Obstetrics and Gynecology, 142*, 670–677.

Lubchenco, L.O. (1970). Assessment of gestational age and development at birth. *Pediatric Clinics of North America, 17*, 125–145.

Matilainen, R., Heinonen, K., Siren-Tiusanen, H., Jokela, V., & Launiala, K. (1987). Neurodevelopmental screening of in utero growth-retarded prematurely born children before school age. *European Journal of Pediatrics, 146* (5), 453–457.

Maulik, D., & McMellis, D. (1987). Doppler ultrasound measurements of maternal-fetal hemodynamics. *Reproduction and Perinatology Medicine Series, 8*.

Minkowsky, A. (1973). Le retard de croissance intrauterine (Local hospital revue). Paris: *Hopital Port Royal, Revue*. 7–31.

Ounsted, M., Moar, V., & Scott, W.A. (1981). Perinatal morbidity and mortality in small-for-date babies: The relative importance of some maternal factors. *Early Human Development, 5*, 367.

Patterson, R.M., & Pouliot, M.R. (1987). Neonatal morphometrics and perinatal outcome: Who is growth retarded? *American Journal of Obstetrics and Gynecology, 157* (3), 691–693.

Patterson, R.M., Prihoda, T.J., Gibbs, C.E., & Wood, R.C. (1986). Analysis of birth weight percentile as a predictor of perinatal outcome. *Obstetrics and Gynecology, 68*, 459–463.

Prechtl, H., & Beintema, D. (Eds.). (1964). The neurological examination of the full term newborn infant. *Little Club Clinics in Developmental Medicine No. 12*. London: William Heinemann Medical Books Ltd.

Prechtl, H.F.R. (1982). Assessment methods for newborn infants: A critical evaluation. In P. Stratton (Ed.), *Psychology of the human newborn* (pp. 21–52). New York: John Wiley & Sons.

Quaschino, S., Spinillo, A., Stola, E., Pesando, P.C., Gancia, G.P., & Rondini, G. (1986). The significance of ponderal index as a prognostic factor in a low birth weight population. *Biologic Research in Pregnancy and Perinatalogy, 7* (3), 121–127.

Rantakallio, P. (1985). A 14 year follow-up of children with normal and abnormal birth weight for their gestational age. *Acta Paediatrica Scandinavica, 74* (1), 62–69.

Reece, E.A., Goldstein, I., Pilu, G., & Hobbins, J.C. (1987). Fetal cerebella growth unaffected by intrauterine growth retardation: a new parameter for prenatal diagnosis. *American Journal of Obstetrics and Gynecology, 157* (3), 632–638.

Rosso, P., & Winick, M. (1974). Intrauterine growth retardation. A new systematic approach based on the clinical and biochemical characteristics of this condition. *Journal of Perinatalogy Medicine, 2*, 147–156.

Roux, J.M. (1971). Studies on cellular development in the suckling rat with IUGR. *Biology of the Neonate, 18*, 290–297.

Sabbagha, R.E. (1978). Intrauterine growth retardation:

Antenatal diagnosis by ultrasound. *Obstetrics and Gynecology, 52*, 252.

Sabbagha, R.E., Barton, B.A., Barton, F.B., Kingas, E., Orgill, J., & Turner, H.J. (1976). Sonar biparietal diameter II. Predictive of three fetal growth patterns leading to a closer assessment of gestational age and neonatal weight. *American Journal of Obstetrics and Gynecology, 126*, 485–490.

Sweet, A.Y. (1986). Classification on the low-birth-weight infant. In M.H. Klaus & A.A. Fanaroff (Eds.), *Care of the high-risk neonate* (pp. 69–95). Philadelphia: W.B. Saunders.

Teng, E.L., Harel, S., Hartzler, J., Shapira, Y., Quilligan, E., & Van der Meulen, J.P. (1976). Relations between birth weight and learning ability in young rabbits. *Biology of the Neonate, 29*, 207–215.

Tenovou, A., Kero, P., Korvenranta, H., Piekkala, P., Sillanpaa, M., & Erkkola, R. (1988). Developmental outcome of 519 small for gestational age children at the age of 2 years. *Neuropediatrics, 19* (1), 41–45.

Thomas, A., Chesni, Y., & Saint-Anne Dargassies, S. (1960). The neurological examination of the infant. In R.C. MacKeith, P.E. Polani, & E. Clayton-Jones (Eds.). *Little Club Clinics in Developmental Medicine No. 1.* London: William Heinemann Medical Books Ltd.

Van Marthens, E., Harel, S., & Zamenhof, S. (1975). Experimental intrauterine growth retardation. A new animal model for the study of altered brain development. *Biology of the Neonate, 26*, 221–231.

van Vliet, M.A.T., Martin Jr., C.B., Nijhuis, J.G., & Prechtl, H.F.R. (1985). Behavioural states in growth-retarded human fetuses. *Early Human Development, 12*, 183–197.

Vladimiroff, J.W., Tonge, H.M., & Stewart, P.A. (1986). Doppler ultrasound assessment of cerebral blood flow in the human fetus. *British Journal of Obstetrics and Gynaecology, 93*, 471–475.

Walsh, S.W. (1985). Preeclampsia: An imbalance in placental prostacyclin and thromboxane production. *American Journal of Obstetrics and Gynecology, 152*, 335–340.

Westwood, M., Kramer, M.S., Munz, D., Lovett, J.M., & Watters, G.V. (1983). Growth and development of the full-term non asphyxiated small-for-gestational-age newborns: Follow-up through adolescence. *Pediatrics, 71* (3), 376–382.

Wigglesworth, J.S. (1964). Experimental growth retardation in the foetal rat. *Journal of Pathology and Bacteriology, 88*, 1–13.

Winick, M. (1971). Cellular changes during placental and fetal growth. *American Journal of Obstetrics and Gynecology, 109*, 166–176.

Yagel, S., Zacut, D., Igelstein, S., Palti, Z., Hurwitz, A., & Rosen, B. (1987). Ponderal index as a prognostic factor in the evaluation of intrauterine growth retardation. *American Journal of Obstetrics and Gynecology, 157*, 415–419.

Chapter 15

Neural Induction and Developmental Disorders of the Nervous System

HARVEY B. SARNAT, M.D., F.R.C.P. (C)
University of Washington, Seattle

T HE TERM *INDUCTION* IS THE INFLUENCE OF one developing tissue upon the differentiation of another. The induced target tissue always forms a different structure at maturity than the inducer itself becomes. Induction occurs at the time of gastrulation and the initial stages of induction are between the differentiating germ layers. The mesoderm is particularly influential upon the differentiation of neurectoderm from the general surface ectoderm, a process known as *neural induction*. In more advanced stages of early embryogenesis, induction occurs within a germ layer. An example is the optic cup, a neuroectodermal derivative, inducing the overlying surface ectoderm to form a lens placode and cornea rather than simply more epidermis.

Formation of the neural tube and maturation of the neuroepithelium is induced by the notochord, a derivative of the primitive streak and node. Mesodermal cells are formed by the primitive streak and egress through it to form masses on either side of the neural tube that soon become segmented as *somites*. From these somites, the dermatomes (primordium of the dermis of the skin), myotomes (incipient muscles), and sclerotomes (progenitors of the bony vertebrae) are formed, and these somites and the notochord together are termed the *chor-*

damesoderm. The notochord may act through other parts of the chordamesoderm, sclerotomal cells in particular, to induce neural tube maturation (Figure 1). Extracellular matrix proteins such as laminin and fibronectin actively separate the neurectoderm from the undifferentiated surface ectoderm that will form the epidermis (Poelmann et al., 1990).

Specificity in neural induction rests not with the inducer but rather with receptors on the surfaces of target cells (Duprat, Gualandris, Kan, Saint-Jeannet, & Boudannaoui, 1987; Grunz, 1985; Tiedemann, 1986). Inducers are generally peptides, small proteins, or carbohydrate-containing compounds such as proteoglycans. These molecules need not penetrate the cell being induced to trigger maturation, but simply must contact or attach to its outer surface.

The inductive process is intimately linked to the actual structure of the plasma membrane of the competent target tissue and the presence of possible receptor sites. Structural modification of the membrane of target cells prior to induction, such as molecular changes produced by lectins which have specific affinities for different carbohydrates, strongly inhibits neural induction (Duprat, Gualandris, & Rouge, 1982). This inhibition is reversible, and after a period of waiting about 20 hours while the normal

---

This chapter was supported by a grant to Dr. Harvey B. Sarnat by the M.S.I. Foundation of Alberta.

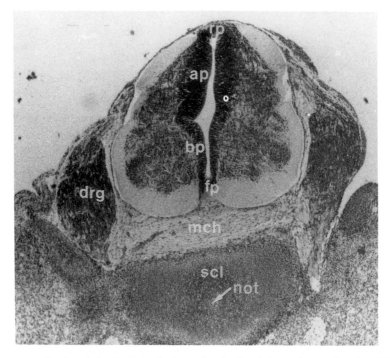

Figure 1. Transverse section through the developing lumbar region of a 6-week human fetus to show the relationships of the notochord (not) and spinal cord. A sclerotome (scl) is forming a vertebral body around the notochord and loose mesenchyme (mch) is interposed between it and the spinal cord. The notochord induces the neural tube to mature. The floor plate (fp) and roof plate (rp) ependyma differentiate early, whereas the neuroepithelium of the alar plate (ap) and basal plate (bp) differentiate later, allowing more mitotic proliferation of neuroblasts at the lateral sides of the central canal and contributing to its vertical slit-like shape in the fetus. The neural crest tissue has already separated from the neuroepithelium in the region of the roof plate and is forming dorsal root ganglia (drg). Hematoxylin-eosin. × 25.

membrane structure is restored by the new synthesis of glycoconjugates, induction may then proceed (Duprat et al., 1987; Gualandris, Rouge, & Duprat, 1983). An extracellular matrix rich in fibronectin and other glycoconjugates containing carbohydrates such as galactose, mannose, glucose, and fructose spreads over the inner surface of the ectodermal layer (Nieuwkoop, Johnen, & Albers, 1985) and plays a fundamental role in the morphogenetic movements during gastrulation (Boucaut et al., 1985), but is not required for the neural inductive process itself (Duprat & Gualandris, 1984). Neural induction is therefore an epigenetic phenomenon and is inextricably linked to complex interactions between cells requiring the recognition of external signals by the plasma membrane of the target cell. A chain of intracellular events is initiated that determines the differentiation of the cell along neural lines

(Duprat et al., 1987). The competent target tissue already possesses the potential and necessary capacities for neurulation.

Many unrelated foreign molecules may mimic the natural inducer and initiate their differentiation, creating a great potential for teratogenesis by substances to which an embryo or early fetus might be exposed and are toxic because of this capacity of acting as a substitute for the natural inducer. Thus, malformations of the developing nervous system may be induced by an abnormally formed notochord or chordamesoderm, or by the exogenous influence of substances that become teratogens by triggering neural induction at a time other than the time which was genetically programmed, thereby interrupting the normal sequence of development.

The early period of neural induction is the differentiation of neurectoderm from undifferentiated surface ectoderm. A later period of neural induction is the regional maturation of the ependyma from the primitive neuroepithelium of the neural tube. The floor plate is the first region to differentiate. It is located in the ventral midline of the spinal central canal, fourth ventricle, and cerebral aqueduct of the mesencephalon, immediately opposite the notochord, with only a loose mesenchyme intervening (Figure 1). If a segment of notochord from a chick embryo is homotopically transplanted to the region lateral to the developing neural tube at another segmental level, two floor plates are formed at that level, the normal floor plate opposite the natural notochord and a second, heterotopic floor plate on the lateral surface of the central canal induced by the ectopic notochord implant (van Straaten, Hekking, Wiertz-Hoessels, Thors, & Drukker, 1988). The remainder of the neuroepithelium lining the central canal remains undifferentiated and continues to exhibit a high rate of mitotic activity, whereas both floor plates are composed of fetal ependymal cells and mitotic activity is arrested. If a semiporous membrane is inserted between the notochord and the neural tube, a floor plate still forms, but if a nonpermeable substance or other tissue is interposed, the notochord is no longer able to induce the floor plate to differentiate from the neuroepithelium, demonstrating that the inducer is a diffusible molecule rather than a migrating cell or cytoplasmic extension.

The phenomenon of neural induction was discovered by Spemann and Mangold (1924) by demonstrating an interaction between different regions of the amphibian gastrula—the blastopore lip acts as the inducer and the target is the presumptive ectoderm dorsal to it. It was subsequently demonstrated that the process of neural induction is universal in embryonic vertebrates and occurs in most invertebrates as well. The hypothesis has been reconfirmed and proved by many independent investigators using many species. Details of the process are provided in several reviews (Brachet, 1985; Duprat et al., 1987; Nieuwkoop et al., 1985; Sarnat, 1992a).

DISTURBANCES OF NEURAL INDUCTION DUE TO A DEFECTIVE NOTOCHORD

The embryonic notochord occasionally becomes duplicated or longitudinally divided, a condition known as the *split notochord syndrome* (Bentley & Smith, 1960). The split notochord develops in the stage of the primitive streak when cells are already committed to germ layers; earlier abnormal division prior to gastrulation results in identical twinning (in animals with indeterminate, radial cleavage patterns including humans) or, if the unprogrammed division is incomplete, variable degrees of Siamese twinning occurs with duplication of some embryonic parts and sharing of others. The fusion of siamese twins is in the midline and usually follows a rostrocaudal or caudorostral gradient. The reason for the splitting of the primitive streak is not evident in most cases. Such duplication or splitting may occur at any level, but most often involves the posterior portion of the unsegmented notochord. Meningomyelocele or a simple meningocele may be associated (Ebisu et al., 1990), but is not always present. Duplication of the notochord may lead to neural induction of two complete spinal cords over several segments, a condition known as *diplomyelia* and associated with severe deformity of the bony spine, variable myelopathy, and radiculopathy (Roessmann, 1985; Sarnat, 1992a). If diplomyelia does not occur, a single spinal cord may show duplication of dorsal and/or ventral horns (Vinters & Gilbert, 1981). At more rostral levels, duplication of the pituitary gland or other midline structures of the brain may occur (Roessmann, 1985).

More commonly, the spinal cord is truly split, the two halves being separated by a septum of sequestered mesodermal tissue that differentiates as fibrous connective tissue, fat, cartilage or bone, the pathogenesis of *diastematomyelia*. This condition becomes progressive due to less rapid growth of neural tissue than the vertebral column, with progressive tethering of the spinal cord and myelopathy or stretching of nerve roots as the child continues to grow. Lipomas may be associated (Mann, Khosla, Gulai, & Malik, 1984). Not only mesenchyme, but also endodermal tissue from the embryonic yolk sac may become entrapped between the two halves of the split notochord and the split spinal cord, creating a fistula to the surface of the back or a sequestration of endodermal tissue within the spinal canal (intramedullary or extramedullary) that differentiates as intestinal mucosa and becomes a *neurenteric (enterogenous)* cyst or, less commonly, differentiates as bronchial epithelium to become a *neurobronchial cyst* (Bentley & Smith, 1960; Ho & Tiel, 1989; Mizuno, Fiandaca, Nishio, & O'Brien, 1988; Sarnat, 1992b; Vinters & Gilbert, 1981). The concept developed in the late 19th century that the neurenteric cyst results from persistence of the embryonic neurenteric canal is erroneous. The neurenteric canal is a hypothetical communication between the yolk sac (which becomes the gastrointestinal tract) and the space (the amniotic sac in reptiles, birds, and mammals) overlying the neural placode. This communication passes through the blastopore, or primitive pit, the incipient anus of the deuterostomes. It may exist briefly in lower chordates such as amphioxus and perhaps amphibians, but probably does not form even transiently in avian and mammalian embryos and cannot be invoked to explain any human embryopathies. Because neurenteric cysts produce mucin and secretory products as do the normal mature intestinal mucosal cells, they have an extremely variable clinical presentation and may be silent for years, then manifesting as either mass lesions compressing the spinal cord or brainstem, or producing radiculopathy. The mucus secretions of the goblet cells may cause a chemical meningitis if the neurenteric cyst ruptures and its contents exude into the spinal canal.

In the split notochord syndrome, mesodermal tissues of the developing splanchnomesoderm may become entrapped between the halves of the forming vertebral bodies. The splanchnomesoderm normally becomes the mesenteries. Entrapment by a split notochord results in inability of the bowel to rotate during fetal life and a volvulus forms. Children presenting with congenital malrotation of the bowel should therefore have careful imaging studies of the spine and neurological examination because the volvulus may be due to a split notochord syndrome.

Sacral agenesis, absence or hypoplasia of the sacrum, and sometimes a variable number of lumbar, thoracic, or even cervical vertebral bodies, are probably due to a defective notochord. Neural induction is often abnormal as well, so that the neural tissue of the spinal cord is severely disorganized (Sarnat, 1992a; Sarnat, Case, & Graviss, 1976; Towfighi & Housman, 1991). Clinical neurological deficits involve ventral roots and spare dorsal roots, which are derived from neural crest tissue and are less dependent upon notochordal induction; primary amyoplasia or absence of muscle is often associated because the same defective chordamesoderm that fails to form sclerotomes for the development of vertebrae also fails to form myotomes for muscle development in the corresponding segmental distribution, usually sacral. Autonomic deficiencies including neurogenic bladder are variable (Sarnat et al., 1976).

The Klippel-Feil deformity, in which usually cervical vertebrae are "fused," is really a failure of segmentation of the sclerotomes, but is not due to a split notochord and is not associated with spinal cord or nerve root abnormalities.

ROLE OF THE FETAL EPENDYMA IN BRAIN DEVELOPMENT

The ependyma is often perceived as a mere lining of the ventricular system, more decorative than functional, though perhaps possessing a minor physiological role as a supplement to the choroid plexus for the secretion and reabsorption of cerebrospinal fluid and as an adjunct specialized locally in the infundibular region for the transport of hypothalamic hormones. Even if the functions of the mature ependyma are understated, the fetal ependyma is still a much more dynamic structure with unique functions in ontogenesis (Sarnat, 1992c).

The embryonic ependyma develops in precise temporal and regional sequences initiated as the final phase of neural induction by the notochord (Sarnat, 1992a). The floor plate and roof plate in the midline of the spinal cord and brainstem differentiate as early as 6 weeks gestation in humans, whereas the ependyma associated with zones of thick "germinal matrix" around the lateral ventricles does not differentiate until 22 weeks gestation. Unlike the monotonous uniform simple cuboidal epithelium found in the adult brain, ependymal cells begin their fetal life as a pseudostratified columnar epithelium, form long radial processes from their basal surfaces, and produce a variety of soluble molecules that influence axonal growth cone projections in developing tracts. Thus, the fetal ependyma is not only an active metabolic and secretory structure of the developing central nervous system, but also one which influences the course of cerebral maturation.

Primitive neuroepithelial cell nuclei move to and fro within their own cytoplasmic extensions that span the ventricular zone, but nearly all mitotic activity occurs at the ventricular surface (Sauer, 1935; Figure 2). The fetus has relatively large ventricles, in part because of a need for a wide surface area for mitotic dispersal and also to avoid cellular crowding. It is advantageous for the fetus to delay the differentiation of the neuroepithelium as long as possible because a requisite number of generations of neuroblasts must be produced within a finite period to provide the number of neurons required for mature function (Smart, 1972). An ependyma differentiating at the ventricular surface prevents further mitoses and effectively arrests neuronogenesis. The central canal of the fetal spinal cord is a vertical slit because of continued cellular proliferation in the lateral walls but lack of mitoses beneath the floor and roof plates due to early ependymal differentiation.

Another important role of the ependyma in the development of the nervous system is in the guidance of axonal growth cones. The tips of

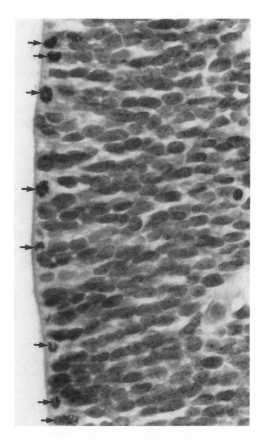

Figure 2. Primitive neuroepithelium lining the lateral ventricle of a 12-week human fetus. Frequent mitoses (arrows) are seen at the ventricular surface and an ependyma is not yet differentiated. This is a pseudostratified columnar epithelium and all cells have a thin cytoplasmic process extending to the ventricular wall, although it is not easily seen with this stain. Hematoxylin-eosin. × 500.

growing axons consist of a continuously changing reorganization of the membrane, microtubules, and cytoskeletal filaments such as actin, so that a series of slender, finger-like extensions (filopodia) with membranes between them (veils) probe a path of axonal trajectory (Goldberg & Burmeister, 1989; Norris & Kalil, 1990). Cell–cell interactions mediated by cell adhesion molecules direct the axon in the final phases as it approaches the target cell with which it will form a synapse. Cell–matrix interactions help form the path by providing an extracellular substrate, such as laminin or fibronectin, to which the axons may adhere and by which the extending filopodia may pull themselves along. The direction of axons along their course, particularly in long projections that ascend or descend the neuraxis, is mediated by small, diffusible molecules that either attract or repel axonal growth cones. The long basal processes of fetal ependymal cells that extend into the cerebral parenchyma superficially resemble radial glial fibers, but are structurally different and functionally very different. They do not serve as guides for the migration of neuroblasts, but rather extend among and between developing long tracts and other regions of axonal growth to influence the course of these fiber projections (Figure 3). Fetal ependymal cells and their basal processes produce several diffusible molecules that influence the course of fibers. For example, the roof plate of the spinal cord differentiates early and projects its ependymal fibers in the dorsal midline to create a dorsal median septum (Figure 4). This septum prevents the aberrant decussation of ascending

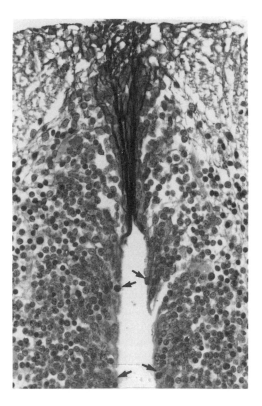

Figure 4. Dorsal third of neural tube of an 8-week human fetus. The roof plate ependymal cells are well differentiated and their processes extend in the midline to the surface of the developing spinal cord to form a dorsal median septum that prevents the aberrant decussation of developing dorsal column axons. The neuroepithelium of the lateral walls of the spinal central canal is undifferentiated and mitotic figures are seen (arrows). Glial fibrillary acidic protein. ×250. (From Sarnat, H.B. [1992b]. Regional differentiation of the human fetal ependyma: Immunocytochemical markers. *Journal of Neuropathology and Experimental Neurology, 51*, 58–75; reprinted by permission.)

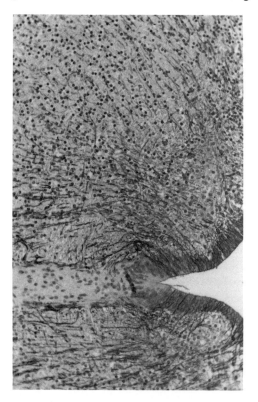

Figure 3. Floor of the fourth ventricle of an 8-week human fetus, showing long extensions of ependymal cells radiating ventrally among developing long paramedian tracts. These ependymal processes produce diffusible molecules that help guide growing axons. The floor plate ependyma is selectively nonreactive with this immunocytochemical stain. Glial fibrillary acidic protein. ×100.

axons of the developing dorsal columns, the fasciculus gracilus and fasciculus cuneatus, by producing a glycosaminoglycan molecule *keratan sulfate* that strongly repels axonal growth cones (Snow, Steindler, & Silver, 1990). Keratan sulfate is found not only in the nervous system, but also in other parts of the fetal body where innervation is not needed or wanted, such as the epiphyseal plates of growing bones and the epidermis to prevent the growth of nerves through the fetal skin (Snow et al., 1990); its presence in ependymal cells prevents axons from entering the ventricular system (Sarnat, 1992b). Keratan sulfate, in developing neural arches of vertebrae, ensures that spinal nerve roots exit only through the intervertebral foramina where keratan sulfate is selectively absent, helping to form the segmental organization of the spinal cord (Tosney & Oakley, 1990). The notochord also produces trypsin, a substance that inhibits the migration of neural crest cells and helps direct the pathway of developing nerve roots (Pettway, Guillory, & Bronner-Fraser, 1990).

The dorsal and ventral median septae are chemical rather than physical barriers to axonal growth. Commissural fibers of the spinal cord easily pass through the ventral median septum formed by the floor plate ependyma, demonstrating an incompletely understood selectivity that permits the passage of some axons while repelling others. In addition to the several glycosaminoglycans and proteoglycans that repel axonal growth cones, other diffusible mole-cules synthesized in fetal ependymal cells attract growth cones. Examples are the several known nerve growth factors, and probably S-100 protein, that have a very restricted distribution in the fetal ependyma (Sarnat, 1992b; Figure 5). These diffusible molecules that direct growing axons disappear from ependymal cells with maturation of the nervous system, and are absent in the adult. The basal ependymal processes also retract after they are no longer needed. Fetal ependymal cells produce a variety of intermediate filament proteins such as vimentin, cytokeratins, and glial fibrillary acidic protein (Figure 6), none of which persist in adult life. These proteins have a restricted and temporally predictable regional distribution in the human fetal ependyma (Sarnat, 1992b).

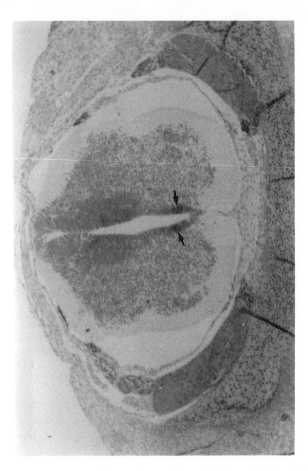

Figure 5. Restricted distribution of S-100 protein (arrows) in the ventral part of the neuroepithelium of the basal plate in the developing spinal cord of a 7-week human fetus. × 25.

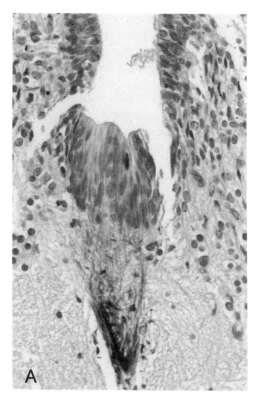
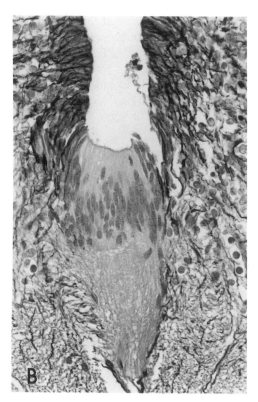

Figure 6. Ventral part of developing spinal cord in a 12-week human fetus. A) Vimentin is expressed in floor plate cells and their processes but also in ependymal cells of the basal plate. B) Glial fibrillary acidic protein is expressed in basal plate ependymal cells but not in the floor plate. The fetal ependyma shows consistent regional differences in immunoreactivity, reflecting different functions of various regions. × 500. (From Sarnat, H.B. [1992b]. Regional differentiation of the human fetal ependyma: Immunocytochemical markers. *Journal of Neuropathology and Experimental Neurology, 51*, 58–75; reprinted by permission.)

The floor plate is a particularly important and unique part of the fetal ependyma because it appears to serve as an anteroposterior gradient organizer of the developing central nervous system (Yamada, Placzek, Tanaka, Dodd, & Jessell, 1991). It is the only part of the ependyma where retinoic acid is produced (Wagner, Thaller, Jessell, & Eichele, 1990). Retinoid-binding proteins and retinoic acid receptors are strongly expressed in the preotic region of the hindbrain and also in mesenchymal cells of the primitive streak (Ruberte, Dolle, Chambon, & Morriss-Kay, 1991). Retinoic acid, in excess, causes an anteroposterior transformation of the neural tube, so that in amphibian tadpoles, severe cerebral hypoplasia and microcephaly result, and the optic cups are small and poorly formed (Durston et al., 1989).

Finally, the fetal ependyma may also play a role in neuroblast migration, not by providing guide fibers for neuroblasts, but rather in regulating the differentiation and maturation of radial glial cells of the subventricular zone. The disappearance of certain intermediate filament proteins from maturing fetal ependymal cells occurs shortly after the completion of neuroblast migration and coincides with the transformation of radial glial cells to mature astrocytes (Sarnat, 1992b).

DISTURBANCES OF NEURONOGENESIS DUE TO FAULTY INDUCTION

If the ependyma is induced to differentiate too early, neuronogenesis is arrested and the required number of neurons is never achieved. The result is diffuse cerebral hypoplasia if the arrest occurs in the first 12 weeks, or less extreme hypoplasia of the brain and microcephaly if the arrest occurs somewhat later in gestation when only the last few cycles of neuroepithelial mitoses are abolished (Sarnat, 1992a; Figure 7). Imaging studies of full-term neonates that show a thin cerebral mantle and generalized ventriculomegaly, but no major architectural alterations, are sometimes misinterpreted as cerebral cortical "atrophy" rather than hypoplasia.

Precocious induction of the ependyma to differentiate may be due to faulty genetic programming, as in some chromosomal diseases, an abnormally developed notochord that emits induction signals too early, or exogenous substances that behave as teratogens by mimicking normal induction signals.

DISTURBANCES OF CEREBRAL ORGANIZATION DUE TO A FAULTY EPENDYMA

Holoprosencephaly is a severe cerebral malformation of early gestation characterized by absence or hypoplasia of median and some paramedian structures of the brain and midline

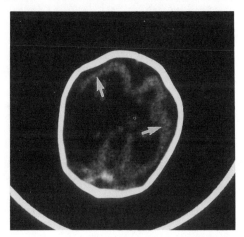

Figure 7. Computed axial tomographic image of the brain of a microcephalic full-term infant whose twin with a separate placenta was delivered stillborn at 17 weeks gestation. The live infant has no congenital anomalies of other organs and chromosomes are normal. The image shows a very thin cerebral mantle (arrows), no midline defects, large ventricles and a wide extra-axial space. This condition of cerebral hypoplasia is probably the result of arrested mitotic activity in the cerebral neuroepithelium at 14- to 18-weeks gestation. The most likely explanation is maternal exposure to a toxin or drug that behaved as a teratogen by inducing precocious differentiation of the ependyma and thus preventing the further generation of neuroblasts. There is no evidence of a genetic defect.

fusion of other paramedian structures, in a rostrocaudal gradient. Additional disturbances of developmental processes involve neuroblast migrations and axonal projections (Leech & Shuman, 1986; Sarnat, 1992a). In its most extreme form, holoprosencephaly is accompanied by midfacial hypoplasia, or even cyclopia. Affected children have severe neurological handicaps including mental retardation, spastic diplegia, epilepsy, and special sensory deficiencies. There is a strong association of holoprosencephaly with chromosomal diseases, particularly 13-15 trisomy, with other genetic disorders, and with maternal diabetes mellitus. Many other cases are transmitted as an autosomal recessive trait.

The ependyma in holoprosencephaly is always very abnormal; many regions are poorly developed, gaps occur through which germinal matrix cells herniate into the ventricles, and proliferations and rosettes of ependymal cells occur in the subventricular region within the cerebral tissue (Sarnat, 1992a). The pathogenesis of this malformation of the brain is not completely understood, but it is thought to be a disorder of neural induction of the *lamina terminalis*, the plate that closes the anterior neuropore of the neural tube and gives origin to the forebrain. If a floor plate fails to form, or is defective, a weak polarizing gradient could result in hypoplasia of midline structures and apparent fusion of paramedian structures that is the unique characteristic of holoprosencephaly. Furthermore, an abnormal ependyma lateral to the floor plate with impaired metabolic activity for the synthesis of diffusible molecules that direct axonal growth cones, could result in abnormal axonal projections and possibly adversely affect neuroblast migrations. In a cyclopian mutant of the zebrafish, the floor plate ependyma fails to form; this may be an animal model of human holoprosencephaly (Hatta, Kimmel, Ho, & Walker, 1991). In some human fetuses with holoprosencephaly, the rostral end of the notochord and its derivatives are abnormal (Müller & O'Rahilly, 1989), although these results are not yet conclusive. Evidence is accumulating that holoprosencephaly is a disorder of neural induction that causes the fetal ependyma to differentiate and function abnormally, and that the ependymal deficiencies contribute to the pathogenesis of the complex cerebral malformations.

Retinoic acid helps establish anteroposterior gradients in many tissues of both mesodermal and ectodermal origin. Retinoid compounds, such as vitamin A, cause metaplasia in mouse and chick embryos, changing keratinizing squamous epithelium to ciliated secretory epithelium and scale-producing epithelium of the feet to feather-producing skin (Johnson & Scadding, 1991). A single dose of a retinoid administered to embryonic mice in early gestation causes spina bifida and the Chiari malformation (Marin-Padilla & Marin-Padilla, 1981). The mechanism probably involves effects on mesenchymal tissues that lead to defective somite formation and disparity of growth between ventral and dorsal regions of developing vertebrae, but primary effects on the neuroepithelium or its derivatives cannot be excluded (Alles & Sulik, 1990). These effects might include the fetal ependyma and the floor plate in particular as a target.

Aberrant axonal projections are complicating features of many dysgeneses of the nervous system and sometimes occur as isolated anomalies that have major or minor clinical expression in neurological function. The pathogenesis is not documented in most cases, but the ependyma usually receives little attention in neuropathological examinations except that minor abnormalities might be noted as "incidental findings." Hydrocephalus is always accompanied by gaps in the ependyma as the ventricles enlarge, and ependymal cells in such a situation often migrate to the subependymal regions where they form small rosettes and clusters. In the fetal brain, these abnormally arranged ependymal cells retract their basal processes and probably become metabolically inactive. Whether these changes in the ependyma contribute to clinical neurological disabilities and chronic developmental problems is unknown at this time, but presents a testable hypothesis for both animal and postmortem human studies. The role of the fetal ependyma in disturbances of brain development will surely be clarified in the near future.

REFERENCES

Alles, A.J., & Sulik, K.K. (1990). Retinoic acid-induced spina bifida: Evidence for a pathogenic mechanism. *Development, 108,* 73–81.

Bentley, J.F.R., & Smith, J.R. (1960). Developmental posterior enteric remnants and spinal malformations: The split notochord syndrome. *Archives of Diseases in Childhood, 35,* 76–86.

Boucaut, J.C., Darribere, T., Li, S.D., Boulekbache, H.S., Yamada, K.M., & Thiery, J-P. (1985). Evidence for the role of fibronectin in amphibian gastrulation. *Journal of Embryology and Experimental Morphology, 89*(Suppl.), 211–227.

Brachet, J. (1985). *Molecular cytology/cell interactions.* New York: Academic Press.

Duprat, A.M., & Gualandris, L. (1984). Extracellular matrix and neural determination during amphibian gastrulation. *Cell Differentiation, 14,* 105–112.

Duprat, A.M., Gualandris, L., Kan, P., Saint-Jeannet, J.P., & Boudannaoui, S. (1987). Neural induction [Review]. *Archives d'Anatomie, de Microscopie, et de Morphologie Experimentale, 75,* 211–227.

Duprat, A.M., Gualandris, L., & Rouge, P. (1982). Neural induction and the structure of the target cell surface. *Journal of Embryology and Experimental Morphology, 70,* 171–187.

Durston, A.J., Timmermans, J.P.M., Hage, W.J., Hendriks, H.F.J., de Vries, N.J., Heidelveld, M., &

Nieuwkoop, P.D. (1989). Retinoic acid causes an anteroposterior transformation in the developing central nervous system. *Nature, 340,* 140–144.

Ebisu, T., Odake, G., Fujimoto, M., Ueda, S., Tsujii, H., Morimoto, M., & Sawada, T. (1990). Neurenteric cysts with meningomyelocele or meningocele. Split notochord syndrome. *Child's Nervous System, 6,* 465–467.

Goldberg, D.J., & Burmeister, D.W. (1989). Looking into growth cones. *Trends in Neuroscience, 12,* 503–506.

Grunz, H. (1985). Information transfer during embryonic induction in amphibians. *Journal of Embryology and Experimental Morphology, 89,* 349–364.

Gualandris, L., Rouge, P., & Duprat, A.M. (1983). Membrane changes in neural target cells studied with fluorescent lectin probes. *Journal of Embryology and Experimental Morphology, 77,* 183–200.

Hatta, K., Kimmel, C.B., Ho, R.K., & Walker, C. (1991). The cyclops mutation blocks the specification of the floor plate of the zebrafish central nervous system. *Nature, 350,* 339–341.

Ho, K-L., & Tiel, R. (1989). Intraspinal bronchogenic cyst: Ultrastructural study of the lining epithelium. *Acta Neuropathologica, 78,* 513–520.

Johnson, K.J., & Scadding, S.R. (1991). Effects of vitamin A and other retinoids on the differentiation and morphogenesis of the integument and limbs of vertebrates. *Canadian Journal of Zoology, 69,* 263–273.

Leech, R.W., & Shuman, R.M. (1986). Holoprosencephaly and related midline cerebral anomalies [Review]. *Journal of Child Neurology, 1*, 3–18.

Mann, K.S., Khosla, V.K., Gulai, D.R., & Malik, A.K. (1984). Spinal neurenteric cyst: Association with vertebral anomalies, diastematomyelia, dorsal fistula, and lipoma. *Surgical Neurology, 21*, 358–362.

Marin-Padilla, M., & Marin-Padilla, M.T. (1981). Morphogenesis of experimentally induced Arnold-Chiari malformation. *Journal of the Neurological Sciences, 50*, 29–55.

Mizuno, J., Fiandaca, M.S., Nishio, S., & O'Brien, M.S. (1988). Recurrent intramedullary enterogenous cyst of the cervical spinal cord. *Child's Nervous System, 4*, 47–49.

Müller, F., & O'Rahilly, R. (1989). Mediobasal proscencephalic defects, including holoproscencephaly and cyclopia, in relation to the development of human forebrain. *American Journal of Anatomy, 185*, 391–414.

Nieuwkoop, P., Johnen, A., & Albers, B. (1985). *The epigenetic nature of early chordate development: Inductive interaction and competence.* Cambridge: Cambridge University Press.

Norris, C.R., & Kalil, K. (1990). Morphology and cellular interactions of growth cones in the developing corpus callosum. *Journal of Comparative Neurology, 293*, 268–281.

Pettway, Z., Guillory, G., & Bronner-Fraser, M. (1990). Absence of neural crest cells from the region surrounding implanted notochords in situ. *Developmental Biology, 142*, 335–345.

Poelmann, R.E., Gittenberger-de Groot, A.C., Mentink, M.M.T., Delpech, B., Girard, N., & Christ, B. (1990). The extracellular matrix during neural crest formation and migration in rat embryos. *Anatomy and Embryology, 182*, 29–39.

Roessmann, U. (1985). Duplication of the pituitary gland and spinal cord. *Archives of Pathology and Laboratory Medicine, 109*, 518–520.

Ruberte, E., Dolle, P., Chambon, P., & Morriss-Kay, G. (1991). Retinoid acid receptors and cellular retinoid binding proteins: II. Their differential pattern of transcription during early morphogenesis in mouse. *Development, 111*, 45–60.

Sarnat, H.B. (1992a). *Cerebral dysgenesis: Embryology and clinical expression.* New York: Oxford University Press.

Sarnat, H.B. (1992b). Regional differentiation of the human fetal ependyma: Immunocytochemical markers. *Journal of Neuropathology and Experimental Neurology, 51*, 58–75.

Sarnat, H.B. (1992c). Role of human fetal ependyma. *Pediatric Neurology, 8*, 163–178.

Sarnat, H.B., Case, M.E., & Graviss, R. (1976). Sacral agenesis: Neurologic and neuropathologic features. *Neurology, 26*, 1124–1129.

Sauer, F.C. (1935). Mitosis in the neural tube. *Journal of Comparative Neurology, 62*, 377–405.

Smart, I.H.M. (1972). Proliferative characteristics of the ependymal layer during the early development of the spinal cord in the mouse. *Journal of Anatomy, 111*, 365–380.

Snow, D.M., Steindler, D.A., & Silver, J. (1990). Molecular and cellular characterization of the glial roof plate of the spinal cord and optic tectum: A possible role for a proteoglycan in the development of an axon barrier. *Developmental Biology, 138*, 359–376.

Spemann, H., & Mangold, H. (1924). Über Inducktion von Enbryonalanlagen durch Implantation aftfrember Organisatoren (On induction of embryonic primordia through tissue organizers). *Wilhelm Roux Archives der Entwicklung, 100*, 599–638.

Tiedemann, H. (1986). The molecular mechanism of neural induction: Neural differentiation of *Triturus* ectoderm exposed to Hepes buffer. *Roux's Archives of Developmental Biology, 195*, 399–402.

Tosney, K.W., & Oakley, R.A. (1990). The perinotochordal mesenchyme acts as a barrier to axon advance in the chick embryo: Implications for a general mechanism of axonal guidance. *Experimental Neurology, 109*, 75–89.

Towfighi, J., & Housman, C. (1991). Spinal cord abnormalities in caudal regression syndrome. *Acta Neuropathologica, 81*, 458–466.

van Straaten, H.W.M., Hekking, J.W.M., Wiertz-Hoessels, E.J.L.M., Thors, F., & Drukker, J. (1988). Effects of the notochord on the differentiation of a floor plate area in the neural tube of the chick embryo. *Anatomy and Embryology, 177*, 317–324.

Vinters, H.V., & Gilbert, J.J. (1981). Neurenteric cysts of the spinal cord mimicking multiple sclerosis. *Canadian Journal of Neurological Sciences, 8*, 159–161.

Wagner, M., Thaller, C., Jessell, T., & Eichele, G. (1990). Polarizing activity and retinoid synthesis in the floor plate of the neural tube. *Nature, 345*, 819–822.

Yamada, T., Placzek, M., Tanaka, H., Dodd, J., & Jessell, T.M. (1991). Control of cell pattern in the developing nervous system: Polarizing activity of the floor plate and notochord. *Cell, 64*, 635–647.

Chapter 16

Development of the Brain
Experience Affects the Structure of Neurons, Glia, and Blood Vessels

WILLIAM T. GREENOUGH, PH.D., CHRISTOPHER S. WALLACE, B.S.,
ADRIANA A. ALCANTARA, M.A., BRENDA J. ANDERSON, M.S., NICHOLAS HAWRYLAK, M.C.,
ANITA M. SIREVAAG, PH.D., IVAN JEANNE WEILER, PH.D.,
AND GINGER S. WITHERS, M.A.
University of Illinois at Urbana-Champaign

THIS CHAPTER FOCUSES ON WHAT IS KNOWN about brain development through the use of animal models and especially through the use of a procedure in which animals are reared or subsequently exposed to environments that provide experience beyond the laboratory norm. The authors present findings supporting these conclusions regarding experience-dependent neuronal plasticity:

1. Providing the opportunity to learn in such a complex environment leads to increases in the number of cerebral cortical synapses and in dendritic field dimensions.
2. An orchestrated series of changes in glial architecture and in the vascular network accompanies the changes in synaptic number and neuronal form.
3. These effects are not restricted to early development.
4. Synaptic addition appears to be associated with learning, rather than demands of activity.
5. Molecular mechanisms through which experience may rapidly induce changes in neuronal structure are currently under study.

This discussion of the role of animal models in understanding brain development begins with a consideration of the levels within the organism at which brain plasticity can be studied, which are indicated in Table 1. When studying humans, of course, excluding autopsy samples, researchers are limited to accessible behavior and a few noninvasive measures of nervous system electrical and metabolic activity. Animal research provides access to all of the levels depicted in Table 1, and, as will be shown, there is substantial evidence for influences of behavioral experience on all of these levels in the developing brain. That the brain is plastic to experience in all these dimensions is nearly universally accepted among neuroscientists today; in the late 60s and early 70s, such concepts were radical or revolutionary and data such as those presented here were widely disbelieved.

EFFECTS OF REARING ENVIRONMENT COMPLEXITY ON NEURONAL DEVELOPMENT

One of the earliest indications of the plasticity of the developing, and later the adult, brain was

Preparation of this chapter and work not previously reported was supported by MH35321, MH40631, AG10154, ONR N0014-89-J-1556, Center grant NSF BNS-8821219 from the National Science Foundation, and training grant HD07333. We thank Valerie Kilman, Krystyna Isaacs, Christine Collins, and James Black for assistance with research reported here.

Table 1. Examples of levels at which experience-dependent plasticity can be examined

Level of organization	Triggering event	Process(es) invoked	Outcome
Behavior	Interaction with the environment	Learning and memory	Adaptive behavior
Nervous system	Sensory stimulation	Regional plasticity	Refined function
Cellular	Input pattern and modulatory state	Integration of synaptic inputs and cell state	Associative response properties
Molecular	Selective activation of receptors, channels, modulatory factors	Regulation of biochemical pathways	Altered cellular activity

the report of Rosenzweig, Krech, Bennett, and Diamond (1962) and Bennett, Diamond, Krech, and Rosenzweig (1964) that portions of the cerebral cortex grew thicker and heavier in animals living in a complex, toy-filled "enriched" environment similar to that depicted in Figure 1. (The authors prefer the term *environmental complexity*, or EC, to avoid giving the impression that the environment is richer than would likely be experienced by feral rats.) Hebb (1947) and his students (e.g., Forgays & Forgays, [1952]; Hymovitch, [1952]) had previously shown that rats reared in this way learned mazes and other complex tasks faster than standard laboratory cage-reared rats. (The authors use the terms *individual cage*, or IC, and *social cage*, or SC, to refer to rats reared in standard laboratory cages.) The authors have similarly found rats reared in EC for 30 days following weaning (at 25–30 days of age) to be superior in learning mazes and other complex appetitively motivated tasks, relative to SC or IC rats (e.g., Greenough, Yuwiler, & Dollinger, 1973).

It should be noted that, to the extent this has been examined, direct physical interaction with the environment is necessary for both the behavioral and the gross brain effects that have been described. Animals housed, for example, inside the complex environment but in cages that prevent their interaction with it do not show the brain weight or behavioral effects (Ferchmin, Bennett, & Rosenzweig, 1975). Direct interaction with the environment may be required for human infants to develop properly as well. For example, the work of Bertenthal,

Campos, and Barret (1984) suggests that cognitive and emotional development may rely on environmental interaction derived from self-produced locomotion.

To determine whether these gross changes in cortical dimensions reflected changes at the level of neuronal structure, Volkmar and Greenough (1972) and Greenough and Volkmar (1973) measured the dendritic processes of neurons stained by the Golgi technique in EC, SC, and IC rats reared in these environments for 30 days following weaning. The simple hypothesis was that, if the acquisition of information from experience involved alterations in the connections among neurons (i.e., the synapses) this should be reflected in the structure of dendrites, the recipients of virtually all excitatory input to cerebral cortical neurons. Results for the projected dendritic length of a fairly heterogeneous class of cells, stellate neurons from layer IV of visual cortex, are shown in Figure 2. These results reflect fairly closely the magnitude of the average difference among groups across the four classes of cells studied, a difference of 20%–25% between EC and IC rats, with SC rats intermediate but closer to the ICs. Similar results for male rats have been obtained by others, while environmental effects upon female rats are somewhat smaller (Juraska, 1984).

An important question was whether the differences in dendrites really indicated differences in the number of synapses per neuron. To assess this, Turner and Greenough (1985) measured the density of synapses and neuronal nuclei in the visual cortex of similarly reared rats,

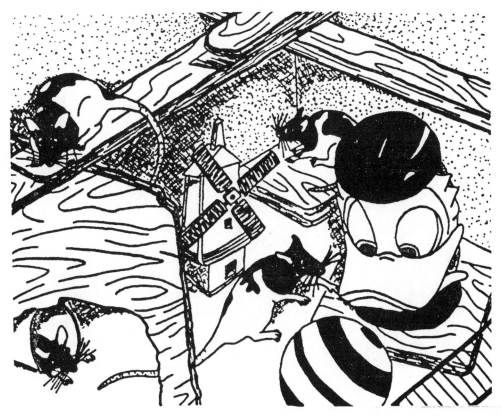

Figure 1. Drawing of rats exploring a complex environment. Groups of EC rats interact with each other as they explore a novel arrangement of objects. (From Black & Greenough, 1986.)

employing stereological formulas that used geometric estimates to correct for expected group differences in the sizes of neuronal nuclei (Diamond, Lindner, & Raymond, 1967) and synapses (West & Greenough, 1972). As the right panel of Figure 3 indicates, these results closely supported the dendritic results: EC and IC rats differing by about 20%–25%, with SC rats intermediate but closer to (and not statistically different from) ICs.

Figure 3 shows another very important result. The left panel indicates that synapse density is not different for the three groups of rats, and the center panel shows that what differs is the density of neurons. For a variety of reasons, the authors are certain that neurons are *not* dying in the EC rats, but that they are being pushed apart by changes in the other tissue surrounding them. Part of the tissue pushing the neurons apart, of course, consists of the new synapses and the dendrites and axons from

which they form. However, there are other changes in the non-neuronal supporting tissue as well. The changes described below, taken with the fact that synaptic density stays nearly constant despite a 20%–25% increase in synapse number, suggest that each synapse brings with it nearly equivalent demands for the support provided by astrocytic glia and vasculature.

PLASTICITY OF NEURONAL SUPPORT COMPONENTS: ASTROCYTES AND BLOOD VESSELS

Astrocytes, defined here as cells with astrocyte morphology (a large number of fine processes radiating from a soma) and immunoreactive to an antibody to glial fibrillary acidic protein, exhibit a two-phase response to exposure to the complex environment at weaning (Sirevaag & Greenough, 1991). The first phase consists of hypertrophy, depicted in Figure 4a. Astrocytic

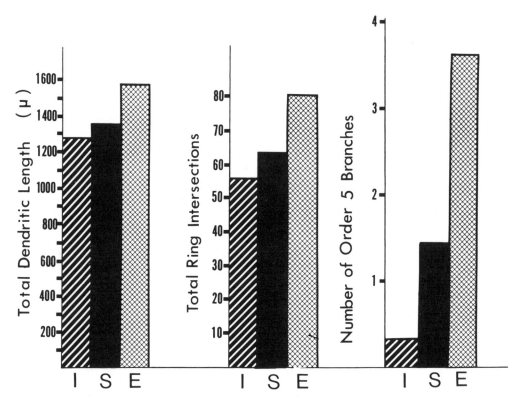

Figure 2. Results from dendritic measurements on Golgi-stained Layer IV stellate cells. Weanling rats housed for 30 days in a complex environment (E) have larger dendritic fields containing more higher-order branches than littermates housed in a social condition (S), or individual cage (I). This result demonstrates the substantial role of experience in the development of cerebral cortex. (From Greenough, W.T., Volkmar, F.R., & Fleischmann, T.B. [1976]. In D.I. Mostofsky [Ed.], Behavioral control and modification of physiological activity [pp. 220–245]. Englewood Cliffs, NJ: Prentice Hall. Copyright © 1976 by Prentice Hall; reprinted by permission.)

processes were quantified using a stereological method for estimating surface density, the amount of astrocyte surface per unit volume of cortical tissue. This measure was used because much of the function of astrocytes—the maintenance of tissue ionic and acidic balance and the uptake of extracellular neurotransmitter released during synaptic activity—is done through transport mechanisms at the cell surface. Figure 4a shows that the average surface area of astrocytes increased in EC rats over the first 30 days of postweaning housing. With continuing environmental demand, astrocytes apparently enter another phase of response. Figure 4b shows that the number of astrocytes increases in the EC rats. This result shows two things. First, neurons do not exist in a vacuum; changes in neuronal function require adjustment by other components of the brain. Second, just as the question of age-dependent effects of experience on *neurons* is of interest, the question of whether *other support components* of the tissue exhibit sensitivity during particular periods of life is important as well. While some answers to the question for neurons and for blood vessels are available, the capacity for astrocytes to grow or proliferate throughout the life span has not yet been assessed.

In contrast to earlier, methodologically flawed reports to the contrary (Diamond, Krech, & Rosenzweig, 1964), the authors' work indicates dramatic proliferation of capillaries in rats placed in a complex environment at weaning. The density of capillaries in the tissue increases, such that the distance from the nearest capillary to any point in the tissue is shorter (Black, Sirevaag, & Greenough, 1987). This is accomplished by the extension of new capillary branches through the tissue (Sire-

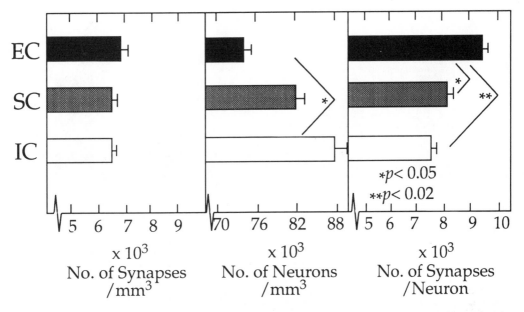

Figure 3. Results from a direct examination of synaptic and neuronal density in upper visual cortex of rats reared for 30 days after weaning in a complex environment (EC), social condition (SC), or individual cages (IC). The panel on the right shows an increase in the number of synapses per neuron in EC rats, a result that confirms predictions from previous Golgi studies of dendritic length (see Figure 2 and text). The middle panel shows a decreased neuronal density in EC cortex, a spatial dilution reflecting the hypertrophy of glial and vascular elements and the addition of synapses. The left-hand panel shows that synaptic density is not statistically different between EC, SC, and IC, possibly suggesting a maximum number of synapses that can be metabolically supported within a given brain volume. (From Turner, A.M., & Greenough, W.T. [1985]. Differential rearing effects on rat visual cortex synapses. I. Synaptic and neuronal density and synapses per neuron. *Brain Research, 329*, 195–203. Copyright © 1984 by Elsevier/North Holland; reprinted with permission.

vaag, Black, Shafron, & Greenough, 1988). The relative increase in the amount of capillary is far greater than that in synapses. As Figure 5 indicates, the number of capillaries is substantially greater in EC rats, an increase of about 50% in "volume fraction," that proportion of total brain volume taken up by blood vessels. This increase is much greater than the 20%–25% increase in synapse number in the same brain region, suggesting that the function of new capillary growth is not just to meet the metabolic needs of the new synapses but that there is an overall increase in neuronal activity associated with the complex environment. As will be shown, the capacity to generate new vasculature declines with age.

AGE-DEPENDENCE OF BRAIN RESPONSES TO ENVIRONMENTAL COMPLEXITY

The degree to which these changes are limited to sensitive periods of development is of ob-

vious theoretical and applied interest. To what extent is rehabilitation possible following a relatively deprived early environment? The answer seems to differ for different tissue components. Neurons appear to retain structural plasticity in adulthood at a level that is little diminished from that seen at the age of weaning. Uylings, Kuypers, Diamond, and Veltman (1978) first noted visual cortex dendritic branching increases in adult EC rats. Subsequently, Juraska, Greenough, Elliott, Mack, and Berkowitz (1980) found that 145-day-old rats housed for 12 weeks in the EC environment exhibited increased visual cortical dendritic branching, compared to rats housed in the IC condition. The dendritic growth seemed essentially as robust at that seen in weanlings. Similarly, Green, Greenough, and Schlumpf (1983) reported nearly comparable results for 15-month-old "middle-age" rats. Synaptic plasticity has been examined only in young adult rats (Greenough et al., in preparation) but likewise remains robust at this age. In 24-month-

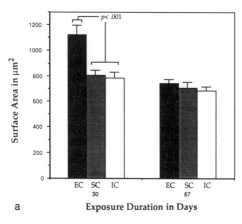
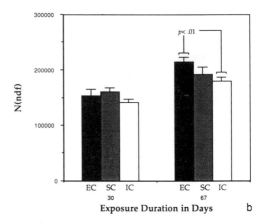

a   Exposure Duration in Days   Exposure Duration in Days   b

Figure 4. Structural response of astrocytes in visual cortex of rats reared for 30 or 67 days after weaning in a complex environment (EC), social condition (SC), or individual cages (IC). Astrocytes were stained with an antibody to GFAP (glial fibrillary acidic protein), a unique marker of astrocytes. Panel 4a shows that surface area per astrocyte is increased significantly after 30 days of exposure, but paradoxically appears decreased at 67 days. Panel 4b explains this result by demonstrating that glial number has actually increased between 30 and 67 days, such that in ECs the addition of new smaller astrocytes has the effect of reducing the average size. Taken together, these findings indicate a two-phase response by astrocytes of initial hypertrophy followed by proliferation. (From Sirevaag, A.M., & Greenough, W.T. [1991]. Plasticity of GFAP-immunoreactive astrocyte size and number in visual cortex of rats reared in complex environments. *Brain Research, 540,* 273–278.)

old rats, however, visual cortex dendritic branching was little affected by environmental complexity (Black, Parnisari, Eichbaum, & Greenough, 1986). The cerebellum, a sensorimotor region of the hindbrain that is also sensitive to developmental environmental complexity (Floeter & Greenough, 1979; Pysh & Weiss, 1979) and that deteriorates significantly in aging brain (Glick & Bondareff, 1979; Rogers, Silver, Shoemaker, & Bloom, 1980; Rogers, Zornetzer, Bloom, & Mervis, 1984), retains sensitivity to complex environment experience in elderly rats; while there was an overall tendency for loss of Purkinje neuron dendritic branches in rats between 2 years and 29 months of age, the formation of new branches in the cerebellar cortex of EC rats significantly offset the deterioration (Greenough, McDonald, Parnisari, & Camel, 1986). Thus, for neuronal plasticity, there is little indication of a sensitive period linked to early development. This result, taken with other indications that the adult brain can rapidly generate new synapses (e.g., Chang & Greenough, 1984) and that the rate of synapse formation may be higher in the brain of EC rats (Greenough, Hwang, & Gorman, 1985), led Black and Greenough (1986) to propose that much of postweaning and adult synaptogenesis was

"experience-dependent," driven by the need to store information.

Cerebral cortical vascular plasticity shows a quite different developmental pattern from that of neurons. While young adult rats retain a capacity to generate new vessels in the visual cortex, capillary density just barely keeps up with the increased volume of brain tissue in the EC rats; there is no density increase of the sort seen in postweaning ECs (Black, Zelazny, & Greenough, 1991). In "middle age," while the capacity to generate some new vessels is still evident, vasculature no longer keeps up with increasing cortical volume; in 2-year-old rats, no capillary plasticity is evident (Black, Polinsky, & Greenough, 1989). Under different conditions of demand, *cerebellar* cortical vasculature retained robust plasticity in response to both learning and physical exercise at mature adulthood, 10 months of age (Black, Isaacs, Anderson, Alcantara, & Greenough, 1990; see below). Thus, in general, vascular plasticity is somewhat more tied to a developmental sequence of decreasingly sensitive periods. To the extent that the weanling rat placed in a complex environment represents normal feral rat development, laboratory rats reared in standard cages will be irrevocably "developmentally disadvantaged," unable to benefit optimally

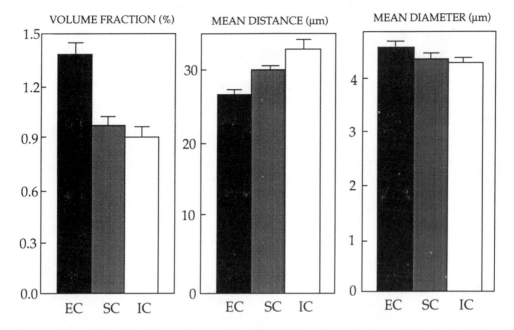

Figure 5. Response of capillaries in the visual cortex of rats reared for 30 days after weaning in a complex environment (EC), social condition (SC), or individual cages (IC). The left-hand panel presents the "volume fraction" of blood, or the percent of a given tissue volume occupied by capillary lumens, for all three groups. EC rats increased blood volume fraction by about 50%, indicating that substantial adaptation of the vascular system accompanies synaptic addition. A decrease in the mean distance between capillaries in ECs (middle panel) indicates that experience increases capillary density. A final adaptation of brain vasculature to the demands of experience is an increase in the mean diameter of EC capillaries, allowing more blood to be delivered per capillary. (From Black, J., Sirevaag, A.M., & Greenough, W.T., [1987]. Complex experience promotes capillary formation in young visual cortex. *Neuroscience Letters, 83*, 351–355; reprinted with permission.)

from later life experience due to the failure to establish a normal cortical vascular system. One can certainly imagine conditions under which the circumstances evident in this animal model might be manifest in humans.

The life span responsiveness of astrocytes to behavioral experience has not yet been studied. It is known that astrocytes hypertrophy, and in some cases proliferate, in response to injury of the brain (Janeczko, 1989; Topp, Faddis, & Vijayan, 1989). Moreover, the authors know that astrocytic surface density increases when long-term potentiation is induced (an electrophysiological animal model of the memory process) in the dentate gyrus of adult rats (Isaacs, Marks, Sirevaag, Chang, & Greenough, 1989). Similarly, astrocytic volume fraction increases in the hippocampus following "kindling," an animal model of epilepsy that has sometimes been proposed as a model of learning (Hawrylak, Chang, & Greenough, 1989). Thus, there is good reason to expect lifetime plasticity of astrocytes in response to behavioral experi-

ence, while the issue of special developmental sensitivity remains unanswered.

ARE THESE EFFECTS DUE TO AGGREGATE NEURONAL ACTIVITY OR TO LEARNING?

The authors have suggested elsewhere that the experience-driven synaptic changes are due to learning (e.g., Greenough, 1985). This was based upon reports that dendritic field alterations occur following training of adult rats on mazes and motor learning tasks (e.g., Greenough, Juraska, & Volkmar, 1979) including within-subject preparations in which differences could not be attributed to general hormonal or metabolic activity (Chang & Greenough, 1982; Greenough, Larson, & Withers, 1985). (The possibility that EC effects arise from stress or stress-related hormonal changes has also been largely ruled out; see Black, Sirevaag, Wallace, Savin, & Greenough [1989] and Black, Sirevaag, & Greenough [1991].) However, in all of these experiments, there was a confound between neural firing and synaptic activity and learning: the region in which learning occurred was likely to have undergone more neuronal activity than the control region that was not learning (or learning less). Hence, it remained possible that the neurons were responding in much the same way that a muscle does when it is repeatedly activated in exercise—growing larger with the addition of new dendrites and synapses. Similarly, whether the vascular and glial changes were independently driven by activity, by learning, or simply by responses to the changes in neurons remained an open question.

One study sheds light on both of these questions (Black et al., 1990). One group of "acrobat" (AC) rats learned motor skills by negotiating a series of elevated pathways leading to a food reward. Pathways included loose hanging ropes, narrow beams, a link chain, and a variety of other obstacles that became increasingly complicated and difficult over 1 month of training. Two other groups controlled for physical and neuronal activity: a voluntary exercise group (VX) with running wheels available from their cages, and a forced exercise group (FX) that ran on a treadmill. Both groups traversed far more distance than the AC group. A final inactivity control (IC) group remained in their cages, except for brief daily handling done to equalize this factor across groups. After 30 days of these conditions, the density of vasculature was examined, as well as the number of synapses per neuron in the cerebellar paramedian lobule, a region intensively involved in forelimb motor activity. As Figure 6 indicates, the exercise conditions appeared to place heavy demands upon the neurons of the paramedian lobule; vascular density was significantly higher in the VX and FX animals than in the AC and IC groups. In contrast, the number of synapses per neuron was elevated in the AC motor learning group, with the exercise and inactivity groups equivalent, indicating that the exercise groups were unchanged in the number of synapses. The interpretation seems clear cut: when animals were required to learn new motor skills, they formed new synapses;

when they were required (or chose) to engage in sustained motor (and cerebellar) activity, they formed new capillaries. In addition to indicating the association of synapse formation with learning, this result highlights the fact that the brain is responding in the most appropriate way to all experimental conditions. In short, **brain adaptation** to behavioral needs can be exhibited as synapse formation or capillary formation, depending upon the circumstances. It is important to realize how much emphasis is placed on "pure" learning, to the exclusion of other forms of behaviorally significant plastic change in the brain.

CELLULAR AND GENETIC MECHANISMS SUPPORTING PLASTIC NEURAL ADAPTATION

The following material is somewhat more technical than the rest of the chapter, but needs to be included for completeness, and contains information of which those interested in human behavioral development should be aware. A particularly interesting issue is the manner in which learning-related neuronal activity becomes translated into changes in the structure of neurons. (For that matter it would be equally interesting to know how learning-unrelated neuronal activity gets translated into changes in the structure of capillaries.) Gene expression, one of the most fundamental ways in which all cells of the body adjust to changes in demands placed upon them, involves the activation of genes in the nucleus of the cell. Messenger RNA (mRNA) is transcribed from the genes and codes for proteins produced outside the nucleus in the cytoplasm. Synapse, dendrite, and capillary formation would almost certainly require the net synthesis of new proteins, which constitute essential elements of their structure. There are many mechanisms by which cellular events can trigger gene expression. *Second messengers*, such as cyclic adenosine monophosphate, can activate cellular cascades leading to the activation of select genes. (*First messengers* would include inputs to neurons, such as neurotransmitters and hor-

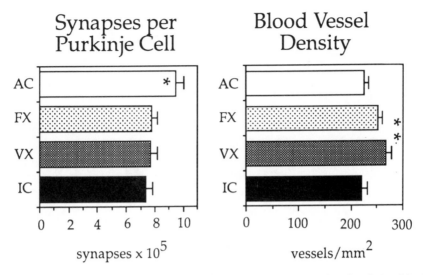

Figure 6. Changes in synapses per Purkinje cell and in blood vessels of rats exposed to 30 days of acrobatic training (AC), forced treadmill exercise (FX), voluntary running wheel exercise (VX), or inactivity (IC). Rats that learned acrobatic skills showed an increase in the number of synapses per Purkinje cell compared to both inactivity and exercise controls (panel 6a). Conversely, blood vessel density was increased in both exercise conditions, but not in the acrobatic or inactivity groups. Taken together, these results indicate that the cerebellum adapts differently to the demands of learning (synaptic addition) than repetitive activity (increased blood supply). (From Black et al., 1990.)

mones that activate second messenger systems.) In some cases, the activation of groups of genes appears to be orchestrated by *third messengers*, genes that respond very early in a cascade of cellular responses and whose protein returns to the nucleus in order to activate a second set of genes. The function of these "immediate early genes," some of which include genes for transcription factors initially isolated from malignant tumors, is depicted in Figure 7.

Two of these transcription factors, Fos and *zif-268* (a "zinc finger" nuclear binding protein), have been investigated, both of which are induced in the brain by stimuli ranging from electrical stimulation (Cole, Saffen, Baraban, & Worley, 1989) to behavioral experience (Anokhin, Mileusnic, Shamakina, & Rose, 1991; Mello, Vicario, & Clayton, 1991). Alcantara, Saks, and Greenough (1991) have found that a Fos immunoreactive product is produced in Purkinje cells in the cerebellar paramedian lobule and adjacent regions very rapidly following the first session of learning in a reaching task. The expression is *patchy*, mirroring the patchy nature of sensorimotor representation in this region (Shambes, Gibson, & Welker, 1978). Expression of Fos is much reduced by

the third session of training, at which time the animals seem to have acquired reaching skills.

Wallace, Withers, Weiler, and Greenough (1991), following up on the finding that dendritic branching differences are detectable within 4 days after weanling rats are placed in a complex environment (Wallace, Kilman, Withers, & Greenough, in press), examined *zif-268* mRNA expression in 4-day EC weanlings using a cDNA probe (complementary DNA, which selectively binds the targeted mRNA). Preliminary analyses of 11 sets of EC-IC littermate pairs indicated dramatically greater binding in the visual cortex of the EC rats.

While considerable work will be necessary to determine if and how these patterns of selective gene expression are related to the transformation of information encoded in neural activity to information encoded in neural structure, these findings begin to suggest ways in which neurons may accomplish the task. Many of these transcription factors have been described and more seem to be on the way; which of them, if any, are actually involved in changes in nerve cell structure remains to be determined.

A final cellular-level finding with regard to translating activity patterns into brain struc-

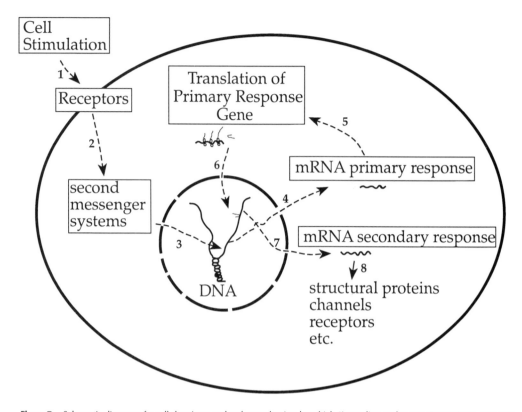

Figure 7. Schematic diagram of a cell showing a molecular mechanism by which "immediate early genes," or "primary response genes" might be involved in the process of structural modification. 1) Extracellular signals reach the cell by way of receptors embedded in the cell membrane. 2) Binding of signals, such as molecules of neurotransmitter, growth factors, or hormones, affects the activity of second messenger systems within the cell. 3) Altered second messenger activity induces the transcription of primary response DNA in cell nucleus. 4) Messenger RNA (mRNA) transcribed from primary response genes enters the cytoplasm where it is translated (5) into a protein transcription factor. These transcription factors then return to the nucleus to bind directly onto specific regions of other genes, thereby activating their expression (7). Potentially, the proteins specified by those genes are involved in structural modification (8).

tural patterns deserves mention because it potentially allows for localized change in the circuit diagram of the brain—something that would seem to be more difficult to accomplish via general activation of genes very distant within the nerve cell from a particular synapse and dendrite. Weiler and Greenough (1991) have found that the depolarization (activation similar to nerve impulses) of *synaptoneurosomes* (synapses that have been isolated from most of the rest of the neuron *in vitro*) can initiate local protein synthesis. While the particular proteins synthesized, or their functions, are not known, this finding provides a mechanism by which neural activity could initiate synaptic structural change very rapidly at a specific location within the cell without an immediate

need for cytoplasmic transport from the cell body. Later consequences of the longer loop of gene expression might serve to confirm or embellish the effects of the early local protein synthesis; perhaps, for example, by stabilizing a newly formed synapse. Thus far, this pathway has only been examined in pre-weanling rats.

ADDITIONAL CONCLUSIONS

While the data-related conclusions from this chapter appear in the first paragraph, there may be more general principles that those studying child development can learn from these animal model studies. The first, a slight restatement, is that there are many ways in which the brain responds to experience during life span development; the previous strong tendency to focus just upon changes in neurons may have limited our perspectives. Second, not all experience-sensitive processes share the same developmental time course; it may be more possible to "catch up" from deficiencies in some components than in others. Whether the net effect of this might be worse in some cases than not catching up at all (e.g., encoding information in many new connections but retaining a blood supply that becomes overloaded; see Smith, 1984), the ability to catch up in some things is probably of positive value. Third, it is necessary to think less in terms of *learning* and more in terms of *brain and behavioral adaptations to environmental demands* in order to get a full perspective on the effects of experience. The formation of new capillaries in a cerebellum overworked by exercise can be considered every bit as behaviorally essential as the formation of new synapses in learning new skills. The brain simply adapts as best it can to the demands the organism's behavior places on it, and learning is just one form of adaptation. Finally, although the theoretical implications remain unclear, it is important to realize that genes *are* relevant to behavior. In at least some cases (probably many) in both development and adulthood, genes are activated specifically in response to a behavioral experience or need. Detailed understanding of how this happens is almost within our grasp, and it seems likely that both developmental and adult behavioral flexibility depend upon processes as fundamental as gene expression.

REFERENCES

Alcantara, A.A., Saks, N.D., & Greenough, W.T. (1991). Fos is expressed in the rat during a forelimb reaching task. *Society for Neuroscience Abstracts, 17*, 141.

Anokhin, K.V., Mileusnic, R., Shamakina, I.Y., & Rose, S.P.R. (1991). Effects of early experience of c-*fos* gene expression in the chick forebrain. *Brain Research, 544*, 101–107.

Bennett, E.L., Diamond, M.C., Krech, D., & Rosenzweig, M.R. (1964). Chemical and anatomical plasticity of brain. *Science, 146*, 610–619.

Bertenthal, B., Campos, J., & Barret, K. (1984). Self-produced locomotion: An organizer of emotional, cognitive, and social development in infancy. In R. Emde & R. Harmon (Eds.), *Continuities and discontinuities in development* (pp. 175–210). New York: Plenum.

Black, J.E., & Greenough, W.T. (1986). Induction of pattern in neural structure by experience: Implications for cognitive development. In M.E. Lamb, A.L. Brown, & B. Rogoff (Eds.), *Advances in developmental psychology* (Vol. 4, pp. 1–50). Hillsdale, NJ: Lawrence Earlbaum Associates.

Black, J.E., Isaacs, K.R., Anderson, B.J., Alcantara, A.A., & Greenough, W.T. (1990). Learning causes synaptogenesis, whereas motor activity causes angiogenesis, in cerebellar cortex of adult rats. *Proceedings of the National Academy of Sciences (USA), 87*, 5568–5572.

Black, J.E., Parnisari, R., Eichbaum, E., & Greenough, W.T. (1986). Morphological effects of housing environment and voluntary exercise on cerebral cortex and cerebellum of old rats. *Society for Neuroscience Abstracts, 12*, 1579.

Black, J.E., Polinsky, M., & Greenough, W.T. (1989). Progressive failure of cerebral angiogenesis supporting neural plasticity in aging rats. *Neurobiology of Aging, 10*, 353–358.

Black, J., Sirevaag, A.M., & Greenough, W.T. (1987). Complex experience promotes capillary formation in young visual cortex. *Neuroscience Letters, 83*, 351–355.

Black, J.E., Sirevaag, A.M., Wallace, C.S., Savin, M.H., & Greenough, W.T. (1989). Effects of complex experience on somatic growth and organ development in rats. *Developmental Psychobiology, 22*, 727–752.

Black, J.E., Zelazny, A.M., & Greenough, W.T. (1991). Capillary and mitochondrial support of neural plasticity in adult rat visual cortex. *Experimental Neurology, 111*, 204–209.

Chang, F.L.F., & Greenough, W.T. (1982). Lateralized effects of monocular training on dendritic branching in adult split-brain rats. *Brain Research, 232*, 283–292.

Chang, F.L.F., & Greenough, W.T. (1984). Transient and enduring morphological correlates of synaptic activity and efficacy change in the rat hippocampal slice. *Brain Research, 309*, 35–46.

Cole, A.J., Saffen, D.W., Baraban, J.M., & Worley, P.F. (1989). Rapid increase of an immediate early gene messenger RNA in hippocampal neurons by synaptic NMDA receptor activation. *Nature, 340*, 474–476.

Diamond, M.C., Krech, D., & Rosenzweig, M.R. (1964). The effects of an enriched environment on the histology of the rat cerebral cortex. *Journal of Comparative Neurology, 123*, 111–120.

Diamond, M.C., Lindner, B., & Raymond, A. (1967). Extensive cortical depth measurements and neuron size increases in the cortex of environmentally enriched rats. *Journal of Comparative Neurology, 131*, 357–364.

Ferchmin, P.A., Bennett, E.L., & Rosenzweig, M.R. (1975). Direct contact with enriched environments is required to alter cerebral weights in rats. *Journal of Comparative and Physiological Psychology, 88*, 360–367.

Floeter, M.K., & Greenough, W.T. (1979). Cerebellar plasticity: modification of Purkinje cell structure by differential rearing in monkeys. *Science, 206*, 227–229.

Forgays, D.O., & Forgays, J.W. (1952). The nature of the effect of free-environments experience in the rat. *Journal of Comparative and Physiological Psychology, 45*, 322–328.

Glick, R., & Bondareff, W. (1979). Loss of synapses in the cerebellar cortex of the senescent rat. *Journal of Gerontology, 34*, 818–822.

Green, E.J., Greenough, W.T., & Schlumpf, B.E. (1983). Effects of complex or isolated environments on cortical dendrites of middle-aged rats. *Brain Research, 264*, 233–240.

Greenough, W.T. (1985). The possible role of experience-dependent synaptogenesis, or synapses on demand, in the memory process. In N.M. Weinberger, J.L. McGaugh, & G. Lynch (Eds.), *Memory systems of the brain: Animal and human cognitive processes* (pp. 77–103). New York: Guilford Press.

Greenough, W.T., Hwang, H.-M., & Gorman, C. (1985). Evidence for active synapse formation, or altered postsynaptic metabolism, in visual cortex of rats reared in complex environments. *Proceedings of the National Academy of Science (USA), 82*, 4549–4552.

Greenough, W.T., Juraska, J.M., & Volkmar, F.R. (1979). Maze training effects on dendritic branching in occipital cortex of adult rats. *Behavioral and Neural Biology, 26*, 287–297.

Greenough, W.T., Larson, J.R., & Withers, G.S. (1985). Effects of unilateral and bilateral training on dendritic branching in occipital cortex of adult rats. *Behavioral and Neural Biology, 44*, 301–314.

Greenough, W.T., McDonald, J.W., Parnisari, R.M., & Camel, J.E. (1986). Environmental conditions modulate degeneration and new dendrite growth in cerebellum of senescent rats. *Brain Research, 380*, 136–143.

Greenough, W.T., Sirevaag, A.M., Kilman, V.L., Hess, U., Wallace, C.S., Black, J.E., & Hwang, H.-M.F. (in preparation). Synapse number per neuron in occipital cortex following exposure of adult rats to a complex environment.

Greenough, W.T., & Volkmar, F.R. (1973). Pattern of dendritic branching in occipital cortex of rats reared in complex environments. *Experimental Neurology, 40*, 491–504.

Greenough, W.T., Yuwiler, A., & Dollinger, M. (1973). Effects of post-trial eserine administration on learning in "enriched" and "impoverished" reared rats. *Behavioral Biology, 8*, 261–272.

Hawrylak, N., Chang, F-L., & Greenough, W.T. (1989). Astrocytic response to in vivo kindling of the hippocampus. *Society for Neuroscience Abstracts, 15*, 779.

Hebb, D.O. (1947). The effects of early experience on problem-solving at maturity. *American Psychologist, 2*, 306–307.

Hymovitch, B. (1952). The effects of experimental variations on problem solving in the rat. *Journal of Comparative and Physiological Psychology, 45*, 313–321.

Isaacs, K.R., Marks, A., Sirevaag, A.M., Chang, F.-L., & Greenough, W.T. (1989). Long-term potentiation alters glial processes in the dentate gyrus. *Society for Neuroscience Abstracts, 15*, 610.

Janeczko, K. (1989). Spatiotemporal patterns of the astroglial proliferation in rat brain injured in the post-mitotic stage of postnatal development: a combined immunocytochemical and autoradiographic study. *Brain Research, 485*, 236–241.

Juraska, J.M. (1984). Sex differences in dendritic response to differential experience in the rat visual cortex. *Brain Research, 295*, 27–34.

Juraska, J.M., Greenough, W.T., Elliott, C., Mack, K., & Berkowitz, R. (1980). Plasticity in adult rat visual cortex: An examination of several cell populations after differential rearing. *Behavioral and Neural Biology, 29*, 157–167.

Mello, C., Vicario, D.S., & Clayton, D.F. (1991). Song induces "immediate early" gene expression in songbird forebrain. *Society for Neuroscience Abstracts, 17*, 1050.

Pysh, J.J., & Weiss, M. (1979). Exercise during development induces an increase in Purkinje cell dendritic tree size. *Science, 206*, 230–232.

Rogers, J., Silver, M.A., Shoemaker, W.J., & Bloom, F.E. (1980). Senescent changes in a neurobiological model system: cerebellar Purkinje cell electrophysiology and correlative anatomy. *Neurobiology of Aging, 1*, 3–11.

Rogers, J., Zornetzer, S.F., Bloom, F.E., & Mervis, R.E. (1984). Senescent microstructural changes in rat cerebellum. *Brain Research, 292*, 23–32.

Rosenzweig, M.R., Krech, D., Bennett, E.L., & Diamond, M.C. (1962). Effects of environmental complexity and training on brain chemistry and anatomy: A replication and extension. *Journal of Comparative and Physiological Psychology, 55*, 429–437.

Shambes, G.M., Gibson, J.M., & Welker, W. (1978). Fractured somatopy in granule cell tactile areas of rat cerebellar hemispheres revealed by micromapping. *Brain, Behavior and Evolution, 15*, 94–140.

Sirevaag, A.M., Black, J.E., & Greenough, W.T. (1991). Astrocyte hypertrophy in the dentate gyrus of young male rats reflects variation of individual stress rather than group environmental complexity manipulations. *Experimental Neurology, 111*, 74–79.

Sirevaag, A.M., Black, J., Shafron, D., & Greenough, W.T. (1988). Direct evidence that complex experience increases capillary branching and surface area in visual cortex of young rats. *Developmental Brain Research, 43*, 299–304.

Sirevaag, A.M., & Greenough, W.T. (1991). Plasticity of GFAP-immunoreactive astrocyte size and number in visual cortex of rats reared in complex environments. *Brain Research, 540*, 273–278.

Smith, C.B. (1984). Aging and changes in cerebral energy metabolism. *Trends in Neuroscience, 7*, 203–208.

Topp, K.S., Faddis, B.T., & Vijayan, V.K. (1989). Trauma-induced proliferation of astrocytes in the brains of young and aged rats. *Glia, 2*, 201–211.

Turner, A.M., & Greenough, W.T. (1985). Differential rearing effects on rat visual cortex synapses. I. Synaptic and neuronal density and synapses per neuron. *Brain Research, 329*, 195–203.

Uylings, H.B.M., Kuypers, K., Diamond, M.C., & Veltman, W.A.M. (1978). Effects of differential environments on plasticity of dendrites of cortical pyramidal neurons in adult rats. *Experimental Neurology, 62*, 658–677.

Volkmar, F.R., & Greenough, W.T. (1972). Rearing complexity affects branching of dendrites in the visual cortex of the rat. *Science, 176*, 1445–1447.

Wallace, C.S., Kilman, V.L., Withers, G.S., & Greenough, W.T. (in press). Increases in dendritic length following a brief period of differential housing in weanling rats, *Behavioral and Neural Biology.*

Wallace, C.S., Withers, G.S., Weiler, I.J., & Greenough, W.T. (1991). Expression of the Immediate Early Gene

Zif–268 influenced by brief exposure to environmental complexity in the occipital cortex of weanling rats. *Third IBRO World Congress of Neuroscience Abstracts*, 25–48.

Weiler, I.J., & Greenough, W.T. (1991). Protein translation in synaptoneurosomal polyribosomes is triggered by de-polarization. *Molecular and Cellular Neurosciences, 2,* 305–314.

West, R.W., & Greenough, W.T. (1972). Effect of environmental complexity on cortical synapses of rats: Preliminary results. *Behavioral Biology, 7,* 279–284.

Index

Page numbers followed by "f" indicate figures; those followed by "t" indicate tables.